Orthopedic Surgery in Patients with Hemophilia

Horacio A. Caviglia • Luigi P. Solimeno
Editors

Orthopedic Surgery in Patients with Hemophilia

Foreword by
Pier Mannuccio Mannucci

Springer

Editors
Horacio A. Caviglia
Department of Orthopedics
Hemophilia Foundation and
General Hospital de Agudos
"Juan A. Fernandez"
Buenos Aires, Argentina

Luigi Piero Solimeno
Hemophilic Arthropathy Treatment Centre
"Maria Grazia Gatti Randi"
Milan, Italy

Coordinator
Gianluigi Pasta
Department of Orthopedics and Traumatology
Angelo Bianchi Bonomi Hemophilia and
Thrombosis Center
IRCCS Maggiore Hospital
Mangiagalli and Regina Elena Foundation
Milan, Italy

ISBN 978-88-470-1564-7
e-ISBN 978-88-470-0854-0

Springer is a part of Springer Science+Business Media
springer.com

Printed in Italy
Springer-Verlag Italia S.r.l. – Via Decembrio 28 – I-20137 Milan

Foreword

Hemophilia A and B are lifelong inherited X-linked bleeding disorders, caused by the deficiency of factor VIII (FVIII) or IX (FIX) in plasma. The clinical hallmark of hemophilias is bleeding into the joints and muscles, which can occur spontaneously in the severe forms of the diseases (FVIII/FIX < 1 IU/dl). The joints more frequently involved are the ankles, knees, and elbows, and the recurrence of joint bleeding leads to the formation of 'target' joints. The final consequence of repeated hemarthroses is the development of hemophilic arthropathy, characterized by synovial hypertrophy, cartilage destruction, and bone damage with stiffness, pain, and ultimately permanent disability.

With this as background it is clear that orthopedic specialists and physiotherapists play a very important role in the framework of the global care offered to hemophiliac patients. Nowadays the cornerstone of hemophilia care is represented by primary prophylaxis aimed at preventing chronic arthropathy. However, the contribution of skilled orthopedic specialists and physiotherapists is crucial to achieve good outcomes, particularly in adult patients who are already suffering from hemophilic arthropathy. The development and availability of efficacious clotting factor concentrates over the last four decades has enabled surgeons to safely manage surgery in haemophiliac patients. On the other hand, between the late '70s and '80s the increasing use of plasma-derived concentrates that were non virus inactivated caused transfusion-transmitted diseases (hepatitis and acquired immunodeficiency syndrome (AIDS), which has greatly affected the generation of adult hemophiliacs who developed arthropathy and now need major orthopedic procedures such as joint replacement. Moreover, the recent availability of hemostatic agents able to initiate the coagulation cascade despite the presence of inhibitors has allowed extension of surgical indications to this problematic subset of patients. In the light of these and many other considerations, patients with hemophilia represent a challenge for orthopedic specialists, because in comparison with the general population they show a different pathogenesis of their arthritis, have different surgical indications, require different surgical techniques to ensure local hemostasis, need dedicated post-operative care, and more frequently develop complications.

We all hope that the new generation of children with hemophilia will benefit worldwide from the widespread use of prophylaxis with no need for orthopedic care, but this ideal goal is far from being realized, since almost 70–80% of those with hemophilia in the world have, as yet, no access to any replacement therapy. Until it is available for all, it is hoped that this book will provide a useful reference for those involved in the treatment of hemophilia and orthopedic surgeons who are dedicated to this challenging disease.

Verona, April 2008

Professor Pier Mannuccio Mannucci
Director of Angelo Bianchi Bonomi
Hemophilia and Thrombosis Center
Department of Internal Medicine and
Medical Specialties
IRCCS Maggiore Hospital
Mangiagalli and Regina Elena Foundation
Milan, Italy

Preface

Severe hemophilia is a lifelong inherited bleeding disorder characterized by recurrent joint bleeding, which results in chronic, painful, and disabling arthropathy. Since the 1990s, the greater availability of safe and effective clotting factor concentrates has allowed satisfactory results to be achieved in hemophilia care. Unfortunately, up to 70–80% of hemophiliacs worldwide, particularly in developing countries, still have no access to adequate replacement therapy and consequently frequently develop musculoskeletal complications with severe impairment of their quality of life. Therefore, the role of the orthopedic surgeon becomes crucial in the management of such patients.

This book aims to elucidate peri-operative and operative management of hemophiliac patients. It focuses on surgical techniques in order to give both fundamental and specialized information to those involved with hemophilia treatment worldwide, and to give useful advice to any orthopedic surgeon who is working in this challenging field.

April 2008 The Editors

Contents

Section III Non-surgical Procedures

Section IV Upper Limb

Section V Lower Limb

Section VI Bone Defects

Section VII Traumatology

Conclusions

Contributors

Abhisek Bhattarai
Department of Orthopedic Surgery, Nepal Medical College Teaching Hospital, Kathmandu, Nepal

Roberto Bernal-Lagunas
Mexican Hemophilia Association, Mexico City, Mexico

Hernan Blanchetiere
Orthopedics and Traumatology Department,
"Juan A. Fernandez" Hospital, Buenos Aires, Argentina

Horacio A. Caviglia
Department of Orthopedics, Hemophilia Foundation and General Hospital de Agudos "Juan A. Fernandez", Buenos Aires, Argentina

Freddy Chakal
Department of Orthopedics, Municipal Blood Bank of Caracas, Caracas, Venezuela

M. Zaki Choudhury
Department of Orthopaedic Surgery, Royal Free Hospital, London, UK

Jorge Daruich
Liver Section of Clinicas San Martín Hospital,
School of Medicine, Buenos Aires University, Buenos Aires, Argentina

Ana Laura Douglas Price
Department of Orthopedics and Traumatology, "Juan A. Fernandez" Hospital, Buenos Aires, Argentina

Federico Fernández-Palazzi
Orthopedic Unit National Hemophilia Treatment Centre, Municipal Blood Bank of Caracas, Caracas, Venezuela

Gustavo Galatro
Department of Orthopedics and Traumatology, "Juan A. Fernandez" Hospital, Buenos Aires, Argentina

Vincent K. Garg
Hemophilia Care Centre, Lions Hospital and Research Centre, New Friends Colony, New Delhi, India

Marvin Gilbert
Department of Orthopedics, Mount Sinai Medical Center, New York, NY, USA

Nicholas Goddard
Department of Orthopaedic Surgery, Royal Free Hospital, London, UK

Michael Heim
Department of Orthopedics and Rehabilitation, Israel National Hemophilia Centre, Tel Hashomer Hospital, Israel

Cyro Kanabushi
University Hospital of Paraná, Paraná, Brazil

Clayton N. Kraft
Orthopaedics and Traumatology, Klinikum Krefeld, Krefeld, Germany

Floris P.J.G. Lafeber
Van Creveldkliniek, National Hemophilia Treatment Centre, Department of Rheumatology and Clinical Immunology, University Medical Centre Utrecht, Utrecht, The Nederlands

Adolfo Llinás
Department of Orthopedics and Traumatology and Hemophilia Treatment Center, Fundación Santa Fe de Bogotá, Fundación Cosme y Damián, Bogotá, Colombia

Paulo J. Llinás Hernández
Department of Orthopedics and Traumatology, Fundación Valle del Lili, Cali, Colombia

Emilia Lozej
Department of Orthopedics, CTO Hospital, University of Milan, Italy

James V. Luck Jr.
Orthopedics-Hemophilia Treatment Center, Orthopedic Hospital, Los Angeles, CA; UCLA and Orthopedic Hospital, Department of Orthopedics, David Geffen School of Medicine, University of California Los Angeles, CA, USA

Maria Elisa Mancuso
Angelo Bianchi Bonomi Hemophilia and Thrombosis Center, Department of Internal Medicine and Medical Specialties, IRCCS Maggiore Hospital, Mangiagalli and Regina Elena Foundation, Milan, Italy

Estela Manero
Liver Section of Clínicas San Martín Hospital, School of Medicine, Buenos Aires University, Buenos Aires, Argentina

Shubhranshu S. Mohanty
King Edward Memorial Hospital, Parel, Mumbai, India

Miguel Moreno
Orthopedics and Traumatology Department,
"Juan A. Fernandez" Hospital, Buenos Aires, Argentina

Noemi Moretti
Orthopedics and Traumatology Department, "Juan A. Fernandez" Hospital, Buenos Aires, Argentina

S.M. Javad Mortazavi
Orthopedic Surgery, Imam University Hospital Hemophilia Centre, Tehran University of Medical Sciences, Tehran, Iran

Kathy Mulder
Musculoskeletal Committee, World Federation of Hemophilia, and Physiotherapist, Manitoba Bleeding Disorders Program, Health Sciences Center, Winnipeg, Manitoba, Canada

Pablo Nuova
Orthopedics and Traumatology Department, "Juan A. Fernandez" Hospital, Buenos Aires, Argentina

Luciano da Rocha Loures Pacheco
Hemophilia Centre, University Hospital of Paraná, Paraná, Brazil

Alfredo Parietti
Anesthesiology Area of the Therapeutical and Diagnostical Gastroenterology Centre, Buenos Aires, Argentina

Gianluigi Pasta
Department of Orthopedics and Traumatology, Angelo Bianchi Bonomi Hemophilia and Thrombosis Center, IRCCS Maggiore Hospital, Mangiagalli and Regina Elena Foundation, Milan, Italy

Enrique Pener
Orthopedics and Traumatology Department, "Juan A. Fernandez" Hospital, Buenos Aires, Argentina

Maurício Alexandre de Meneses Pereira
University Hospital of Paraná, Paraná, Brazil

Olivia Samantha Perfetto
Hemophilic Arthropathy Treatment Centre "Maria Grazia Gatti Randi", Milan, Italy

Paolo Radossi
Haemophilia Center and Hematology, Transfusion Service, Castelfranco Veneto, Italy

Salvador Rivas
Orthopedic Unit, National Hemophilia Centre, Caracas, Venezuela

Emérito Carlos Rodríguéz-Merchan
Orthopedic Unit, La Paz University Hospital, and University Autonoma, Madrid, Spain

Goris Roosendaal
Van Creveldkliniek, National Hemophilia Treatment Centre, Department of Rheumatology and Clinical Immunology, University Medical Centre Utrecht, Utrecht, The Nederlands

Elena Santagostino
Hemophilia Outpatient Clinic, Angelo Bianchi Bonomi Hemophilia and Thrombosis Center, Department of Internal Medicine and Medical Specialties, IRCCS Maggiore Hospital, Mangiagalli and Regina Elena Foundation, Milan, Italy

Nadir Şener
SB Goztepe Hospital, Department of Orthopedics and Traumatology, Istanbul, Turkey

Axel Seuser
Department of Orthopedics, Kaiser Karl Clinic Bonn, Bonn, Germany

Mauricio Silva
Outpatient Medical Center, Hemophilia Treatment Center, Orthopedic Hospital, Los Angeles, CA; UCLA/Orthopedic Hospital Department of Orthopedics, David Geffen School of Medicine, University of California Los Angeles, CA, USA

Mahesh Prasad Shrivastava
Department of Orthopedic Surgery, Nepal Medical College Teaching Hospital, Kathmandu, Nepal

Muhammad Tariq Sohail
Department of Orthopedic and Spine Surgery, Services Hospital, Services Institute of Medical Sciences, Lahore, Pakistan

Luigi P. Solimeno
Hemophilic Arthropathy Treatment Centre "Maria Grazia Gatti Randi", Milan, Italy

Victoria Soroa
Department of Orthopedics and Traumatology, "Juan A. Fernandez" Hospital, Buenos Aires, Argentina

Giuseppe Tagariello
Haemophilia Center and Hematology, Transfusion Service, Castelfranco Veneto, Italy

Ömer Taşer
Orthopedic Surgery, Medical Faculty of Istanbul Topkapi, Istanbul, Turkey

Gaetano Torri
Department of Orthopedics, CTO Hospital, University of Milan, Milan, Italy

Remzi Tözün
Istanbul Medical Faculty, Department of Orthopedics and Traumatology, Istanbul, Turkey

Nosrat Vatani
Department of Orthopedics and Traumatology, "Juan A. Fernandez" Hospital, Buenos Aires, Argentina

Rafael Viso
Department of Orthopedics, Municipal Blood Bank of Caracas, Caracas, Venezuela

Thomas A. Wallny
Department of Orthopedics, University Hospital, Bonn, Germany

Hussain Warraich Wazahat
Department of Orthopedic and Spine Surgery, Services Hospital, Services Institute of Medical Sciences, Lahore, Pakistan

Jerome Wiedel
Anschutz Outpatient Pavillion, Department of Orthopedics, University of Colorado Health Sciences Centre, Aurora, CO, USA

List of Abbreviations

AES	ascitic-edematous syndrome
AIDS	acquired immune deficiency syndrome
ALP	alkaline phosphatase
ALT	alanine aminotransferase
AO/ASIF	Arbeitsgemeinschaft für Osteosynthesefragen/Association for the Study of Internal Fixation (Group)
AP	anteroposterior
aPCC	activated prothrombin complex concentrate
AST	aspartate transaminase
BU	Bethesda unit
BZD	benzodiazepine
CPM	continuous passive movement/motion
CT	computerized tomography
CVAD	central venous access device
DDAVP	1-desamino-8-d-arginine vasopressin (desmopressin)
DIC	disseminated intravascular coagulation
EDH	extension/de-subluxation hinge
EEG	electroencephalogram
EMG	electromyogram
ESR	erythrocyte sedimentation rate
FDA	Food and Drug Administration
FEIBA	factor VIII inhibitor bypassing agent
GABA	γ-aminobutyric acid
GAG	glucosaminoglycan
GGT	γ-glutamyl transferase
HA	hyaluronic acid
HAART	highly active antiretroviral therapy
HBV	hepatitis B virus
HCV	hepatitis C virus
HDP	hydroxymethane diphosphonate
HEDP	hydroxyethylidene diphosphonate
HIV	human immunodeficiency virus
IL-1	interleukin-1
ITI	immune tolerance induction

MDP	methylene diphosphonate
MNC	mononuclear cell
MRI	magnetic resonance imaging
PCC	prothrombin complex concentrate
PH	portal hypertension
RBC	red blood cell
rFVIIa	recombinant activated factor VII
THA	total hip arthroplasty
THR	total hip replacement
TJA	total joint arthroplasty
TKA	total knee arthroplasty
TNF-α	tumor necrosis factor-α
TPS	thiopental
WFH	World Federation of Hemophilia

Chapter 1
Professor Henri Horozowski. In Memoriam

Michael Heim

The acquisition of an orthopedic specialty is a very difficult challenge in Israel. The specialization course extends over 6 years, and includes two examinations. The initial examination takes place after 3 years in training, and the final one after the entire study period. It is with a great degree of sadness that I came to the realization that there are young, qualified orthopedic surgeons at the beginning of their professional lives who have grown and graduated from Tel Hashomer hospital without having ever seen Professor Henri Horozowski. This new generation has grown up in the shadow of the previous boss, having heard, and still hearing stories about Henri, but never having had the opportunity to be in direct contact with him. The present senior staff members, including myself, had the honor of growing with Henri, for we all served and started our specialization under Professor Farine, Henri being his deputy.

Professor Farine retired and unfortunately died as a result of a motor vehicle accident a few years after Henri succeeded him in becoming the director of orthopedic services.

- What are the qualities required to become a boss?
- What transpires in the mind of a successful orthopedic surgeon with a huge and flourishing private practice, which makes him want to take on additional responsibility at the hospital and the university?
- What made Henri Horozowski so special?

Growing up in a very busy orthopedic service, in a major hospital, is stressful for every resident. One's work is never done; the casualty department works 24 hours a day, and the inpatient service is constantly dealing with pre- and post-operative cases. Henri, too, had grown up in this system and never forgot the anguish and exhaustion that residents feel. He was always there to lend a helping hand and provide assistance and guidance, never insisting that others do things that he himself was not prepared to do. One never hesitated to call him for advice or assistance. Even if he was not on call duty, one always felt sure that he would provide guidance. This comforting knowledge was reinforced by the fact that he emanated a feeling of dependability.

Then there were the department staff meetings where a junior resident was given a topic to present, and members of the department added additional infor-

H.A. Caviglia, L.P. Solimeno (eds.), *Orthopedic Surgery in Patients with Hemophilia.*

mation based on the information provided. Henri took upon himself the task of summing up the evening. He always did so, and quoted references that we had never come across. These were the days prior to internet search modules. Once a few of us decided to check out whether such references in fact existed. We did so, and found them, confirming that Henri had an exceptional memory and abounded in knowledge.

Henri had the vision, more than 20 years ago, to foresee that within the realms of orthopedics there were groups of surgeons entering into subspecialties, and that it was his task to channel the personnel of the department into positions where they would be able to participate in the diversity of the orthopedic world. Young specialists were sent abroad to acquire additional training in the fields of: trauma, pediatrics, joint replacement, oncology, spine, hands, feet, and even bone banking.

Even within these groups there were subdivisions such as shoulder, hip, and knee replacement. These specialization opportunities were mostly the fruits of his endeavors in finding not only suitable placements but also financial support. Henri always accepted visiting students, residents, and specialists with open arms, hoping to enrich their quality of medical practice and adding scope for his team to broaden their visions. This policy led the orthopedic department into arenas of international exposure.

Henri's generosity of spirit was such that he searched for no glory for himself, constantly backing and pushing his staff to the fore.

As the years passed, an understanding developed between us, so that often words became redundant. A simple stare, sigh, or the raising of an eyebrow transmitted the message. I am truly honored that in the last years of Henri's life I became one of his confidants, and, in years to come, facts will be revealed highlighting his involvement in many fields outside the realms of orthopedic surgery. Henri was an energetic person, requiring little sleep. He was a man of deeds rather than words. He was involved in cultural programs, boards of trade, nature preservation, and historical, archeological, geographical, and charitable organizations.

Henri loved the sea and little gave him more pleasure than taking his annual leave, traveling to France with his family, and spending time on a boat, fishing.

Unfortunately he was never able to fulfill his dream – early retirement which would have permitted him to spend more time with his family. Of one thing I am sure, and that is that Henri got the most out of each day that he lived, and that in his short life he managed to create far more than most people ever achieve.

May his dear soul rest in peace.

Section I
Pathogenesis

Chapter 2
Joint Damage as a Result of Hemarthrosis

Goris Roosendaal and Floris P.J.G. Lafeber

The immediate symptoms or "short-term" effects of hemarthrosis are pain, swelling, warmth, and muscle spasm. The "long-term" effects of recurrent joint bleeding are more serious. Repeated episodes of intra-articular bleeding cause damage to the joint, leading to deformity and crippling [1, 2]. However, the delay between joint bleeding and the subsequent joint damage makes it difficult to establish the exact pathogenetic mechanism of blood-induced joint damage.

Recurrent hemarthroses, as occur in hemophilia, lead to specific changes in the synovium and cartilage, which finally result in total destruction of the joint. This process is called hemophilic arthropathy [3–8]. The pathogenetic mechanisms of hemophilic arthropathy are not precisely known.

Several joint disorders result in cartilage damage and changes in synovial tissue; these disorders can be degenerative, such as osteoarthritis, inflammation-mediated, such as rheumatoid arthritis, or blood-induced, such as hemophilic arthropathy. Several mediators are involved in these changes, for example, enzymes, cytokines, and oxygen metabolites. Current theories, which are based on experimental in vitro studies [2, 3] and clinical experience, suggest that the synovium becomes catabolically active because of excessive exposure to blood components, and as a result induces cartilage destruction. Synovial iron deposition, which can easily be detected by magnetic resonance imaging, is suggested to be indicative of the severity of hemophilic arthropathy. However, these theories are based on only a limited number of studies. In comparison to our knowledge about osteoarthritis and rheumatoid arthritis, little is known about the mechanisms of cartilage damage in hemophilic arthropathy. It is possible that the pathophysiology is multifactorial in origin and includes degenerative cartilage-mediated and inflammatory synovium-mediated components.

It is recognized that repeated extravasation of blood into the joint cavity is the factor responsible for synovial and cartilage changes [8, 9]. Synovial changes are thought to precede cartilage changes. Progressive accumulation of iron from red blood cells removed from the joint cavity by synovial macrophages over time, during successive intra-articular hemorrhages, has been postulated to be the trigger for synovial inflammation. This synovial inflammation would ultimately lead to joint damage that becomes evident years after the

H.A. Caviglia, L.P. Solimeno (eds.), *Orthopedic Surgery in Patients with Hemophilia.*

first bleeding episode has occurred [10]. An important characteristic of synovial changes is the deposition of iron (hemosiderin) in the synovium. Experimental hemarthrosis induces synovial changes resembling those seen in patients with hemophilia. The hemosiderin deposits are thought to induce synoviocyte hypertrophy (resulting in villus growth), and neovascularization in the subsynovial layer (resulting in increased vascularity). Another suggested effect of the hemosiderin deposits is an infiltration of the synovial membrane with lymphocytes, although follicles of lymphocytes, which can be seen in the synovial membrane in rheumatoid arthritis, have not been observed. Compared with inflammatory arthropathies like rheumatoid arthritis there are only mild inflammatory changes. Synovial iron deposits as a result of recurrent intra-articular hemorrhages are also found in other joint disorders such as pigmented villonodular synovitis, hemangiomas of the synovial membrane, and hemosiderotic synovitis. These joint disorders all result in joint damage resembling hemophilic arthropathy, which suggests that synovial iron deposits indeed play an important role in the pathogenesis of blood-induced cartilage damage [11, 12]. Accumulation of iron, as a degradation product of hemoglobin, may be a direct stimulus for the proliferation of synoviocytes and attract inflammatory cells; the subsequent production of enzymes and cytokines could lead to the destruction of articular cartilage [13, 14].

In a study of patients with hemophilia who underwent elective orthopedic surgery of the knee, it was found that the synovial tissue in all patients showed areas with a hemosideritic appearance adjacent to areas of normal appearance [15]. This finding provided a model for an analysis of the effect of synovial iron deposits in synovial tissue. The macroscopic appearance corresponded closely to the histological iron deposits and, in addition, to the inflammatory and catabolic activity of the tissues. The results show that the iron deposits at localized sites in the synovium are associated with the production of pro-inflammatory cytokines and an ability to inhibit the formation of human cartilage matrix. This supports the hypothesis that iron plays a leading role in the induction of synovial changes and the consequent production of catabolic mediators that are harmful to articular cartilage. It is not clear whether hemosiderin is directly involved in the stimulation of cytokine production; it seems more likely that phagocytosis by synovial cells and blood macrophages released into the hemarthritic joint leads to the stimulation of cytokine production. However, the inflammatory changes in hemosideritic synovial tissue, as determined histologically, are mild compared with those in tissue with inflammatory joint disease such as rheumatoid arthritis [15, 16]. The potential for damage by hemosideritic synovial tissue underlines the importance of early diagnosis and treatment of chronic synovitis in hemophiliac patients.

In addition to synovial triggering, it has been suggested that intra-articular blood has a direct harmful effect on cartilage before, and independently of, the synovial changes, and that joint damage may occur *before* the synovial inflammation becomes evident; primarily there may be damage of articular cartilage with synovitis as a consequence. These studies demonstrate that the initial process involves cartilage damage as a result of a short encounter between cartilage and blood. Synovial changes (inflammation) are secondary to the process of cartilage damage.

The latter concept is underscored by findings in a human in vitro model of hemarthrosis [17–20]. Biochemical and metabolic analyses showed that subtle but irreversible changes in chondrocyte metabolic activity occurred in human cartilage after a short exposure to blood in vitro. These changes cannot be detected clinically, but they may play a role in the pathogenesis of blood-induced arthropathy. Human articular cartilage consists of a relatively small number of chondrocytes embedded in a relatively large amount of extracellular matrix. This extracellular matrix consists mainly of collagen and proteoglycan. There is a continuous turnover of these matrix components, with a delicate balance between synthesis and breakdown [21]. Several mediators, such as growth factors, enzymes, cytokines, oxygen metabolites, and their natural inhibitors, are involved in maintaining this balance but are also involved in cartilage damage when there is an imbalance between synthesis and breakdown. Results of these studies show that a relatively short exposure (4 days; the expected natural removal time of blood from a human joint) of human cartilage to whole blood in concentrations up to 50% (the blood concentration during hemarthrosis is expected to approach 100%) induces long-lasting damage. There is marked inhibition of matrix formation (proteoglycan synthesis) and increased breakdown, i.e., release of matrix components (proteoglycan release), resulting in a continuing loss of matrix (proteoglycan content). The initial biochemical changes seen in these studies were not accompanied by changes that were either histologically or macroscopically detectable. However, the studies reveal that cartilage changes induced by short-term exposure to whole blood result in continuing inhibition of proteoglycan synthesis, accompanied by a continuing decrease in proteoglycan content. In the long term, histological and macroscopic changes would probably follow.

To acquire more insight into the mechanism of blood-induced cartilage damage, it is crucial to know which blood components are responsible for cartilage changes. Human in vitro studies reveal marked inhibition of proteoglycan synthesis by mononuclear cells (MNCs). This effect of MNCs has been reported before, for instance, in studies of blood from patients with rheumatoid arthritis [22]. The proposed mechanisms include, among others, effects of lysosomal enzymes and catabolic cytokines such as interleukin-1 (IL-1) and tumor necrosis factor-α (TNF-α). However, these effects have been proved to be transient. In vitro studies showed that whole blood induced long-lasting inhibition of proteoglycan synthesis and enhancement of glucosaminoglycan (GAG) release in contrast to isolated components. Only the combination of MNCs and red blood cells (RBCs) revealed effects that were comparable to whole blood. A possible explanation for the irreversible damage caused by this combination is the conversion of oxygen metabolites produced by chondrocytes to toxic hydroxyl radicals, catalyzed by iron from the RBCs, which in turn is triggered by cytokines (e.g., IL-1) produced by the monocytes/macrophages in the MNC population [23–26].

These results, indicating a direct harmful effect of blood on cartilage, do not exclude the important role of reported synovium-induced cartilage damage. In addition to "synovium-related" changes (which are certainly important in the long run), cartilage damage may be induced initially by blood. This cartilage damage may in turn induce inflammatory responses in addition to those induced by hemosiderin. Canine in vivo studies corroborate these theories [27, 28]. These studies were undertaken to test the hypothesis, based on results of in vitro studies, that a short exposure to blood during a single or limited number of bleeding events results in changes that inevitably lead to joint destruction.

Results of these canine in vivo studies show that canine cartilage exposed in vivo to whole blood for a relatively short time (4 days) exhibits long-lasting biochemical and histochemical changes of the cartilage matrix and changes in chondrocyte metabolic activity; these changes occur as well as, although secondary to, changes in the synovium. Recent studies also show that immature cartilage is more susceptible to blood-induced damage than mature articular cartilage [29]. These biochemical changes are predictive of irreversible joint damage in the long term. The changes with respect to loss and total content of proteoglycans were shown to persist for at least 16 days. The total proteoglycan content remained low despite enhanced synthesis of proteoglycans on day 16. The shift from inhibition to stimulation of proteoglycan synthesis from day 4 to day 16, while the decreased proteoglycan content remained low, suggests that the increase in proteoglycan synthesis was an ineffective attempt to repair cartilage. A similar ineffective enhancement of proteoglycan synthesis has also been described for osteoarthritic cartilage.

Swelling of cartilage is an early sign and an important marker of osteoarthritic cartilage, and is believed to be caused by disruption of the collagen network. The cross-linked three-dimensional fibrillar network of collagen is responsible for the tensile strength of cartilage, and disruption of this network by proteolytic enzymes, excessive mechanical loading, and oxygen metabolites will lead to pathologic conditions. In this canine in vivo study [26], a slightly, but statistically significant, higher percentage of degraded collagen was detected in the injected joint compared with the control joint on day 4, indicating that even a short exposure to intra-articular blood can damage the collagen network, with the possibility of a detrimental effect over time. The results of these in vivo studies reconfirm the hypothesis from in vitro studies that hemoglobin-derived iron, together with enhanced hydrogen peroxide production by chondrocytes due to monocyte/macrophage IL-1 stimulation, causes increased formation of hydroxyl radicals, which permanently damages the chondrocytes (apoptosis) [25, 26]. This would suggest that the short exposure to blood itself, and not the synovitis that was evident on day 16, is involved in this collagen-destructive process.

More-recent studies have shown a discrepancy between the long-term effects of blood on cartilage in vivo and in vitro [20]. Short-term in vitro exposure (4 days) of human or canine cartilage to whole blood inhibited proteoglycan synthesis by more than 98% (day 4), an inhibition which lasted until week 10. Short-term in vivo exposure of cartilage to blood also induced adverse changes in cartilage proteoglycan turnover seen shortly after exposure. However, cartilage matrix turnover was shown to have returned to normal 10 weeks after the last injection. Synovial inflammation was absent and no destructive activity was found. A possible explanation for the in vivo recovery after experimental joint bleeding in dogs could be that the observed changes in cartilage only predispose to acute damage, and additional (e.g., mechanical) factors are needed to induce permanent joint damage. In order to confirm this possible explanation, a further study was performed. A limited number of experimental joint bleeds combined with loading of the affected joint were carried out, and the effect on the development of progressive degenerative joint damage was analyzed [30]. In this study the right knees of eight mature beagle dogs were injected with freshly collected autologous blood twice a week over 4 weeks, to mimic a limited number of joint hemorrhages in a short time. To ensure loading of the experimental joint, the contralateral control knee of the animal was fixed to the trunk, for 4 hours per day, 3 days per week. Ten weeks after the last injection, cartilage tissue and synovium were collected from both knees to analyze features of joint degeneration. Cartilage was prepared for analysis of proteoglycan turnover (synthesis, retention, release, and content) and histology, and synovium was prepared for histological analysis. The proteoglycan synthesis rate was significantly increased, which is characteristic of the degenerative cartilage damage seen in osteoarthritis. Release of newly formed proteoglycans (as a measure of retention) and total loss of proteoglycans from the cartilage matrix was increased. Cartilage matrix integrity was adversely changed, as shown by histological damage. Histology also showed signs of synovial inflammation. When loading of the joints was not forced, these effects were not observed 10 weeks after experimental bleeds. These results suggest that, when combined with loading of the affected joint, experimental joint bleeds result in features of progressive degenerative joint damage, whereas similar joint hemorrhages without joint loading do not. This suggests a possible mechanism for joint damage in hemophilia.

These canine in vivo findings concerning the effects of blood on cartilage proteoglycan and collagen are consistent with those of Convery and colleagues [31]. In 14 mongrel dogs they found morphological changes in articular cartilage after 16 weeks of blood exposure; there was a significant decrease in GAG content after only 4 weeks and the total collagen content was significantly altered after 12 weeks. Biophysical analysis of the cartilage surface after 8 weeks showed that the tissue was more deformable and less resistant to shear than the control cartilage. In addition, Parsons et al found in an animal model that the continuous presence of blood in the joint for 10 days resulted in cartilage that was significantly more compliant than normal [32]. They attributed these changes to the loss of proteoglycan. We suggest that intra-articular blood-induced collagen damage is also involved, both mechanisms acting together, and that such changes take place after a short exposure to intra-articular blood.

These studies show that synovitis is involved, but is not the only mechanism in the joint damage caused by intra-articular bleeding. This pathogenetic concept does not contradict the current concept of blood-induced cartilage damage in which synovial changes are thought to play an important role. Several pathological processes are possibly involved, some occurring in parallel and others sequentially.

It can be concluded that the pathogenetic mechanism of hemophilic arthropathy is multifactorial and includes degenerative cartilage-mediated and inflammatory synovium-mediated components. Intra-articular blood first has a direct effect on cartilage, as a result of iron-catalyzed formation of destructive oxygen metabolites (resulting in chondrocyte apoptosis), and subsequently affects the synovium, in addition to hemosiderin-induced synovial triggering. Both processes occur in parallel, and while they influence each other they probably do not depend on each other. This concept resembles the degenerative joint damage found in osteoarthritis as well as the inflammatory processes in rheumatoid arthritis [16]. These processes finally result in a fibrotic and destroyed joint. It is unknown whether, and if so, when, a point of no return is reached. More insight into the mechanisms of hemophilic arthropathy may have consequences for the (prophylactic) treatment of patients with hemophilia. Unraveling these mechanisms as well as defining a possible point of no return is still a subject of research.

References

1. van Creveld S, Hoedemaker PJ, Kingma MJ, Wagenvoort CA (1971) Degeneration of joints in haemophiliacs under treatment by modern methods. J Bone Joint Surg 53:296–302
2. Madhok R, Bennett D, Sturrock RD, Forbes CD (1988) Mechanisms of joint damage in an experimental model of haemophilic arthritis. Arthritis Rheum 31:1148–1155
3. Stein H, Duthie RB (1981) The pathogenesis of chronic haemophilic arthropathy. J Bone Joint Surg 63B:601–609
4. Madhok R, York J, Sturrock RD (1967) Haemophilic arthritis. Ann Rheum Dis 50:588–591
5. Hoaglund FT. Experimental hemarthrosis. The response of canine knees to injections of autologous blood. J Bone Joint Surg 49:285–298
6. Zeman DH, Roberts ED, Shoji H, Miwa T (1991) Experimental haemarthrosis in rhesus monkeys: morphometric, biochemical and metabolic analyses. J Comp Pathol 104:129–139
7. Wolf CR, Mankin HJ (1965) The effect of experimental hemarthrosis on articular cartilage of rabbit knee joints. J Bone Joint Surg Am 47:1203–1210
8. Roy S, Ghadially FN (1966) Pathology of experimental haemarthrosis. Ann Rheum Dis 25:402–415
9. Mainardi CL, Levine PH, Werb Z, Harris ED (1978) Proliferative synovitis in hemophilia: biochemical and morphologic observations. Arthritis Rheum 21:137–144
10. Pelletier J-P, Martel-Pelletier J, Ghandur-Mnaymneh L et al (1985) Role of synovial membrane inflammation in cartilage matrix breakdown in the Pond-Nuki model of osteoarthritis. Arthritis Rheum 28:554–561
11. Abrahams TG, Pavlov H, Bansal M, Bullough P (1988) Concentric joints space narrowing of the hip associated with hemosiderotic synovitis (HS) including pigmented villonodular synovitis (PVNS). Skeletal Radiol 17:37–45
12. France MP, Gupta SK (1991) Non-haemophilic hemosiderotic synovitis of the shoulder. A case report. Clin Orthop 262:132–136
13. Morris CJ, Blake DR, Wainwright AC, Steven MM (1986) Relationship between iron deposits and tissue damage in the synovium: an ultra structural study. Ann Rheum Dis 45:21–26

14. Blake DR, Gallagher PJ, Potter AR et al (1984) The effect of synovial iron on the progression of rheumatoid disease. A histologic assessment of patients with early rheumatoid synovitis. Arthritis Rheum 27:495–501
15. Roosendaal G, Vianen ME, Wenting MJG et al (1998) Iron deposits and catabolic properties of synovial tissue from patients with haemophilia. J Bone Joint Surg 80B:540–545
16. Roosendaal G, Van Rinsum AC, Vianen ME et al (1999) Haemophilic arthropathy resembles degenerative rather than inflammatory joint disease. Histopathology 34:144–153
17. Roosendaal G, Vianen ME, van den Berg HM et al (1997) Cartilage damage as a result of hemarthrosis in a human in vitro model. J Rheumatol 24:1350–1354
18. Roosendaal G, Vianen ME, Marx JJM et al (1999) Blood induced joint damage: a human in vitro study. Arthritis Rheum 42:1025–1032
19. Lafeber FP, Vander Kraan PM, van Roy JL et al (1993) Articular cartilage explant culture; an appropriate in vitro system to compare osteoarthritic and normal human cartilage. Connect Tissue Res 1993;29:287–299
20. Hooiveld MJJ, Roosendaal G, Van den Berg HM et al (2003) Blood-induced joint damage: long-term effects in vivo and in vitro. J Rheumatol 30(2):339–344
21. Niibayashi H, Shimizu K, Suzuki et al (1995) Proteoglycan degradation in hemarthrosis. Intraarticular, autologous blood injection in rat knees. Acta Orthop Scand 66:73–79
22. Van Roon JA, van Roy JL, Lafeber FP, Bijlsma JW (1996) The stimulation of mononuclear cells from patients with rheumatoid arthritis to degrade articular cartilage is not modulated by cartilage itself. Clin Exp Rheumatol 14(2):177–182
23. Bates EJ, Lowther DA, Handley CJ (1984) Oxygen free-radicals mediate an inhibition of proteoglycan synthesis in cultured articular cartilage. Ann Rheum Dis 43:462–469
24. Burkhardt H, Schwingel M, Menninger H et al (1986) Oxygen radicals as effectors of cartilage destruction. Direct degradative effect on matrix components and indirect action via activation of latent collagenase from polymorphonuclear leukocytes. Arthritis Rheum 29:379–387
25. Hooiveld MJJ, Roosendaal G, Wenting M et al (2003) Short-term exposure of cartilage to blood results in chondrocyte apoptosis. Am J Pathol 162(3):943–951
26. Hooiveld MJJ, Roosendaal G, van den Berg HM et al (2003) Hemoglobin-derived iron-dependent hydroxyl radical formation in blood-induced joint damage: an in vitro study. Rheumatology 42:784–790
27. Roosendaal G, TeKoppele JM, Vianen ME et al (1999) Blood induced joint damage: a canine in vivo study. Arthritis Rheum 42:1033–1039
28. Roosendaal G, TeKoppele JM, Vianen ME et al (2000) Articular cartilage is more susceptible to blood-induced cartilage damage at young age than old age. J Rheumatol 27:1740–1744
29. Hooiveld MJJ, Roosendaal G, Vianen M et al (2003) Immature articular cartilage is more susceptible to blood-induced damage than mature articular cartilage: an animal in vivo study. Arthritis Rheum 48(2):396–403
30. Hooiveld MJJ, Roosendaal G, Jacobs K et al (2004) Experimental joint bleeds, combined with loading of the joint initiates degenerative joint damage: a possible mechanism in hemophilic arthropathy. Arthritis Rheum 50(6):2024–2031
31. Convery FR, Woo SL, Akeson WH, Amiel D et al (1976) Experimental hemarthrosis in the knee of the mature canine. Arthritis Rheum 19:59–67
32. Parsons JR, Zingler BM, McKeon JJ (1987) Mechanical and histological studies of acute joint hemorrhage. Orthopedics 10:1019–1026

14. Blake DR, Gallagher PJ, Potter AR et al (1984) The effect of synovial iron on the progression of rheumatoid disease. A histologic assessment of patients with early rheumatoid synovitis. Arthritis Rheum 27:495–501
15. Rosenthal CJ, Vincent MJ, Manning MBG et al (1998) Iron deposits and catabolic properties of synovial tissue from patients with haemophilia. J Bone Joint Surg 80B:540–545
16. [illegible]

Section II

Peri-operative Management of Hemophiliac Patients

Chapter 3

Conservative or Surgical Treatment? Motion Analysis Can Help Decide

Axel Seuser

Introduction

Patients with hemorrhagic diatheses such as hemophilia A and B, and von Willebrand syndrome frequently develop spontaneous bleeding, especially in the musculoskeletal system. Although the incidence of joint bleeding has been significantly reduced over the last 30 years through the consistent use of prophylaxis and clotting factor replacement, and the clinical manifestations of this patient population in the area of orthopedics have undergone radical transformation in recent years, these patients are still at risk from joint dysfunction due to bleeding [1]. An ongoing multicenter study involving motion analysis in children with hemophilia aged 3 to 18 years was launched $2^1/_2$ years ago. Fourty-hundred knee joints have been analyzed to date. The study showed age-dependent kinematic development of the knee joint, with patterns that differed in terms of coordination (treadmill walking) and strength (knee bends). In addition to these age-dependent criteria, another biomechanical criterion pertaining to motion analysis also became apparent which was entirely independent of age: the roll and glide pattern of the knee joints. Whereas a regression coefficient of 0.59 was estimated with reference to age for knee bends, and a value of 0.54 for gait, the age correlation of the score for internal knee joint kinematics was 0.05 [2–6].

Physical Fundamentals

According to Schumpe [7], an optimum roll–glide pattern (Fig. 3.1) is due to all the structures surrounding and forming the knee, such as joint shape, capsular ligament apparatus, menisci, and muscle. In the presence of strain in a closed chain such as knee bending or during gait, there is naturally a higher roll component, which ensures that forces are transferred perpendicularly to the cartilage surface. There is also a continuous alternation of contact surfaces, which optimizes the nutrition supply to the cartilage and minimizes cartilage overuse.

H.A. Caviglia, L.P. Solimeno (eds.), *Orthopedic Surgery in Patients with Hemophilia.*

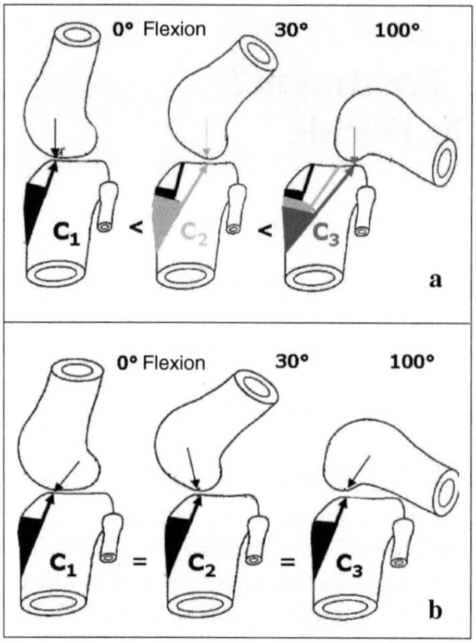

Fig. 3.1 a Rolling: loading angle C changes, loading is perpendicular, loading area changes, good for cartilage and function! **b** Gliding: loading angle C is constant, sagittal forces, more loading for cartilage, more strain for ligaments!

Brief Pathogenesis of Knee Joint Bleeding

When spontaneous bleeding into the knee joint occurs, the changes that take place include effects on the action of the muscles surrounding the knee. Even minor irritation and inflammation increases the tension in the flexor muscles of the leg, and in electomyogram (EMG) studies the contractility of the extensor muscles decreases in response to increasing intra-arterial pressure, starting with the vastus medialis [8]. This inevitably affects the internal kinematics of the knee, which in turn is manifest in the roll and glide pattern.

Three-Dimensional Functional Analysis (Fig. 3.2)

Function tests have been conducted on hemophiliac patients in Bonn on a regular basis since 1979. The measuring system developed at the Department of Biomechanics and Biophysics at the University of Bonn (original ultrasound topometry) is an acoustic measurement technique for non-contact three-dimensional spatial measurement. It is based on the measurement of the run times of regularly emitted ultrasound impulses. The ultrasound impulses of transmitters attached to the body to be measured are recorded by receivers installed at fixed spatial locations. The run times are used to determine the distances from the transmitters to the receivers. The latter are converted by computer to rectangular cartesian coordinates,

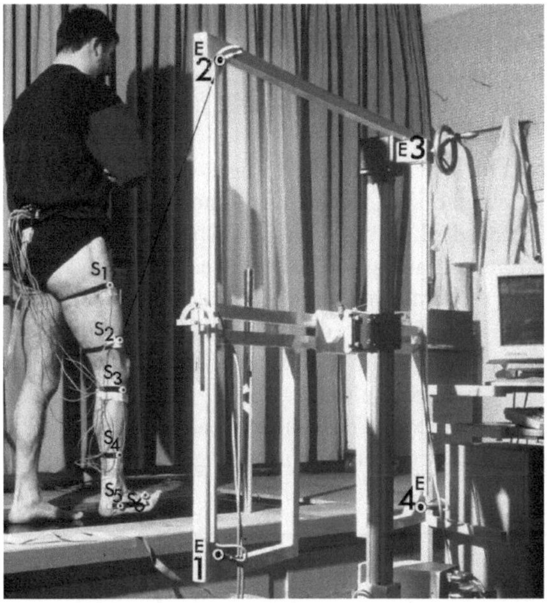

Fig. 3.2 Gait analysis of the right knee on a treadmill with the ultrasound topometer. *S*, ultrasound transmitters; *E*, ultrasound receivers

and represented in online graphics on the terminal, for the various projections. Two ultrasound-measuring transmitters are each attached above and below the knee joint to measure the roll and glide pattern of the joint. The results are evaluated using a special software program that calculates the roll and glide motion on the basis of tibial position during knee bends. The angle that the tangent occupies on the trajectory of movement with the axis of the lower leg transmitter is determined. The roll is defined as a permanent change of the tangential angle of the tibia versus the knee curvature angle in an upward direction. Glide is expressed in a consistent tangential angle of the tibia during knee bends. Point-by-point load distribution, such as takes place during rolling, is no longer present, and pressure increases on the same unvarying contact sites between the femur and tibia. Increasing forces from a sagittal direction impose an added strain on the cartilage. Negative roll is characterized by a decreasing tangential angle of the tibia during knee bends, and resembles the motion made by car tires when the vehicle drives up a steep hill and skids backwards with spinning wheels [9–13].

Results in Hemophiliac Patients

We have now conducted roll–glide measurements in almost 1000 knees of patients of various ages and joint conditions. The results did not correlate with the patients' subjective rating, with the clinical examination, or with the radiological picture. Nor did morphological magnetic resonance imaging (MRI) changes correlate with the roll and glide action.

The multicenter pediatric study has now produced initial prospective remeasurements in children before, with, and without physiotherapy. A trend is apparent from the results, suggesting that physiotherapy brings about a significant improvement in gait analysis score, knee bend score, and the roll and glide mechanism [7, 9, 14].

Earlier studies in patients with differently affected knees produced similar results. Patients with hemophilia deviated significantly from normal levels, with reduced roll components and increased glide components. After repeated knee bends, in some cases a very different roll and glide pattern was quantified as an expression of unstable internal joint motion. The curves tended to be much more irregular. Depending on the extent of kinematic disturbance, the profiles displayed various degrees of negative roll against the respective direction of motion. This can be demonstrated by two examples.

The subjectively and objectively more impaired right knee of patient WL (Fig. 3.3) showed a significantly uncoordinated profile with a high glide component.

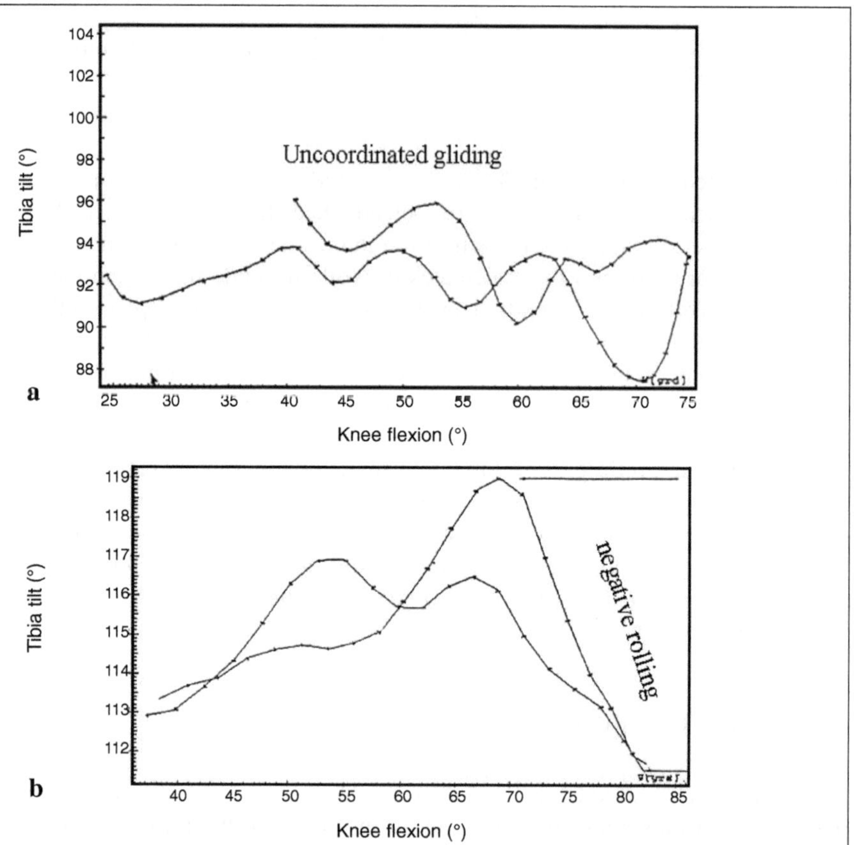

Fig. 3.3 a Right knee of patient "WL" (Pettersson score 12) shows varying gliding motion. **b** left knee (Pettersson score 0) shows rolling between 50°; and 70°; and negative rolling from 70°; to 80°

The minor roll component was unsteady, sometimes present only at the start of motion, sometimes in mid-motion, and sometimes at the end of a movement. A brief increase in the roll component alternated with pure glide or indeed a negative roll against the direction of movement (Fig. 3.3, top); the left knee (Fig. 3.3, bottom), which was completely unimpaired by bleeding, seemed entirely normal at clinical examination. The Pettersson score [15] was 0, but the roll and glide mechanism was changed similarly to that in the impaired contralateral side, although not to the same extent. The roll component never rose above 8°, even when the strain was increased. In contrast to the impaired right side, the concentric phase in the left leg with a predominantly quadriceps function was more affected by change than the eccentric phase, with a predominantly hamstring action. In both the eccentric and the concentric phase, the roll component was mainly at the start of the motion, in some cases after a short initiation of movement with a higher glide ratio. Negative roll components were also measured. This patient had never received suitable physiotherapy.

Other patients demonstrated adequate kinematics with a sufficiently large roll component, low glide components, and steadier profiles, despite a high Pettersson score (8) and a subjectively and clinically poor state (Fig. 3.4). These patients had received regular but not very systematic physiotherapy.

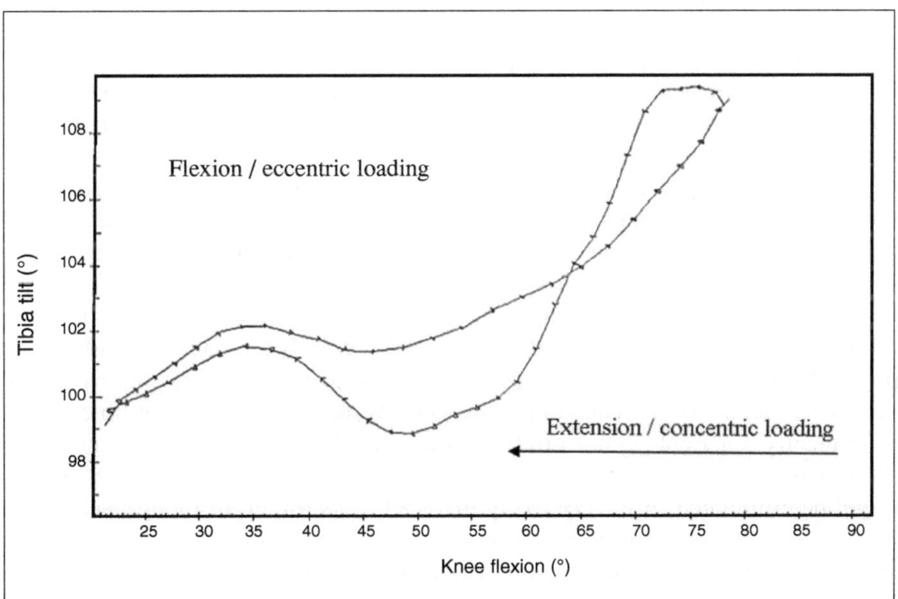

Fig. 3.4 Good roll pattern through whole range of motion. Right knee with hemarthropathy and Pettersson score 8

Discussion

The value of three-dimensional functional analysis in assessing the necessity of surgery depends on the nature of the planned intervention [16]. This does not apply to interventions required for synovial control in the presence of synovitis and an increased risk of bleeding; rapid action is necessary in such cases [17, 18]. If physiotherapy, antiphlogistic treatment, intra-articular cortisone administration, and synoviorthesis are unsuccessful, early synovectomy should be performed by transarthroscopic or open technique.

Implantation of an artificial knee joint [19, 20] or other morphologically and structurally modifying interventions in the knee joint might, however, benefit from motion analysis and measurement of roll and glide action. This needs to be discussed from a short-term and a long-term perspective.

In patients with a physiological roll and glide action, it is safe to assume that the polycentricity of the knee joint is preserved and determined by the muscles. The more the roll component declines, or indeed gives way to a negative roll, the closer the knee approaches a monocentric pattern of motion. In the latter case, the muscles may lose their importance and the motion of the knee joint may be determined solely by the bone tissue or the shrunken capsule. However, the terminal kinematic status of the knee joint as a monocentric joint does not always correlate with the radiological picture. For example, we have seen knee joints with a low Pettersson score (6–8) that were markedly monocentric in terms of kinematics. Conversely, we have seen knee joints with a Pettersson score of 8–12 that displayed adequately large roll components and were thus polycentric. Measurements before and after therapy have shown that the function of a monocentric joint barely responds to improved muscular guidance. Surgery is usually the best solution here. Capsular atrophy should be ruled out beforehand as a potential cause. Manual treatment methods followed by muscle strengthening may restore the internal joint mechanics.

In contrast, the polycentric joint is still amenable to conservative training therapy and physiotherapy. A highly individual knee-related physiotherapeutic and training therapy program can be drawn up on the basis of the data measured.

Long-term prevention of a surgical procedure would be possible for many children if motion analysis studies were performed across the board. All the children in our prospective multicenter study who regularly followed individualized physiotherapy recommendations [21] were able to significantly improve their kinematic status. This means that knee joint dysfunction that is not objectively or clinically apparent — but produces strain on the wrong areas and increases the risk of bleeding into the knee joint and hemarthropathy with every step — might be eliminated. It is very likely that such impairment of motion accompanies the subject through the growing years and into adulthood, with the excess strain making the knee joint more vulnerable to bleeding and the associated hemarthrotic sequelae.

Summary

Biomechanical motion analysis can be used to analyze the internal kinematics of the knee joint on the basis of roll and glide patterns. This facilitates the initiation of appropriate joint-based therapeutic concepts and monitoring of the patient's response to treatment. It has been shown that a joint that is less involved clinically and radiologically tends to adapt in kinematic terms to the more severely involved contralateral side. Detailed concentric and eccentric stress phase analysis is a good basis for identifying and providing specific treatment for muscle imbalance. Clinical and radiological diagnostic procedures do not constitute a basis for drawing conclusions regarding functional motion sequences in the knee joint. Long-term kinematic monitoring has shown that individual treatment programs can help to improve internal kinematics and thus help to preclude joint interventions later on. Adequate pain management should never be neglected. A study in more than 100 hemophiliacs in Bonn showed that people with hemophilia tend to suffer in silence [22].

References

1. Seuser A, Oldenburgh J, Brackmann HH (1999) Pathogenese, Diagnose und orthopädische Therapie der hämophilen Gelenkarthropathie. In: Hämostaseologie: Molekulare und zelluläre Mechanismen, Pathophysiologie und Klinik. Springer, Berlin, pp 198–209
2. Seuser A, Wallny T, Schumpe G et al (2003) Motion analysis in children with hemophilia. In: Rodríguez-Merchán EC (ed) The haemophilic joints: new perspectives. Blackwell Publishing Ltd, Oxford, pp 155–162
3. Seuser A, Schulte-Overberg U, Wallny T et al (2002) In: Scharrer I, Schramm W (eds) Functional analysis as a basis for optimizing physiotherapy in hemophilic children. 33rd Hemophilia Symposium, Hamburg
4. Seuser A, Wallny T, Schumpe G et al (2003) Motion analysis in children with haemophilia. In: Rodríguez-Merchán EC (ed) The haemophilic joints new perspectives. Blackwell Publishing Ltd, Oxford, p 155
5. Seuser A (2004) The young haemophilic knee – a 3D motion analysis multi centre study. Haemophilia 10(3):79–87
6. Seuser A, Schumpe G, Brackmann HH, Wallny T (2004) Functional disorders and treatment modalities in hemophilic children. In: 34th Hemophilia Symposium, Hamburg 2003. Springer Medizin Verlag, Heidelberg, pp 232–237
7. Schumpe G, Hallbauer T, Seuser A (1990) Application of an ultrasonic measuring system to determine internal muscle and constraining forces. In: Goh JCH, Nather A (eds) Proceedings of the Sixth International Conference on Biomedical Engineering in Singapore. BAC Printers, Singapore, pp 127–131
8. Bittscheidt W, Hofmann P, Schumpe G (1978) Elektromyographische Untersuchung an der Oberschenkelmuskulatur bei hämophilem Kniegelenkerguss und bei Reizzuständen des Kniegelenkes. Z Orthop 116:56–60
9. Seuser A, Hallbauer T, Schumpe G (1992) 3D Gang-und Bewegungsanalyse des Kniegelenkes beim medizinischen Muskelaufbautraining. In: Proceedings zum Europäischen Symposium über klinische Gangananlyse, Zürich (Laboratorium für Biomechanik der ETH Zürich Hrsg). Hans Beusch, Schlieren/Schweiz, pp 192–195

10. Seuser A, Schumpe G, Eickhoff HH et al (1993) Analyse der Kniekinematik bei Patienten mit Hämarthopathie beim Leg Press Training. In: Scharrer I, Schramm W (eds) 24th Hämophilie-Symposium, Hamburg. Springer Berlin Heidelberg, pp 150–157
11. Seuser A, Schumpe G, Eickhoff H et al (1994) Gait analysis of the hemophilic knee with different shoes and inlays. In: Ambriz R (ed) Abstracts of the XXI International Congress of the World Federation of Hemophilia, Mexico City, p 144
12. Seuser A, Wallny T, Klein H et al (1997) Gait analysis of the hemophilic ankle with silicone heel cushion. Clin Orthop 343:74–80
13. Seuser A, Wallny T, Schumpe G et al (2000) Biomechanical research in haemophilia. In: Rodríguez-Merchán EC, Goddard NJ, Lee CA (eds) Musculoskeletal aspects of haemophilia. Blackwell Science, Oxford, pp 27–36
14. Seuser A, Klein H, Wallny T et al (1998) Biomechanical basics of medical training therapy for hemophiliacs. In: Lee CA, Kessler CM (eds) Abstracts of the 23rd International Congress of the World Federation of Hemophilia 4(3)
15. Wallny T, Lahaye L, Brackmann HH et al (2002) Clinical and radiographic scores in haemophilic arthropathies: how well do these correlate to subjective pain status and daily activities. Haemophilia 8:802–808
16. Hallbauer T, Seuser A, Schumpe G (1992) Beispiel der Notwendigkeit einer dreidimensionalen Analyse des Gangbildes zur weiteren Therapieplanung bei einer mehrfach knieoperierten Patientin. In: Proceedings zum Europäischen Symposium über klinische Gangananlyse, Zürich (Laboratorium für Biomechanik der ETH Zürich Hrsg). Hans Beusch, Schlieren/Schweiz, pp 196–199
17. Fernández-Palazzi F (1990) Radioactive synoviorthesis in haemophilic haemarthrosis. In: Hämäläinrn M, Hagena F-W, Schwägerl W, Teigland J (eds) Revisional surgery in rheumatoid arthritis. Rheumatology 13:251–260
18. Eickhoff HH, Brackmann HH, Koch W (1990) Orthopädische Therapie der hämophilen Kniegelenksarthropathie unter besonderer Berücksichtigung der operativen Arthroskopie. In: Landbeck G, Scharrer I, Schramm W (eds) 21st Hämophilie-Symposium, Hamburg. Springer, Berlin Heidelberg New York
19. Greene WB, Degnore LT, White GC (1990) Orthopaedic procedures and prognosis in hemophilic patients who are seropositive for human immunodeficiency virus. J Bone Joint Surg 72:2–11
20. Luck JV, Kasper CK (1989) Surgical management of advanced hemophilic arthropathy. Clin Orthop 242:60–82
21. Seuser A, Kurme A, Wallny T et al (2002) Sport and physical fitness recommendations for young hemophiliacs. In: Scharrer I, Schramm W (eds) Functional analysis as a basis for optimizing physiotherapy in hemophilic children. 33rd Hemophilia Symposium, Hamburg
22. Wallny T, Hess L, Seuser A et al (2001) Pain status of patients with severe haemophilic arthropathy. Haemophilia 7:453–458

Chapter 4
Orthopedic Surgery in HIV-Positive Hemophiliac Patients

Giuseppe Tagariello and Paolo Radossi

Introduction

The introduction, more than 20 years ago, of pro-coagulant concentrates in the treatment of hemophilia A and B brought about a real advance which permitted a rapid normalization of the coagulation time. The even more extraordinary fact is that this coagulation time, normalized in a few minutes, can be maintained for hours or days, depending on the clinical necessities of the patients and of the treatment programs.

Hemophiliac haemorrhages in any part of the body, whether spontaneous, post-traumatic or surgical, were managed in this way. At the same time, it was hoped for a definitive solution to the more important symptom: haemorrhagic arthropathy. The facts did not completely satisfy the expectations. By normalizing the coagulation time the haemarthroses are less violent, of shorter duration, but their unpredictability and capacity to reoccur over a period of many years have not been eliminated [1].

Unfortunately, commercial concentrates transmitted infections such as hepatitis and human immunodeficiency virus (HIV), which dramatically changed the life of the hemophiliac community [2] and are still heavily affecting patients and doctors dealing with this disease.

It is well known that patients with hemophilia can exhibit severe joint destruction in adult life as a result of recurrent hemarthrosis. This is often multi-articular, affecting the shoulders, elbows, hips, knees, and ankles [3–5]. Meanwhile, in some countries the widespread use of early "on-demand" or prophylactic therapy has reduced the long-term joint damage in patients with hemophilia [6, 7]. However, a vast proportion of patients, most of them now older than 30 years, have lived a significant part of their life without the possibility of effective replacement therapy. For these patients, surgery often becomes the only option to improve their quality of life.

Over the last decades, joint replacement has became the gold standard for end-stage hemophilic arthropathy. One of the limitations or concerns about a

H.A. Caviglia, L.P. Solimeno (eds.), *Orthopedic Surgery in Patients with Hemophilia.*

surgical approach in these patients is that a proportion are HIV positive, with an associated reduction in life expectancy and increased risk of post-operative infections.

In our opinion the points to consider for major surgery in patients with hemophilia and HIV should be:

1. Who should undergo surgery?
2. Is there a basic blood test that should be carried out before performing surgery?
3. Are some types of surgery safer than others?
4. Risks related to bleeding
5. Risks in relation to the progression of HIV-related disease
6. Risks of infection following surgery

Fortunately, over recent years, patients with HIV have been treated with efficacious antiviral therapy which has improved their life expectancy, and a proportion of those patients with orthopedic problems have been evaluated for surgery and subsequently operated on. Thanks to these therapies, in the last few years we have been dealing with patients who have been treated for nearly a decade with highly active antiretroviral therapy (HAART) [8, 9]. This is a relatively new cohort of patients as the majority of studies on surgery in hemophilia have included either patients who were not yet infected with HIV (before the 1980s), or HIV-infected patients with limited life expectancy because of the absence of an effective therapy such as HAART.

Are the general criteria for considering major surgery in patients with HIV the same as for HIV-negative hemophiliacs or non-hemophiliac patients? Additional problems may be presented by co-morbidity with hepatitis C virus (HCV) infection and the higher risk of bleeding, not only because of hemophilia, but also, as recently reported, because of the protease inhibitors included in the HAART cocktail [10].

Although HIV infection is considered a disease that causes immune suppression, the methods used to measure this alteration in the immune system are limited. In fact they are quite similar to the analyses performed to follow up patients with HIV infection, which are based simply on the CD4 lymphocyte blood level and/or on the viral load in the serum. The majority of papers describing this approach select patients using a cut-off for CD4 of 200/mm^3 and a very low viral load; however, when the CD4 level is over this limit, the rate of infection in these patients also seems to be higher than in HIV-negative patients. The rate of infection in these patients varies widely, but Ragni et al [11] reported an infection rate of 26% when CD4 was below 200/mm^3, and Hinks et al [12] reported a rate of 36% when a re-implantation was performed. This level of infection is much higher than in either the general population or non-HIV hemophiliac patients. One of the factors facilitating infection in hemophiliacs could be the frequent administration of intravenous drugs, which can easily introduce microbes to seed a prosthesis.

This paper aims to review the experience of total joint arthroplasty (TJA) in patients with hemophilia and HIV. Total hip and knee arthroplasties (THA, TKA) are commonly used, although other joints have also been replaced.

Total Joint Replacement: An Overview

A report by Wiedel et al. [13] in 1989 of 97 TKAs in 76 patients with hemophilia showed a progressive increase in acute infections and, although the HIV status of the patients was not always reported, the authors noted a higher risk of infections in HIV-positive patients. In 1990, Kjaersgaard-Andersen et al described results of 13 TKAs in nine patients with hemophilia [14]; one was HIV positive at the time of surgery and died 3 months later. Two other patients subsequently died from acquired immune deficiency syndrome (AIDS), and the authors expressed concern that surgery may facilitate infections. In 1993, Teigland et al reported 15 TKAs in 15 patients, and three patients died of AIDS [15]. Greene et al reviewed the effect of HIV status on the immune system and recommended that surgery should be avoided if the CD4 count was below $200/mm^3$ [16]; they also observed that patients with a low CD4 count were at an increased risk of post-operative infection and more rapid progression to AIDS. Gregg-Smith et al reported six cases of septic arthritis in patients with hemophilia, and considered that there may be a high risk of secondary infection in HIV-positive patients with a TKA [17]. On the other hand, in 1994 Birch et al published a study of 15 TKAs in patients with severe hemophilia; eight were HIV positive but only one developed a deep infection which occurred 5 years after the TKA, following a dental infection — the same organism was identified at both sites [18]. Therefore Birch et al supported the use of TKA. They did not consider there was adequate evidence to deny HIV-positive patients a TKA if it was clinically indicated. So the questions at that point were: can we offer total joint replacement to HIV-positive patients without additional risk of infection or progression of HIV-related disease? And, do we have blood tests that are able to predict a faster progression of HIV-related disease? Phillips et al investigated the effect of orthopedic surgical procedures on the CD4 count in a group of HIV-positive and HIV-negative patients with hemophilia [19]. They established that the CD4 count did not decline more quickly in HIV-positive patients following surgery. From a different point of view, Silva et al [20] reported that the CD4 count at the time of TKA surgery in eight HIV-positive patients who developed an infection was similar to that of the 33 HIV-positive patients who did not develop one.

However, in the early 1990s there was a marked decrease in orthopedic surgery in patients with HIV; this may have been related to the fear of exposing staff to HIV, concerns about an increase in infections, or the cost–benefit ratio of performing an expensive operation in patients with a potentially shorter life. Lofqvist et al reported on six TKAs in patients with hemophilia, and one became infected [21]. Astermak et al also reported that surgery in HIV patients with hemophilia does not represent a risk factor for progression to AIDS in terms of

CD4 decline [22]. Regarding the question of post-surgical infections, several papers have reported they are not related to the faster progression of HIV-related disease, and Unger et al reviewed the results of 15 HIV-positive hemophilic patients who had undergone 26 TKAs [23]. The HIV status of three patients was not known at the time of surgery, but all other patients were HIV positive at the time of the operation. The mean follow-up was 4.4 years (1 to 9). Radossi et al [24] have reported the experience of our institute of a total of 79 arthroplasties in 66 hemophiliacs performed between 1987 and 2005, with a mean follow-up of 8 years: 10 patients were HIV positive and the rate of infection was 20% despite the presence of a CD4 count over $200/mm^3$; these results are in keeping with several other studies [25–27]. A large retrospective survey from 115 centres in 37 US states carried out by Ragni et al concluded that the post-operative infection rate in HIV-positive hemophiliacs with a CD4 count under $200/mm^3$ was much greater than in a normal population [11]. Eight of the 27 (29%) knee arthroplasties became infected. In particular, the results demonstrated that knee arthroplasties were three times more likely to develop post-operative infection than non-arthroplasty procedures. Overall, these results suggest that TKA may have a very high risk of post-operative infection in HIV-positive hemophiliac patients with a CD4 count of less than $200/mm^3$. Ragni et al also highlighted the importance of early and vigorous treatment when an infection is suspected, and antibiotic prophylaxis should be recommended when surgery is to be performed in HIV-positive patients. It should be remembered that an infected prosthesis will require a revision arthroplasty or a joint arthrodesis. Both salvage procedures may again increase the risk of new infections. In a large multicenter study, Hicks et al reported the outcome of 102 replacement arthroplasties in 73 HIV-positive patients from eight specialist hemophilia centres [12]. Of these, 91 were primary procedures. The mean age of the patients at surgery was 39 years, and the median follow-up time was five years. The overall rate of deep sepsis was 18.7% for primary procedures and 36.3% for revisions. This is a much higher rate of infection than that seen in normal populations.

However, as stated by Rodríguez-Merchán et al in 2002 [28], there is a certain contrast between papers — some encourage surgery but some emphasize that the procedures increase the risk of infection, while others [21, 22] conclude that there seems to be no evidence to suggest an acceleration in the rate of CD4 lymphocyte decline in HIV-positive patients with hemophilia as a result of elective joint surgery. In the same paper, Rodríguez-Merchán et al describe the personal experience of 37 TKAs in 26 men, 17 of whom were HIV positive; of these, nine have died from complications of AIDS. The mean survival time for HIV-positive patients was 113.8 months (9.6 years) after surgery, with a range of 3 to 16 years. HIV-positive patients tolerated surgery well and there was no significant decline in the HIV wellness scale.

In a recent paper (2005), Powell et al determined the incidence of deep infection rates following total knee and hip arthroplasties in HIV-seropositive and HIV-seronegative persons with hemophilia [29]. Fifty-one primary joint replacements were performed on 32 patients. Thirty prostheses were placed in patients who were HIV seropositive prior to surgery (n = 14) or seroconverted later (n = 16). Deep infections developed in five (9.8%) of 51 replacement joints. There were two infections during 204.15 joint-years without HIV infection, and three infections during 205.28 joint-years with HIV infection. The incidence rate of joint infection was not increased with HIV and these authors conclude that HIV infection is not a contraindication to knee or hip replacement arthroplasty in the appropriate clinical setting. This is also supported by Habermann et al [30] who recently reported that total hip replacement performed in a specialized hemophilia center is a safe procedure. Most of the studies discussed in the text are summarized in Table 4.1.

Conclusion

Despite the wide variety of prostheses and protocols, TKA and THA deep infection rates in the general population are consistently reported to be 1–2% and <1% respectively [31–33]. However, infection rates in patients with hemophilia are reported to be much higher, ranging from 7% to 26.5% [11–30]. The highest risks are thought to be in those with HIV infection and CD4 counts below 200/mm^3 when a re-implantation is necessary [11, 12]. The paper by Powell et al. [29] reports an overall 9.8% infection rate following primary TJR in persons with hemophilia, irrespective of HIV status, which is comparable with previously reported rates in patients with hemophilia; it should be remembered that the study by Ragni et al [11] was carried out before the introduction of HAART which has improved the immunity of HIV-infected persons.

Despite the general idea that patients with hemophilia and HIV infection but not AIDS can undergo major surgery without additional risks of progression to AIDS, the general experience for joint infections is that hemophiliacs and HIV-infected patients have a higher infection rate than the general population irrespective of their HIV status, if thir CD4 level is over 200/mm^3.

For TJR, additional risk factors might be represented by (1) the duration of the operation, (2) the use of cement, and (3) the use of tourniquets. In most papers these data are not available, and the difference between early and late infections is not stated, which is relevant as recently reported by Zimmerli et al [33]. In fact, early infections are due to intra-operative and peri-operative management, they occur in the first 24 months after surgery and are usually acquired during implantation of the prosthesis. Late infections occurring more than 24 months after surgery, on the other hand, are predominately acquired by hematogenous seeding. A major risk factor for this manner of infection in hemophiliacs is represented by the multiple injections necessary for these patients. In fact delayed infections are thought to be transmitted by a hematological route, which might be of special relevance in the case of patients with hemophilia. In a recent study by Giulieri et al [34] on 63 consecutive episodes of infection in non-hemophiliac patients, associated with hip prostheses over a 16-year period, 29% of the cases were early infections, 41% were delayed infections, and 30% were late infections.

Table 4.1 Papers reporting total joint replacement in patients with hemophilia, including those with HIV infection

Reference	Number of arthroplasties	Arthroplasties in HIV+	Infections in HIV+	Follow-up (years)	Died from HIV[a]	Notes[b]
Wiedel et al. 1989 [13]	93 TKA	NA	NA	NA	NA	HIV status is a risk factor, but no information on the number of HIV+ patients
Kjaersgaard-Andersen et al. 1990 [14]	13 TKA	3	NA	NA	3	NA
Teigland et al. 1993 [15]	15 TKA	3	NA	12	3	NA
Birch et al. 1994 [18]	15 TKA	8	1 (13%)	5	NA	NA
Kelley et al. 1995 [25]	34 THA	20	2 (20%	8	7	=
Ragni et al. 1995 [11]	74 orthopedic procedures	74	10 (15%)	NA	NA	CD4 status <200/mm^3 as major risk
Unger et al. 1995 [23]	26 TKA	26	0	9	NA	NA
Lofqvist et al. 1996 [21]	13 THA	NA	2	7	NA	NA
Hicks et al. 2001 [12]	102 TKA/THA	102	19 (18%)	5	NA	*44%* of infections resolved with medical and surgical therapy, re-implantation as major risk factor for infection
Rodríguez-Merchán et al. 2002 [28]	37 TKA	17	2 (22%)	9	NA	Source of infections was identified outside of joint
Norian et al. 2002 [26]	53 TKA	38	NA	NA	13	HIV not related to development of infective hematogenous spread of bacteria during concentrate administration
Sheth et al. 2004 [27]	14 TKA	1	NA	6	1	NA
Silva, Luck JR 2005 [20]	90 TKA	61	11(17%)	NA	NA	NA
Powell et al. 2005 [29]	51 TKA/THA	31	3 (10%)	7	NA	NA
Radossi et al. 2005 [24]	79 TKA/THA	10	2 (20%)	8	2	NA
Habermann et al. 2006 [26]	15 THA	NA	1	11	NA	NA

[a]Number of patients died because of HIV infection during the follow-up
[b]Comments by the authors
NA: not available

There is not enough information in the literature about the start of infection in hemophiliacs to enable an assessment of whether or not they might be considered early or late infections. However, in the case of hemophilia late infection might more often involve a hematogenous route or recurrent hemarthrosis. In these cases we could improve both prophylaxis and early treatment by antibiotic use as well as early "on-demand" treatment or prophylaxis with factor VIII or factor IX concentrates.

As reported by Silva et al [20], the high prevalence of late infection after arthroplasties in hemophiliac patients may be a consequence of an array of factors, including, but not limited to, HIV status, hepatitis C status, hematogenous infections from frequent intravenous self-administration of clotting factor concentrate, or other remote infection sources. A hematogenous source is also suggested by other authors [26], and by the high prevalence of infections observed with bilateral total knee replacement. Prevention of late infection would substantially improve the long-term outcome of TKR in the hemophiliac population. In the hope of reducing the prevalence of late infection, patients should be instructed regarding the importance of meticulous antisepsis during self-infusion, regular medical check-ups, immediate reporting of any signs of infections, and the use of prophylactic antibiotics prior to any other procedures with a potential for contamination, including dental work. The use of short-term prophylactic antibiotics prior to self-infusion should be considered, and it is very important to clearly inform the patient of the higher risks associated with TJR, emphasizing the importance of meticulous attention to post-operative infection-prevention recommendations.

In a recent abstract reported by Ashrani et al [35] at the XXVIII Congress of the World Federation of Hemophilia in Vancouver, among a large cohort of 8042 patients, 24 (0.3%) had a documented joint infection. The knee was most commonly affected (67%) and gram-positive organisms were identified in 84% of cases. Risk factors studied included age, race, hemophilia type and severity, number of joint bleeds, use of central venous access device (CVAD), inhibitor, target joint, invasive procedure, and HIV and HCV infection. In a logistic regression model that included all variables, only increasing age, black race, presence of inhibitor, invasive procedure in the past year, and presence of target joint remained statistically significant. The authors conclude that septic arthritis is an uncommon complication that occurs in hemophiliacs with underlying joint arthropathy and a history of recent invasive procedures, but not with HIV infection. Although the paper describes a higher infection rate in patients who underwent replacement joints, a high proportion occurs in patients without any prosthesis. This observation opens a possible interpretation for patients with hemophilia whose infection rate in the case of prosthesis seems much higher irrespective of the presence of HIV infection.

Traldi et al stated:

In patients with hemophilia and HIV the observations made during and after surgery were identical to those of HIV negative patients who underwent the same *type of surgery. We did not report slowness in cicatrisation or formation of bone tissue, even in the two HIV positive patients who had emergency operations for exposed fracture of the tibia-fibula and fracture of the neck of the thigh bone who had CD4 levels below 100/mm^3 [1].*

In spite of the good hemostasis obtained during and after the intervention, the high rate of infection is probably due to the duration of the more difficult and time-consuming surgery and not to the supposed high risk of bleeding, as the vast majority of hemophiliac patients undergoing surgery have comparable hemostasis to that of the normal population.

As several studies have demonstrated, high rates of infection occur, but analysis of survivors strongly suggests that most patients already diagnosed with HIV infection at the time of surgery should derive many years of symptomatic relief after a successful joint replacement. For this reason, we think that major surgery such as prosthesis is possible in patients with hemophilia, with acceptable risks and good results in terms of quality of life and joint movement improvement.

In summary, TJR provides considerable benefits in the majority of hemophiliac patients, with marked pain relief and improvement in function. The procedure can, however, be associated with a high number of complications. Some complications in early reports may have been due to inadequate factor replacement, although experience suggests that bleeding can occur in spite of high levels of factor replacement and it may represent a further risk factor for seed vehicle infections. Careful counseling and education of both patients and healthcare workers before operating are therefore essential.

References

1. Traldi A, Davoli PG, Gajo GB et al (1993) Surgical treatment of HIV positive patients: the haematological approach.b Proceedings of the IX International Meeting of the Muscular Skeletal Committee of the WFH, Ed. Castelfranco Veneto 73–79
2. Darby SC, Ewart DW, Giangrande PL et al (1995) UK Haemophilia Centre Directors Organisation. Mortality before and after HIV infection in the complete UK population of Haemophiliacs. Nature 377:79–82
3. York J (1991) Musculoskeletal disorders in the haemophilias. Bailliere's Clin Rheumatol 5:197–220
4. Rodríguez-Merchán EC (1996) Effects of haemophilia on articulations of children and adults. Clin Orthop 328:7–13
5. Luck J, Kasper C (1998) Surgical management of advanced hemophilic arthropathy an overview of 20 years' experience. Clin Orthop 242:60–82
6. Nilsson IM, Berntorp E, Lofqvist T, Pettersson H (1992) Twenty-five years experience of prophylactic treatment in severe hemophilia A and B. J Intern Med 232:25–32
7. Plug I, van der Bom JG, Peters M et al (2004) Thirty years of hemophilia treatment in the Netherlands, 1972–2001. Blood 104:3494–500
8. del Amo J, Perez-Hoyos S, Moreno A et al (2006) Trends in AIDS and mortality in HIV-infected subjects with hemophilia from 1985 to 2003: the competing risks for death between AIDS and liver disease. J Acquir Immune Defic Syndr 41:624–31

9. Arnold DM, Julian JA, Walker IR (2006) Association of Hemophilia Clinic Directors of Canada.Mortality rates and causes of death among all HIV-positive individuals with hemophilia in Canada over 21 years of follow-up. Blood 108:460–464
10. Stanworth SJ, Bolton MJ, Hay CR, Shiach CR (1998) Increased bleeding in HIV-positive haemophiliacs treated with antiretroviral protease inhibitors. Haemophilia 4:109–114
11. Ragni MV, Crossett LS, Herndon JH (1995) Postoperative infection following orthopaedic surgery in human immunodeficiency virus-infected hemophiliacs with CD4 counts < or = 200/mm^3. J Arthroplasty 10:716–721
12. Hicks JL, Ribbans WJ, Buzzard B et al (2001) Infected joint replacements in HIV-positive patients with haemophilia. J Bone Joint Surg Br 3:1050–1055
13. Wiedel JD, Luck JV, Gilbert MS (1989) Total knee arthroplasty in the patients with hemophilia: evaluation and long-term results. In Gilbert MS, Greene WB eds Musculoskeletal problems in hemophilia National Hemophilia Foundation, New York, pp 152–157
14. Kjaersgaard-Andersen P, Christiansen S, Ingerslev J, Sneppen O (1990) Total knee arthroplasty in classic hemophilia. Clin Orthop 256:137–145
15. Teigland J, Tjonnfjord G, Evensen S, Charania B (1993) Knee arthroplasty in hemophilia. Acta Orthop Scand 64: 53–56
16. Greene W, DeGnore L, White G (1990) Orthopaedic procedures and prognosis in hemophilic patients who are seropositive for human immunodeficiency virus. Am J Bone Joint Surg Am 1(72):2–11
17. Gregg-Smith S, Pattison R, Dodd C et al (1993) Septic arthritis in haemophilia. J Bone Joint Surg Br 3(75):368–370
18. Birch NC, Ribbans WJ, Goldman E, Lee CA (1994) Knee replacement in hemophilia. J Bone Joint Surg Br (76):165–166
19. Phillips A, Sabin C, Ribbans W, Lee C (1997) Orthopaedic surgery in haemophilic patients with human immunodeficiency virus. Clin Orthop 343:81–78
20. Silva M, Luck JV Jr (2005) Long-term results of primary total knee replacement in patients with hemophilia. J Bone Joint Surg Am 87:85–91
21. Lofqvist T, Sanzen L, Petersson C, Nilsson IM (1996) Total hip replacement in patients with hemophilia. 13 hips in 11 patients followed for 1–16 years. Acta Orthop Scand 67:321–324
22. Astermak J, Lofqvist T, Schulman S et al (1998) Major surgery seems not to influence HIV disease progression in haemophilia patients. Br J Haematol 103:10–14
23. Unger AS, Kessler CM, Lewis RJ (1995) Total knee arthroplasty in human immunodeficiency virus-infected hemophiliacs. J Arthroplasty 10:448–452
24. Radossi P, Bisson R, Petris U et al (2005) Total joint replacement in haemophiliacs: 17 year single institution experience at Castelfranco Venetoexperience. Haematologica 90(Suppl p 393):260
25. Kelley SS, Lachiewicz PF, Gilbert MS et al (1995) Hip arthroplasty in hemophilic arthropathy. J Bone Joint Surg Am 77:828–834
26. Norian JM, Ries MD, Karp S, Hambleton J (2002) Total knee arthroplasty in hemophilic arthropathy. J Bone Joint Surg Am 84(7):1138–1141
27. Sheth DS, Oldfield D, Ambrose C, Clyburn T (2004) Total knee arthroplasty in hemophilic arthropathy. J Arthroplasty 19:56–60
28. Rodríguez-Merchán EC, Wiedel JD (2002) Total knee arthroplasty in HIV-positive haemophilic patients. Haemophilia 8:387–392
29. Powell DL, Whitener CJ, Dye CE et al (2005) Knee and hip arthroplasty infection rates in persons with haemophilia: a 27 year single center experience during the HIV epidemic. Haemophilia 11:233–239
30. Habermann B, Eberhardt C, Hovy L et al (2006) Total hip replacement in patients with severe bleeding disorders: A 30 years single center experience. Int Orthop 20 (Epub ahead of print)
31. Fender D, Harper DW, Gregg PJ (1999) Outcome of Charnley total hip replacement across a single heath region in England. J Bone Joint Surg Br 81:577–581
32. Harris WH, Sledge CB (1990) Total hip and total knee replacement. N Engl J Med 323:801–807

33. Zimmerli W, Trampuz A, Ochsner PE (2004) Prosthetic-joint infections. N Engl J Med 351:1645–1654
34. Giulieri SG, Graber P, Ochsner PE, Zimmerli W (2004) Management of infection associated with total hip arthroplasty according to a treatment algorithm. Infection 32:222–228
35. Ashrani A, Key N, Duffy N et al (2006) Characteristics of and risk factors for septic arthritis in males with hemophilia. Haemophilia 12(Suppl 2)51

Chapter 5
The Liver and Surgery

Jorge Daruich, Estela Manero and Alfredo Parietti

Introduction

Individuals with hemophilia frequently present with infections caused by the hepatitis C (HCV), hepatitis B (HBV), and human immunodeficiency (HIV) viruses. Therefore, the possible need for an anesthetic-surgical procedure must be analyzed carefully in order to determine the presence and severity of hepatic illness, as morbidity and mortality may be increased within this sick group.

Patients with liver disease are more susceptible to bleeding, post-operative infection, and hepatic hypoxia caused by the decreased blood flow to the organ during anesthesia and general surgery. Moreover, they present pharmacokinetic alterations because of the drugs used during the procedure [1–3]. These elements all contribute to a deterioration of hepatic function. The surgical risks depend on several factors: the severity of liver disease, surgical intervention, and type of anesthesia [4–6].

Signs of Chronic Liver Diseases

Chronic liver diseases may present with portal hypertension (PH), with or without ascitic-edematous syndrome (AES), and portosystemic encephalopathy [5, 7, 8].

Portal Hypertension

The causes of PH may be classified according to their localization in: (a) prehepatic (portal and/or esplenic vein thrombosis), (b) intrahepatic (cirrhosis, chronic hepatitis, hepatic carciroma, etc), or (c) post-hepathic (Budd–Chiari syndrome, constrictive pericarditis, etc) sites [5, 6]. In patients with cirrhosis, an upper gastrointestinal endoscopy must be performed in order to investigate the presence of esophageal and/or gastric varicose veins and hypertensive gastropathy. If varicose veins are observed that are at risk of bleeding, appropriate pro-

H.A. Caviglia, L.P. Solimeno (eds.), *Orthopedic Surgery in Patients with Hemophilia.*

phylactic treatment must be performed before the surgical procedure, as their rupture may increase during surgery and the post-operative period, with a high morbidity and mortality as a result of this complication [1, 2].

Ascitic-Edematous Syndrome

The causes that determine the presence of ascites (accumulation of fluid in the peritoneal cavity) may be numerous. They may be broadly classified as: (a) hepatic: alcoholic hepatitis, cirrhosis of any etiology, primary and secondary tumors, etc, (b) hematological: Budd–Chiari syndrome, (c) cardiovascular: constrictive pericarditis, chronic heart failure, (d) peritoneal: tuberculosis, or (e) neoplastic: peritoneal carcinomatosis, lymphoma, and acquired immune deficiency syndrome (AIDS) [9]. Appropriate treatment for AES is important prior to the anesthetic-surgical procedure, because it improves hemodynamic, respiratory, and renal function, reduces infection risk and renal insufficiency and, in abdominal surgery, reduces suture dehiscence. The use of nephrotoxic and nonsteroidal anti-inflammatory drugs (NSAIDs) should be avoided, as they may hasten renal failure [1, 4].

Child–Pugh Score and Surgical Risk

Laboratory tests and physical examination allow an evaluation of the Child–Pugh score and an assessment of surgical risk [10]. The Child–Pugh score is positively related to the surgical risk (Table 5.1).

Table 5.1 Child–Pugh score

	Score		
	1	2	3
Hepatic encephalopathy	Absent	Grades 1 and 2	Grades 3 and 4
Ascites	Absent	Slight	Moderate
Bilirubin (mg/dl)	1–2	2–3	>3
Albumin (g/dl)	3.5	2.8–3.5	<2.8
Prothrombin time (s)	1–4	4–6	>6

The scores 1, 2 and 3 correspond to increasing abnormality for each of the five measured parameters:
Grade A: total score of 5 or 6
Grade B: total score of 7 to 9
Grade C: total score of 10 to 15

The effects of anesthesia and surgery depend on the drugs used, the type of surgical procedure, and the severity of liver disease. Some peri-operative conditions, such as arterial hypertension, infection, or the use of hepatotoxic drugs, may cause liver injury. In patients without liver disease, slight alterations in laboratory test results may occur. These alterations are usually resolved without consequences. However, in patients with previous liver disease there may be a noticeable deterioration of liver function that is clinically relevant [4].

The type of surgery is an important risk factor. Procedures that may cause major blood loss increase the risk of hepatic and renal ischemia [3]. Intra-abdominal operations cause greater reduction in hepatic blood flow than extra-abdominal ones. Gastric, colon, or cholecystectomy surgery has a high mortality rate in patients with dysfunctional cirrhosis. Also, emergency surgery may be more risky than elective surgery. Changes of hepatic blood flow have an impact on the liver's functional capacity as well as on its drug binding and excretion [1, 4].

Steatosis and non-alcoholic steatohepatitis (diseases that frequently present in individuals who are overweight, or have dyslipidemia or diabetes mellitus) do not cause clinically relevant disorders of hepatic function, unless they have progressed to the cirrhotic phase. In these patients, laboratory tests show a normal prothrombin time, aspartate aminotransferase (AST), and alanine aminotransferase (ALP), and normal or slightly raisedγ-glutamyl transferase (GGT). Drug metabolism is normal or slightly altered and this does not have a relevant influence on planning the therapeutic procedure [4].

Patients with cirrhosis are very sensitive to hemodynamic disturbance. Factors that may cause a change in hepatic flow are diverse: hypertension of long duration, postural or instrumental venous compression, liver disease and portal hypertension, injuries, or medicines [2, 7, 9, 11]. Changes in hemodynamics may also affect the metabolism of anesthetic agents.

Patients with cirrhosis have a reduced life expectancy, and anesthetic-surgical procedures may be associated with clinical decompensation [1, 2]. Peri-operative mortality, up to 30 days after surgery, may reach a rate of between 10% and 12%, while the overall morbidity of surgical procedures in cirrhosis is 30%. Factors that may be related to decompensation are a high Child–Pugh score, the presence of AES, increased creatinemia, chronic obstructive pulmonary disease, previous infection, bleeding of the digestive tract, inter-operative hypertension, etc.

On the other hand, the increased prothrombin time in individuals with cirrhosis is associated with a corresponding increase in the morbidity and mortality in patients undergoing surgery of medium complexity, especially when it is raised more than 2.5 times above normal [2, 4, 5]. Thrombocytopenia is found relatively frequently in this type of patient, and necessitates platelet transfusion in order to maintain a blood level of between 80,000 and 100,000 cells/mm^3.

In cases of compensated cirrhosis, activity of the renin–angiotensin system increases progressively in parallel with the hepatic injury, resulting in an increase of water and sodium retention. A hypercaloric salt-free diet that replaces animal proteins by vegetables, with additional prohibition of potassium salt due to the risk of hyperkalemia, are simple changes that will decrease the risk of functional renal failure [9].

In patients with AES, paracentesis with protein replacement and the use of diuretics must be monitored very carefully, as these patients have a highly unstable hemodynamic equilibrium, and very small changes in homeostasis may sometimes induce hepatorenal syndrome [9].

Even though renal disorder occurs most frequently in patients who receive antibiotic therapy with aminoglucosides, it is necessary to make a differential diagnosis with severe tubular necrosis, as the use of these drugs increases the risk of renal toxicity by up to 35% in AES, compared with 3–5% in those with a healthy liver [12].

The worse the hepatic lesion becomes, the higher the degree of cardiovascular repercussion; this is characterized by a decrease in cardiac reactivity and reduced activity of the beta andrenergic receptors, which manifests as ventricular extrasystole and other arrhythmias. The patient with liver disease requires careful assessment and monitoring of the cardiovascular system both preoperatively and during surgery, in order to reduce the risk of post-operative heart failure [13].

Also, patients with severe liver disease demonstrate a low oxygen saturation, even in the absence of a history of smoking or chronic restrictive pulmonary disease. This disorder becomes more acute when the patient is in the supine position. Generally, their carbon dioxide concentration is low because they are permanently in metabolic and respiratory alkalosis. In patients with alcoholic liver disease, a concomitant finding of chronic restrictive pulmonary disease is usual, because of the association with a smoking habit, which affects oxygen exchange. This forces the anesthetist to enhance the peri-operative conditions in order to obtain the best oxygenation level, while taking into account the use of respiratory kinesitherapy, bronchial dilators, antibiotics, and other drugs [7, 8, 11].

Patients with alcoholic liver disease show a raised drug resistance to barbiturates, benzodiazepines, and narcotics, which is caused by induction of microsomal enzymes over long periods of disease. However, as the liver injury progresses, a phenomenon of increased susceptibility to these drugs is noticed: under normal circumstances, benzodiazepines and barbiturates are bound by plasma albumin, but this does not happen in the sick liver, so a given dose will have an increased effect [7, 8].

When choosing an anesthetic for the patient with the liver disease, in addition to considering its metabolic action, the anesthetist must also take into account its effect on hepatic flow. Drugs that are excreted through the liver must be avoided, or they should be administered in small doses, choosing sedative and analgesic drugs with a short half-life to avoid triggering encephalopathy or episodes of delirium [7, 8, 11, 12]. Most intravenous anesthetic agents are metabolized in the liver, but strictly speaking recovery from anesthesia depends more on their method of distribution than on their metabolism. This is apparent with the use of propofol in compensated patients with cirrhosis, in whom the effect of this drug is slightly increased [13], while the effect of thiopental, which does not bind well to plasma proteins, is balanced by an increase in excretion.

There are particular situations where elective surgery is contraindicated because of high morbidity and mortality, such as acute liver failure, acute hepatitis, alcoholic hepatitis, stage C of the Child–Pugh score, or extrahepatic complications such as renal insufficiency, severe hypoxemia, and cardiac insufficiency. Most of these patients die in the immediate post-operative period because of liver insuffuciency or sepsis caused by their susceptibility to infection [1, 2].

Acute hepatic failure is defined as an insufficiency that develops in a previously healthy liver. This disorder becomes evident as a consequence of sudden failure of hepatic function.

Anesthetic-surgical procedures in patients with cirrhosis must be performed by a multidisciplinary team whose members have experience with this type of patient.

Pre-surgical Assessment

Anamnesis

All patients must be questioned carefully with the aim of assessing the presence of risk factors such as alcohol consumption background, time and quantity, drug use, sexual behavior, tattoos, chronic use of drugs (NSAIDs), prior anesthetic-surgical procedures, and other co-morbid factors, such as obesity and diabetes, among others [11].

Physical Examination

The physical examination must include a systematic search for signs of chronic hepatic disease such as hepatomegaly, palmar erythema splenomegaly, parotid hypertrophy, AES, or portosystemic encephalopathy.

Laboratory Tests

Besides the usual routine tests (blood count with platelet recount, urea, creatinine, glycemia, and erythrocyte sedimentation rate (ESR)), the following must be included: bilyrrubin, AST, ALT, ALP, GGT, proteinogram by electrophoresis, serum cholinesterase, prothrombin concentration, cholesterol, and α-fetoprotein. An appropriate interpretation of these tests will indicate the functional hepatic condition. Viral serology should also be tested (Table 5.2) to determine the presence or absence of viral infection and its stage.

Table 5.2 Serological scores of viral hepatitis A, B, and C

Serological score	Interpretation
Anti HAV IgM(+)	Acute Hepatitis A
Anti HAV IgG(+)	Cured Hepatitis A
HBs Ag(+)/anti HBc IgM(+)	Hepatitis B (acute)
HBs Ag(+)/anti HBc IgM(–)/ HBeAg(+) or (–)	Hepatitis B (chronic)
Detectable HBV DNA	Chronic hepatitis (replicative condition)
Anti HBc IgG(+)/anti HBs(+)	Hepatitis B (cured)
Anti HCV(+)/HCV RNA detectable	Hepatitis C (acute or chronic)
Anti HCV(+)/HCV RNA non-detectable	Hepatitis C (cured/false positive/false negative)

Diagnostic Imaging

Diagnostic imaging should principally include an abdominal scan. This examination will detect the presence of slight ascites (not detected in the physical examination), and can evaluate the liver's echogenicity, size, and form, which can be altered in different situations, such as fatty liver, chronic hepatitis, and cirrhosis. Imaging can also reveal signs that are suggestive of portal hypertension. In patients with chronic liver disease, a group with a high incidence of hepatocarcinoma, it should also find any occupying hepatic masses [14].

Anesthetics and Hepatotoxicity

The relationship between drugs and the liver is governed by: (a) the hepatic metabolism of toxic drugs, (b) the effects of liver diseases on the drugs' metabolism, and (c) liver injuries caused by drugs.

Hepatotoxicity caused by anesthetic agents is an issue that has been tackled in much research. Halothane is, beyond any doubt, the agent that has generated most interest. A short time after its introduction into anesthetic practice in 1956, halothane use became widespread, mainly because it is easy to use and not explosive, and so was considered to be a safe anesthetic agent. Its use spread quickly to become usual practice, and after a few years the first hepatotoxicity reports started to appear. These associated halothane with the development of devastating liver failure [15–18]. The studies developed to determine the frequency and type of liver injury caused by this drug, in particular one performed by the National Research Council in the USA in 1965, had a high profile because of their importance and the conclusions that could be made. In fact, the most detailed analysis in this research showed huge errors in the protocol design that ultimately generated major controversy, although some observations were subsequently confirmed. The results of this and other papers allowed a conclusion that the estimated frequency of hepatotoxicity is approximately one case in 10,000 in those exposed for the first time, against up to seven in 10,000 of those who receive it repeatedly [19].

The liver injury caused by halothane is more frequent in adults, obese individuals, and middle-aged women. Examination usually reveals previous exposure to the anesthetic, followed by a late fever, whose cause is not understood. Jaundice without serious complications is frequently manifested in the 14-day post-operative period, whether or not halothane has been used. However, the typical hepatitis syndrome caused by halothane starts with pains and heavy abdominal feelings, followed by, or even associated with, severe liver disease, characterized by fever, itching, nausea, anorexia, and jaundice, although the latter may be the first sign of a clinical manifestation. Once the jaundice has become established, it is evidenced by liver failure, and coagulation and renal function disorders start, as well as digestive bleeding and, finally, encephalopathy that may become liver coma. The histological injury is linked to massive necrosis in those patients who subsequently die, while in benign cases it mimics an acute viral hepatitis with subsequent *restitutio ad integrum*. The necrosis is most apparent in zone 3 of the liver lobule. Aminotransferases increase significantly, reaching levels around 250 times their normal value, although this is not predictive of outcome. ALP is slightly increased. Hyperbilirubinemia is caused by an increase of both indirect and direct fractions of bilirubin. The fall in prothrombin concentration has a predictive value and, if it reaches values of 15% of normal, death usually occurs. Furthermore, bilirubin levels above 20 mg/100 ml, age over 40 years, a short latent period from halothane administration to jaundice, and obesity are considered to be predictive of poor outcome. Anemia is frequently present, while leukocytosis is observed in up to 50% of patients. Eosinophilia is present in 20–50% of cases, and its presence is a suggestive factor for diagnosis. The finding of antibodies in the serum (a test that is not available in many countries), allows confirmation of the diagnosis [19].

Although the process that results in hepatic injury is not defined, it is suggested that the early stage depends on halothane metabolism, and that the metabolite trifluoroacetic chloride affects the microsomal proteins of the hepatic cells, generating neoantigens that cause a response of the immune system (immunological theory). A second hypothesis has been etiologically linked to the injury caused by halothane-induced hypoxia (hypoxia theory). A third hypothesis, which also has its followers and critics, is one that links the injury with the formation of toxic metabolites from the drug [20].

Many researchers believe that hepatic injury is probably the result of a mixed mechanism involving all three hypotheses. This type of lesion has also been associated with other inhaled agents such as methoxyfluorane (not used nowadays), enfluorane, isofluorane, and desfluorane, which also produce trifluoroacetic acid as a facilitator in their metabolism.

Hyperbilirubinemia can also appear after surgery, either as a result of an increase of the bilirubin load or because of reduced hepatic clearance.

Hemolysis, blood transfusions, sepsis, hematoma reabsorption, as well as hypoxemia, and reduced blood flow can also deteriorate hepatic function.

Transitional hypertension or peri-operative shock might cause acute lesions in the third area of the liver (central lobular zone). In these situations, there is frequently a significant increase of aminotranferases, which may reach a value 100 or 200 times the normal level, or even higher. This increase is usually self-limiting, and enzymes return to normal in about 5 or 7 days in patients with normal hepatic function; however, in individuals with compensated hepatopathies, the degree of hepatocellular necrosis might be enough to provoke serious functional disorders [18, 19, 21–23].

To summarize, the evolution of these disorders will depend on the relationship of multiple factors such as the underlying hepatic function, duration of hypoxemia, aggregated infections, hepatotoxicity caused by antibiotics, and also the anesthetic agents used.

Beta-blocking drugs, α_1-receptor blockers, and H_2 blockers reduce blood flow, and conflict with the action of dopamine. This is shown by an increase of circulating catecholamines, cushioned by pharmacological block of the sympathetic nervous system.

The action of the inhaled agents modifies, to a certain extent, the activity of other drugs. One example is ketamine — by either direct or indirect action — which is modified by fentanyl metabolism. Opiate agents such as fentanyl, alfentanil, nalbufin, and morphine, among others, might cause spasms of the sphincter of Oddi, with clinical symptoms that are similar to those of biliary colic. The appearance of a medical profile like this makes it important to consider a differential diagnosis between the adverse effect of these drugs and the presence of bile duct obstruction. In these cases, a scan of the area to decide the subsequent procedure is extremely useful [19, 24, 25].

NSAIDS may produce hepatic changes, which can range from a mild and temporary increase of aminotransferase to acute cytolytic hepatitis, cholestatic or mixed hepatitis, or even chronic hepatitis. The incidence is very low, and the hepatotoxic potential varies from one NSAID to another. These drugs, as already mentioned, may provoke a temporary increase of serum hepatic aminotransferases that will generally return to normal when treatment finishes. The most hepatotoxic NSAIDs are sulindac, diclofenac, and fenbufen, and, to a lesser degree, fenilbutazone, piroxicam, and droxicam [26].

Anesthetic Drugs

A significant number of new anesthetic drugs are being used daily in surgery, and therefore it is important to know their side-effects; it is also valuable to analyze, from a historical perspective, the adverse effects or complications related to anesthetics that are no longer in use.

Benzodiazepines (BZD), which are employed in almost all anesthetic procedures, each have slightly different effects according to their structure and metabolism.

Diazepam, for example, has a long half-life, and its metabolism in the liver produces two metabolites: oxazepam and desmetildiazepam. These metabolites are modified in phases I and II of biotransformation, depending on the predominant hepatic disease. Thus, clearance of the drug is prolonged in individuals with cirrhosis or hepatitis, whereas clearance is not affected in individuals with cholestasis. In addition, cimetidine (rarely used in current medical practice) may modify the P450 2E1 enzyme and increase the sedative effect of the diazepam [19].

Another drug from this group, midazolam (short half-life), is hydrolyzed in the liver and cleared through the kidney. Its action is only modified in critical cases by metabolic activity in phase I of biotransformation. One of its main features is that it is not metabolized by the P4502B6 and 2C9 cytochromes, but by the CYP34A cytochrome. The CYP34A cytochrome turns it into 4-hydroxymidazolam; a small proportion turns into α-hydroxymidazolam, with similar effects on the electroencephalogram (EEG) to those of the original drug, and both are excreted in the urine. There is a group of patients with slow metabolism who have an increased half-life for midazolam. Its cause remains unknown [19, 27].

Lorazepam has an intermediate 3-hour half-life that increases when it is deactivated in phase I of biotransformation in patients with cirrhosis, who show an altered distribution volume. Another BZD, flunitrazepam, also oxidizes in the liver [27].

Similarly, sedative BZDs also have an effect on the brain through the action of γ-aminobutyric acid (GABA) receptors. These receptors are particularly sensitive, depending on the stage of the hepatic disease, since they may be hypertrophic and/or hyperplasic. An incorrect prescription of BZD drugs may result in a hepatic encephalopathy crisis. Using flumazenil as a BZD antagonist may be useful, even though it must be administered cautiously [17].

Barbiturates such as thiopental (TPS) have an ambivalent action depending on the hepatic pathology that modifies their biotransformation (hypoalbuminemia, malnutrition, etc). Their distribution volume is modified by the concentration of the dose. Alcoholic patients are thought to need higher doses, although this opinion is questioned nowadays. Nonetheless, TPS induces liver microsomal enzymes which, through the microsomal enzyme synthetases, may provoke a porphyria crisis [19].

Propofol is a non-barbiturate anesthetic agent from the alkylphenol group, with a short-term effect on the organism. Since it is metabolized not only in the liver phase I of biotransformation but also in the lungs and gastrointestinal tract, its pharmacokinetics are not altered in patients with hepatopathy. An indirect effect may be produced by the presence of propofol oil excipients in long-term administration, which may also affect a previously altered hepatic function. A recently published study suggests that in patients with hepatic injuries, propofol, reduces platelet adhesion and affects patients with hyperlipidemia. Furthermore, propofol has documented antioxidant properties linked to the action of CYP450 2B6. There is controversy about the mechanisms producing these effects, but they are probably related to the plasma concentration of the drug [13, 17, 28, 29].

Etomidate is an imidazole derivative that mainly binds to albumin. It is metabolized by hepatic microsomal enzymes. They cause ester hydrolysis, which determines the formation of an inactive metabolite: a carboxylic acid. To a lesser degree, it is metabolized by plasma esterase. Its half-life, and therefore clearance, is prolonged in hepatic failure. The distribution volume may rise if associated with hypoalbuminemia, thus reducing its binding to proteins [11].

Ketamine chloridrate is a drug that is not often used because of its adverse effects on the central nervous system. Neither its action nor its metabolism are modified during liver failure. Therefore, it is becoming a drug to consider in some special cases. Its biotransformation is complex and uses two hepatic routes: demethylation by cyclohexamine-dependent enzymes — which results in two other metabolites — and hydroxylation of the cyclohexamine. It has been observed that an increase in enzymatic activity after repeated administration of this drug produces tolerance [7, 8, 11].

Opiates, which are frequently used as anesthetics, have a significant effect on the liver. Morphine is a drug from this group that metabolizes in phase II of biotransformation, producing more-powerful metabolites than the original drug, and the more severe the hepatic failure, the more prolonged its activity [7, 8, 11].

Remifentanil's metabolic behavior during a liver transplant is similar to that in a healthy patient and it has no significant action on lung clearance. The use of this drug in intra-operative and post-operative analgesia is common in patients with liver failure, because of its short half-life and because it does not require hepatic metabolism, since it is degraded by blood esterase and other tissues. Fentanil is metabolized by hydrolysis and eliminated in the urine, without being significantly affected in cases of hepatic lesion. Cumulative doses increase the analgesic effect of the drug. Alfentanil, another synthetic opiate, deactivates rapidly in the liver and binds to an acid glycoprotein which is affected when there is a hepatic lesion. In these cases, a reduction in protein binding is observed and an extension of its pharmacological effect. Its metabolism might be inhibited by erythromycin [11, 24, 25].

Sulfentanil, a fentanil analogue, has a prolonged half-life in the elderly. It binds to acid proteins and is widely metabolized in the liver by N-dealkylation. Another weak opiate, tramadol, is demethylated in the liver [7, 11].

Dexemedetomidine, a selective α_2-agonist, is a sedative which has recently appeared on the market. It is used in patients with varying degrees of hepatic lesion, where it has reduced clearance compared to that in healthy individuals, which forces a reduced administration dose in cases of hepatic functional impairment. A transitional increase of the AST, ALT and GGT enzymes is also frequently seen [11].

Respiratory depression caused by opiates is antagonized by a group of drugs such as naloxone, which has a 60–90-minute half-life. Naloxone, as well as nalbufine is also metabolized in the liver, and both are modified depending on the functional conditions of the organ [7].

In summary, if we generally consider the opiates, antagonists, and partial agonists, and the facts that they all clear in the liver and that hepatic failure may result in a reduction in their rate of metabolism, it is still apparent that, in clinical terms, those factors are not significant enough to prevent their use.

Volatile anesthetic agents reduce hepatic blood flow when they actively modify the organism's hemodynamics. Since they are lipid soluble, they become water-soluble compounds in the liver that are disposed of through the bile [30].

Halothane, as mentioned before, is 50% metabolized in the liver by the P450 cythocrome reductase and oxidase pathways. With low oxygen tensions, halothane becomes unstable free radicals, which become volatile metabolites such as chlorodifluoroethane and chlorotrifluoroethane. It is known that halothane induces peroxidation of microsomal lipids in the human liver, when catalyzed by CYP2A6 and CYP3A4, which provokes inhibition in the reductive pathways. Lesions caused by halothane are an example of toxicity by multiple mechanisms, among them hypersensitivity and metabolic idiosyncrasy [15, 16, 18, 19].

Isofluorane and desfluorane produce an intermediate metabolite — trifluoroacetic acid — which sometimes, in a small number of patients, provokes an increase in hepatic enzyme serum levels between 3 and 14 days after surgery; this is observed with these two drugs more frequently than with sevofluorane. They are less likely to produce hepatitis, and undergo less hepatic metabolism than halothane. Repeated exposure to sevofluorane and isofluorane — from 30 to 180 days — will not increase serum concentrations of either hepatic enzyme, or the removal of proteins and glucose in the urine, when compared to that seen with the first exposure to the same agent [15, 18, 21-23, 29, 31–33].

Laboratory tests have shown that nitrous oxide has a very low probability of causing hepatotoxicity [19].

Succinylcholine is metabolized in the liver and degraded by the action of the cholinesterase enzyme. Even though its levels reduce in hepatic disease, they are rarely so low that spontaneous recovery is not possible. If they do drop too low, there is enough enzyme in a plasma unit to hydrolyze the residual succinylcholine [19, 34].

Mivacurium is also rapidly metabolized by butyrylcholinesterase, giving inactive metabolites. All the factors that may cause a reduction of this enzyme will also reduce its rate of metabolism. In the same way, damage to hepatic function significantly reduces its clearance. A comparison between mivacurium and succinylcholine in patients with hepatic disease shows that its activity is related to the pre-existing concentrations of cholinesterase in plasma. This means that the conditions for tracheal intubation with mivacurium at 2 minutes are comparable to those for intubation with succinylcholine at 1 minute [34].

Rapacuronium is another blocker of new-generation drugs. Its short capacity of distribution produces an initial action similar to that of succinylcholine. Its 3 hydroxy active metabolite may cause accumulation, and it is cleared through bile [35, 36].

Rocuronium has a high level of hepatic clearance with altered removal in hepatopathies. It is mainly cleared through bile and partly through the kidney (30%). In hepatic failure it accumulates and does not produce active metabolites [37, 38].

The removal of atracurium and cisatracurium is independent of the liver (because of the Hoffmann reaction and the presence of esterase). It is carried out by hydrolysis and increases in alkalosis, and is delayed by hypothermia. The predictable actions of these drugs make them useful in cases where renal and/or hepatic function are altered. Similar characteristics are observed with vecuronium, which is captured by the liver and cleared by bile, with very little renal activity. Its deactivation is caused more by redistribution than by metabolism [19].

Pancuronium — the steroidal type — is metabolized in the liver, producing metabolites with little activity, but the kidneys are its route of disposal (higher than 50%). As it is removed in the bile, it has a longer half-life in cholestasis, which results in an uncomfortable relaxation [19].

Some diseases influence the pharmacokinetics of local anesthetic agents, by altering mechanisms that affect their distribution and disposal, and so increasing their toxicity. Therefore, hepatic failure alters the rate of biotransformation of lidocaine, extending its half-life. Local anesthetics with amide bonds, such as lidocaine and bipuvacaine, are metabolized in the liver by enzymatic degradation. Both metabolites and non-metabolized drugs are cleared through the urine, and a small amount through feces. Local agents with ester-type bonds, and tetracaine, are hydrolyzed by cholinesterase. This is the reason the duration of action increases with a deficit of cholinesterase or in the presence of atypical cholinesterase [39].

Post-operative cholestasis caused by intrapleural bipuvacaine is still a matter of controversy, since some authors refer to its appearance. However, others have not noticed the development of this adverse effect during recovery, even after intercostal, intrapleural, or intraperitoneal analgesic. Nonetheless, we believe that as its use increases, these differences will be resolved in future years. In any case, this cholestasis is self-limiting and appears to have no long-term consequences [40].

Conclusion

The choice of anesthetic agents, antibiotic therapy, and analgesics is directly related to findings in the presurgical assessment and to the type of surgery to be performed [41].

Presurgical hepatic assessment helps to differentiate three main risk groups: (1) steatosis, steatohepatitis, and chronic hepatitis, (2) compensated hepatic cirrhosis, and (3) decompensated cirrhosis. Those from group 1 have a risk from anesthetic-surgical procedure that is similar to that of healthy people undergoing the same procedures. In those from group 2 (Child–Pugh A cirrhosis), the antibiotic prophylaxis must be strictly controlled, since these individuals are more susceptible to infections. Maintaining stable hemodynamics is vital during and after surgery. An upper gastrointestinal endoscopy before surgery should be performed in these patients, and if there is any risk of bleeding it must be treated before the surgery. The choice of anesthetic and analgesic must be made in accordance with the history of alcohol use and the time course of hepatic metabolism of the drugs — they must be used in lower doses. In group 3 patients (decompensated cirrhosis), it is best not to perform any anesthetic-surgical procedure unless it is strictly necessary, because of their high morbidity and mortality.

Patients with hemophilia and chronic hepatic disease must be evaluated by a multidisciplinary team in order to achieve the best possible results.

References

1. Friedman LS, Maddrey WC (1987) Surgery in the patients with the liver disease. Med Clin North Am 71:453–476
2. Friedman LS (1999) The risk of surgery in patients with liver disease. Hepatology 29:1617–1623
3. Rosenberg PM, Friedman LS (2003) The liver in circulatory failure. In: Schiff ER, Sorell MF, Maddrey (eds) Diseases of the liver, 9th edition. Lippincott-Raven, Philadelphia, pp 1327–1340
4. Patel T (1999) Surgery in the patient with liver disease. Mayo Clin Proc 74:593–600
5. Bruix J, Castells A, Bosch J et al (1996) Resection of hepatocellular carcinoma in cirrhotic patients: prognostic value of preoperative portal pressure. Gastroenterology 111:1018–1022
6. Grace ND, Garcia-Pagan JC, Angelico M et al (2006) Primary prophilaxis for variceal bleeding. De In: Franchis R (ed). Proceedings of the 4th Baveno International Consensus Worshop on Portal Hypertension. Blackwell Publishing Ltd, Oxford, pp 168–200
7. Longnecker DE, Tinker JH, Morgan GE (1998) Principles and practice of anesthesiology, 2nd ed. Mosby, St Louis
8. Prys-Roberts C, Brown BR (1996) International practice of anaesthesia, Butterworth-Heinemann, Oxford
9. Cárdenas A, Ginés P, Rodés J (2003) Renal complications and hepatorenal syndrome. In: Schiff ER, Sorell MF, Maddrey (eds) Diseases of the liver, 9th edition. Lippincott-Raven, Philadelphia, pp 497–512
10. Conn HO (1981) A peek at the Child-Turcotte classification. Hepatology 1:673–676
11. Morgan GE, Mikhail MS (1999) Anestesiología clínica. El Manual Moderno, México
12. Córdoba J, Mínguez B (2008) Hepatic encephlopathy. Semin Liver Dis 28:70–80
13. Dawidowicz AL, Fornal E, Mardarowicz M, Fijalkowska A (2000) The role of human lungs in the biotransformation of propofol. Anesthesiology 93:992–997
14. Schuppan D, Afdhal NH (2008) Liver cirrhosis. Lancet 371:838–851
15. Iwanaga Y, Komatsu H, Yokono S, Ogli K (2000) Serum glutathione S-transferase alpha as a measure of hepatocellular function following prolonged anaesthesia with sevoflurane and halothane in paediatric patients. Paediatric Anaesthesia 10:95–98
16. Inoda Y, Kharasch ED (2001) Halothane-dependent lipid peroxidation in human liver microsomes is catalyzed by cytochrome P4502A6 (CYP2A6). Anesthesiology 95:509–514
17. Chen TL, Wu CH, Chen TG et al (2000) Effects of propofol on functional activities of hepatic and extrahepatic conjugation enzyme systems. Br J Anaesth 84:771–776
18. Darling JR, Sharpe PC, Stiby EK et al (2000) Serum mitochondrial aspartate transaminase activity after isoflurane or halothane anaesthesia. Br J Anaesth 85:195–198
19. Zimmerman HJ (1999) Anesthesic agents. In: Zimmerman HJ (ed) Hepatotoxicity: the adverse effcects of drugs and other chemicals on the liver, 2nd edition. Lippincott Williams & Wilkins, Philadelphia, pp 457–482

20. Zimmerman HJ (1999) Classification of hepatotoxins and mechanims of toxicity. In: Zimmerman HJ (ed) Hepatotoxicity: the adverse effcects of drugs and other chemicals on the liver, 2nd edition. Lippincott Williams & Wilkins, Philadelphia, pp 111–145
21. Bruun LS, Elkjaer S, Bitsch-Larsen D, Andersen O (2001) Hepatic failure in a child after acetaminophen and sevoflurane exposure. Anesthes Analg 92:1446–1448
22. Nishiyama T, Yokoyama T, Hanaoka K (1998) Liver and renal function after repeated sevoflurane or isoflurane anaesthesia. Can J Anaesth 45:789–793
23. Obata R, Bito H, Ohmura M et al (2000) The effects of prolonged low-flow sevoflurane anesthesia on renal and hepatic function. Anesth Analg 91:1262–1268
24. Dumont L, Picard V, Marti RA, Tassonyi E (1998) Use of remifentanil in a patient with chronic hepatic failure. Br J Anaesth 81:265–267
25. Navapurkar VU, Archer S, Gupta SK et al (1998) Metabolism of remifentanil during liver transplantation. Br J Anaesth 81:881–886
26. Zimmerman HJ (1999) Drugs used to treat rheumatic and musculopatic disease. In: Zimmerman HJ (ed) Hepatotoxicity: the adverse effcects of drugs and other chemicals on the liver, 2nd edition. Lippincott Williams & Wilkins, Philadelphia, pp 517–554
27. Zimmerman HJ (1999) Psychotropic and anticonvulsivant agents. In: Zimmerman HJ (ed) Hepatotoxicity: the adverse effcects of drugs and other chemicals on the liver, 2nd edition. Lippincott Williams & Wilkins, Philadelphia, pp 483–516
28. Court MH, Duan SX, Hesse LM et al (2001) Cytochrome P-450 2B6 is responsible for interindividual variability of propofol hydroxylation by human liver microsomes. Anesthesiology 94:110–119
29. Ebert TJ, Arain SR (2000) Renal responses to low-flow desflurane, sevoflurane, and propofol in patients. Anesthesiology 93:1401–1406
30. Friederich P, Benzenberg D, Trellakis S et al (2001) Interaction of volatile anesthetics with human Kv channels in relation to clinical concentrations. Anesthesiology 95:954–958
31. Guitton J, Buronfosse T, Desage M et al (1998) Possible involvement of multiple human cytochrome P450 isoforms in the liver metabolism of propofol. Br J Anaesth 80:788–795
32. Osawa M, Shinomura T (1998) Compound A concentration is decreased by cooling anaesthetic circuit during low-flow sevoflurane anaesthesia. Can J Anaesth 45:1215–1218
33. Hamaoka N, Oda Y, Hase I, Asada A (2001) Cytochrome P4502B6 and 2C9 do not metabolize midazolam: kinetic analysis and inhibition study with monoclonal antibodies. Br J Anaesth 86:540–544
34. Green DW, Fisher M, Sockalingham I (1998) Mivacurium compared with succinylcholine in children with liver disease. Br J Anaesth 81:463–465
35. Fisher DM, Dempsey GA, Atherton DP et al (2000) Effect of renal failure and cirrhosis on the pharmacokinetics and neuromuscular effects of rapacuronium administered by bolus followed by infusion. Anesthesiology 93:1384–1391
36. Duvaldestin P, Slavov V, Rebufat Y (1999) Pharmacokinetics and pharmacodynamics of rapacuronium in patients with cirrhosis. Anesthesiology 91:1305–1310
37. Proost JH, Eriksson LI, Mirakhur RK et al (2000) Urinary, biliary and faecal excretion of rocuronium in humans. Br J Anaesth 85:717–723
38. Proost JH, Eriksson LI, Mirakhur RK et al (2000) Urinary, biliary and faecal excretion of rocuronium in humans. Br J Anaesth 85:717–723
39. Ziser A, Plevak DJ, Wiesner RH et al (1999) Morbidity and mortality in cirrhotic patients undergoing anesthesia and surgery. Anesthesiology 90:42–53
40. Yokoyama M, Ohashi I, Nakatsuka H et al (2001) Drug-induced liver disease during continuous epidural block with bupivacaine. Anesthesiology 95:259–261
41. Power LM, Thackray NM (1999) Reduction of preoperative investigations with the introduction of an anaesthetist-led preoperative assessment clinic. Anaesth Intens Care 27:481–488

Chapter 6

Peri-operative and Post-operative Management of Hemophiliac Patients without Inhibitors

Maria Elisa Mancuso and Elena Santagostino

Introduction

Orthopedic surgery in patients with hemophilia should be planned by the surgeon together with the hemophilia specialist and the physiotherapist, in order to establish a long-term program that integrates surgery with medical and rehabilitative interventions. Orthopedic surgery should be performed in centres that are able to provide hematologic expertise, medical support, and laboratory monitoring of coagulation throughout the period of hospitalization.

Pre-operative Assessment

The pre-operative assessment should include the following:

Definition of the Severity of Coagulation Factor Deficiency

In addition to measurement of the level of the deficient factor in plasma, information should be collected on the current regimen of replacement therapy (i.e., on-demand or prophylaxis). In patients with mild hemophilia A, their factor VIII response after desmopressin administration should be documented in order to consider its potential use to cover minor procedures [1–3].

Information on Inhibitor History and Current Inhibitor Status

The presence of inhibitors makes surgical management problematic. High-dose factor concentrate is required in patients with low-titer inhibitors, while replacement therapy is not effective in the presence of high titers (see Chapter 7). Information on the history of inhibitors should be accurately collected because patients who have had a previous inhibitor could show a suboptimal response to replacement therapy.

H.A. Caviglia, L.P. Solimeno (eds.), *Orthopedic Surgery in Patients with Hemophilia.*

Evaluation of Immunity to Hepatitis A and B

The immune status against hepatitis viruses is usually assessed once a year in order to administer booster doses of vaccinations if necessary [2]. The purpose of vaccination is to protect patients from the risk of blood-borne viral infections associated with the use of blood components or plasma-derived concentrates.

Evaluation of Concomitant Liver Disease

The vast majority of patients with hemophilia who received plasma-derived concentrates manufactured prior to the implementation of effective virucidal procedures were infected with hepatitis viruses (HBV and HCV) [4, 5]. The presence of chronic hepatitis with liver dysfunction, cirrhosis, and thrombocytopenia may account for an increased risk of bleeding. In these cases, fresh-frozen plasma and/or platelet transfusions may be needed in addition to clotting factor concentrates. Moreover, patients with cirrhosis require careful monitoring because of the risk of liver decompensation associated with stressful events such as surgery or infection.

Evaluation of Concomitant HIV Infection

Immunological parameters (CD4+ and CD8+ lymphocyte counts; human immunodeficiency virus (HIV) viremia) should be evaluated to assess the presence of immunodepression that may increase the risk of peri-operative and post-operative infections. It should be remembered that the introduction of highly active antiretroviral therapy (HAART) can minimize this risk [6]. With respect to the bleeding risk, spontaneous and surgery-related bleeding complications have been reported in hemophiliacs treated with protease inhibitors [7].

Choice of Replacement Therapy

There are no specific recommendations for the use of a particular type of concentrate in surgery. It is crucial to estimate the overall amount of concentrate needed to cover the peri-operative and post-operative period (including the rehabilitation program), in order to ensure an adequate stock of concentrate. It would be better to maintain the use of the same concentrate throughout the whole treatment period in order to avoid possible changes in the factor pharmacokinetics and to minimize the risk of inhibitor development. Ideally, the dose regimen for major surgery should be established on the basis of an in vivo recovery and pharmacokinetic study after a single infusion of the chosen concentrate at a fixed dose (in a non-bleeding state after a proper washout period) [3]. Replacement therapy can be delivered by repeated bolus injections or by continuous infusion.

Continuous infusion should be considered for major surgery because it minimizes concentrate use, maintains steady plasma levels avoiding peaks and troughs, and facilitates laboratory monitoring [8]. Nevertheless, potential drawbacks of continuous infusion may be: reduced stability at room temperature after reconstitution, enhanced inactivation due to the interaction with the plastic materials pumps are made of, and bacterial contamination. Hence, it is recommended to considerer this modality of treatment delivery is considered for products that have already been evaluated for use by continuous infusion [9–11]. Minipumps may be useful to facilitate early mobilization and rehabilitation. Finally, patients with mild hemophilia A treated by continuous infusion and exposed to intensive factor VIII treatment should be carefully monitored because some cases of inhibitor development have been reported [12, 13]. If the use of desmopressin has been documented to increase circulating factor VIII to the targeted levels without tachyphylaxis, this drug is preferred [2, 3].

Peri-operative and Post-operative Treatment

Patients are usually admitted 2–3 days prior to surgery in order to undergo all the biochemical and instrumental controls that are useful for the intervention and general anesthesia. Blood is cross-matched according to the normal surgical blood-ordering policy of the hospital, taking into account that patients at high risk of bleeding may need more units than non-hemophiliac patients. The coagulation laboratory should be alerted to the potential need for frequent and/or unscheduled assays. Major orthopedic surgery and joint replacement require plasma factor levels within the normal range, and a trough level of 50 IU/dl should be maintained until healing [14]. Minor surgery can be safely managed with factor levels of at least 30–50 IU/dl maintained for a shorter period, depending on the type of procedure [14].

The first bolus of factor concentrate is administered 15–30 min prior to surgery at a dose established to increase the deficient factor to the targeted level in plasma. A single bolus may be sufficient to ensure hemostasis in some minor procedures for which laboratory monitoring is usually not necessary. On the other hand, the post-infusion recovery should be evaluated before major surgery, and a second bolus of clotting factor concentrate is given after 12–24 h, according to the laboratory result. After major surgery, patients are treated every 12–24 h under daily recovery monitoring until day 6, which often corresponds to discharge, and every 24 h until complete wound healing. If continuous infusion administration is chosen, the loading bolus is usually followed by a fixed infusion rate (3–4 IU/kg/h), and daily factor monitoring allows dose adjustment [15]. After suture removal, individualized prophylactic regimens may be required to avoid bleeding complications during the rehabilitation period.

Finally, a regular follow-up of patients with hemophilia is crucial to establish the definite outcome of surgery and to monitor the long-term evolution of orthopedic status.

References

1. Mannucci PM, Ruggeri ZM, Pareti FI, Capitanio A (1977) 1-Deamino-8-D-Arginine vasopressin: a new pharmacological approach to the management of haemophilia and von Willebrand's disease. Lancet i:869–872
2. Santagostino E, Mannucci PM (2000) Guidelines on replacement therapy for haemophilia and inherited coagulation disorders in Italy. Haemophilia 6:1–10
3. United Kingdom Haemophilia Centre Doctors' Organisation (UKHCDO) (2003) Guidelines on the selection and use of therapeutic products to treat haemophilia and other hereditary bleeding disorders. Haemophilia 9:1–23
4. Fletcher ML, Trowell JM, Craske J et al (1983) Non-A, non-B hepatitis after transfusion of factor VIII in unfrequently treated patients. Br Med J 287:1754–1757
5. Kernoff PBA, Lee CA, Karayanis P, Thomas HC (1985) High risk of non-A, non-B hepatitis after a first exposure to volunteer or commercial clotting factor concentrates: effects of prophylactic immune serum globulin. Br J Haematol 60:469–479
6. Powell DL, Whitener CJ, Dye CE et al (2005) Knee and hip arthroplasty infection rates in persons with haemophilia: a 27 year single center experience during the HIV epidemic. Haemophilia 11:233–239
7. Wilde JT, Lee CA, Collins P et al (1999) Increased bleeding associated with protease inhibitor therapy in HIV-positive patients with bleeding disorders. Br J Haematol 107: 556–569
8. Martinowitz U, Schulman S, Gitel S et al (1992) Adjusted dose continuous infusion of factor VIII in patients with haemophilia A. Br J Haematol 82:729–734
9. Schulman S, Gitel S, Martinowitz U (1994) Stability of factor VIII concentrates after reconstitution. Am J Hematol 45:217–223
10. Schulman S, Varon D, Keller N et al (1994) Monoclonal purified FVIII for continuous infusion: stability, microbiological safety and clinical experience. Thromb Haemost 72:403–407
11. Chowdary P, Dasani H, Jones JA et al (2001) Recombinant factor IX (BeneFix) by adjusted continuous infusion: a study of stability, sterility and clinical experience. Haemophilia 7:140–145
12. Sharathkumar A, Lillicrap D, Blanchette VS et al (2003) Intensive exposure to factor VIII is a risk factor for inhibitor development in mild hemophilia A. J Thromb Haemost 1:1228–1236
13. White B, Cotter M, Byrne M et al (2000) High responding factor VIII inhibitors in mild haemophilia – is there a link with recent changes in clinical practice? Haemophilia 6:113–115
14. Rickard KA (1995) Guidelines for therapy and optimal dosages of coagulation factors for treatment of bleeding and surgery in haemophilia. Haemophilia 1(Suppl 1):8–13
15. Dingli D, Gastineau DA, Gilchrist GS et al (2002) Continuous factor VIII infusion therapy in patients with haemophilia A undergoing surgical procedures with plasma-derived or recombinant factor VIII concentrates. Haemophilia 8:629–634

Chapter 7
Peri-operative and Post-operative Management of Hemophiliac Patients with Inhibitors

Elena Santagostino and Maria Elisa Mancuso

Introduction

In the past, elective orthopedic surgery in hemophilic patients with inhibitors was usually not contemplated because of the high risk of bleeding complications. Thanks to the progress made in the development of bypassing therapies, elective surgery has become feasible; however, only centers that are already experienced can tackle this challenge. A strict collaboration amongst surgeons, hematologists, and physiotherapists is essential for a successful long-term outcome.

Pre-operative Assessment

In addition to the clinical assessment already reported for patients without inhibitors (see Chapter 6), the pre-operative evaluation of hemophiliac patients with inhibitors should be focused on underlying cardiovascular diseases and thrombotic risk factors because bypassing therapy may be associated with thromboembolic complications [1–3], particularly in elderly patients.

Documentation of Inhibitor Titer and Anamnestic Response

Inhibitors modify the pharmacokinetics of the infused clotting factor and can render replacement therapy ineffective. The choice of therapeutic strategy is mainly based on the current inhibitor titer and the information on historical peak titer. Inhibitors are defined as high-responding or low-responding on the basis of the anamnestic response of the antibody to antigenic challenge. An antibody which is persistently ≤ 5 BU (Bethesda units)/ml despite repeated challenge with factor replacement is termed a low-response inhibitor, whereas the term high-response inhibitor is applied to cases where titers have been >5 BU/ml at any time [4]. Inhibitors may be undetectable in high-responding patients not recently exposed to factor VIII/IX, but titers may quickly rise after a new factor exposure.

H.A. Caviglia, L.P. Solimeno (eds.), *Orthopedic Surgery in Patients with Hemophilia.*

Choice of Hemostatic Therapy

Bypassing agents are activated prothrombin complex concentrate (aPCC) and recombinant activated factor VII (rFVIIa), and represent the first choice in patients with high-responding inhibitors [5, 6]. It has to be considered that aPCC contains small amounts of factor VIII and may induce an anamnestic response in some patients [7]. High efficacy rates were reported using either aPCC [7, 8] or rFVIIa [9] in the surgical setting; however, no controlled surgical study has compared these two agents. The main drawback of rFVIIa is the need for frequent infusions due to its very short half-life. Some experiences with the use of rFVIIa by continuous infusion at different dose-rates (15–50 μg/kg/h) have been reported [10–12]; however, the results are difficult to interpret. Treatment delivery of rFVIIa by continuous infusion is not licensed, furthermore, in vitro evidence supports the idea that bolus injections lead to better hemostasis than continuous infusion because thrombin generation is enhanced by peak levels of FVIIa [13, 14].

No bypassing product can guarantee sustained hemostasis, and no laboratory assay is available to predict the efficacy of treatment. For this reason it may be useful to know the patient's clinical response previously obtained using bypassing agents for treatment of bleeding and, in particular, in the setting of surgery.

High-dose factor replacement may neutralize low-titer inhibitors, allowing the desired factor levels for surgery to be achieved and maintained. A preliminary pharmacokinetic study is particularly useful in these cases to establish the optimal dose regimen. Factor replacement therapy represents the first-choice approach for patients with low-responding inhibitors, and it should also be considered in high responders who have a temporarily low inhibitor titer [5, 6]. In the latter, the efficacy of treatment is usually limited to the first post-operative days because of the anamnestic rise of inhibitor titer that often requires that treatment changes to bypassing agents. Continuous-infusion administration is particularly convenient in inhibitor patients on high-dose replacement because it allows reduction of the total amount of factor needed and maintenance of hemostatic factor levels avoiding peaks and troughs.

In particular cases of high-responding, high-titer inhibitors who previously failed using bypassing agents, *extracorporeal immunoadsorption* can be used to decrease inhibitor titers to levels that allow factor replacement therapy [5, 6]. The procedure consists of passing the patient's entire plasma pool through columns containing protein A or anti-human immunoglobulins that bind and trap inhibitors, removing them from the plasma. The procedure may take 24 h preparation and should be repeated until inhibitor titer is <5 BU/ml. The safety of immunoadsorption is generally considered to be good and no column-related side-effects are usually observed [15].

Immune tolerance induction (ITI) represents the only strategy able to eradicate anti-factor VIII/IX antibodies, and is indicated in newly diagnosed patients with inhibitors [5, 6]. Candidates for elective orthopedic surgery are usually adults with longstanding inhibitors who are considered to have poor prognosis for ITI outcome [16]. However, in individual cases ITI may be considered in order to abolish or reduce the inhibitory activity and to allow surgery with guaranteed hemostasis by factor replacement treatment.

Peri-operative and Post-operative Treatment

Patients are usually admitted 2–3 days prior to surgery in order to undergo all the biochemical and instrumental assessments that are useful for the intervention and general anesthesia.

Blood is crossmatched according to the normal surgical blood-ordering policy of the hospital, taking into account that patients at high risk of bleeding may need more units than patients without hemophilia. Washed red blood cells should be preferred to avoid anamnestic response in high-responding patients who have a current low-titer inhibitor treated with bypassing agents.

The coagulation laboratory should be alerted to the potential need for frequent and/or unscheduled assays.

Hemostatic Treatment

High-Dose Factor Replacement

The loading bolus of factor concentrate is administered 15–30 min prior to surgery at a dosage able to neutralize the inhibitory activity and to increase the factor levels to the targeted values; treatment can be continued by administering repeated boluses every 6–12 h, or by continuous infusion [5]. Careful laboratory monitoring is crucial for dose adjustment, during both repeated boluses and continuous infusion administration. Factor recovery should be measured after the loading bolus and monitored at least daily until discharge. An advantage of continuous infusion is the convenience of factor monitoring because samples can be taken at any time on a daily basis. Hospitalization due to major orthopedic procedures usually lasts 10–14 days, so that patients can be discharged when sustained hemostasis is achieved and may be safely maintained, if necessary, continuing replacement treatment at home without the need for frequent laboratory monitoring.

Bypassing Agents

aPCC is usually administered by boluses at a dosage of 75–100 IU/kg. The preoperative bolus is given 15–30 min prior to surgery and, for major procedures, the following boluses should be administered every 8–12 h until day 5 and then every 12 h until day 14 [17]. rFVIIa is administered by boluses at a dose of

90–120 μg/kg. The pre-operative bolus is given 15 min prior to surgery, and the following boluses should be administered every 2 h for the first 24 h; every 3 h on day 2; and every 4 h on days 3–5. If hemostasis is satisfactory, treatment can be continued every 6 h until day 14 [17]. No laboratory monitoring has proved to be helpful for dose optimization of either aPCC or rFVIIa treatment. Factor VII levels measured in plasma have not been shown to correlate with the hemostatic efficacy of rFVIIa [10].

Thromboembolic events, myocardial infarction, and disseminated intravascular coagulation (DIC) have been associated with the use of both agents [1–3]. For this reason, the maximum daily dose of 200 IU/kg of aPCC [3] should never be exceeded and caution is recommended administering high doses of rFVIIa in elderly patients or those with risk factors for thrombosis. DIC screening is useful to monitor activation of the coagulation cascade during bypassing therapy. The association of antifibrinolytic therapy with aPCC should be avoided, while it can be safely administered with rFVIIa [5, 6].

The cornerstone of post-operative management is to avoid bleeding complications, and if bleeding occurs it must be treated without delay. With this aim in mind, early mobilization, which may trigger a bleed, should be individually tailored and started with great caution in patients with inhibitors. In order to reduce the bleeding risk, giving a single concentrate infusion before each physiotherapy session may be considered start of the post-operative rehabilitation program [18]. A further aspect to take into consideration in these challenging patients is the risk of infectious complications. Some case reports suggested that the onset of infections is related to peri-operative/post-operative bleeds [18]; nevertheless, no comparative data are available on the incidence of infectious complications in inhibitor and non-inhibitor hemophiliac patients.

Finally, information on the long-term outcome of orthopedic surgery in inhibitor patients is still scarce, so that a prolonged follow-up is recommended. This information is needed to optimize surgical procedures and improve the selection of candidates for surgery.

References

1. Aledort LM (2004) Comparative thrombotic event incidence after infusion of recombinant factor VIIa versus factor VIII inhibitor bypassing activity. J Thromb Haemost 2:1700–1708
2. Abshire T, Kenet G (2004) Recombinant factor VIIa : review of afficacy, dosing regimens and safety in patients with congenital and acquired factor VIII and IX inhibitors. J Thromb Haemost 2:899–909
3. Ehrlich HJ, Henzl MJ, Gomperts ED (2002) Safety of factor VIII inhibitor bypass activity (FEIBA): 10-year compilation of thrombotic adverse events. Haemophilia 8:83–90
4. White GC II, Rosendaal F, Aledort LM et al (2001) Recommendations of the Scientific Subcommittee on Factor VIII and Factor IX of the Scientific and Standardization Committee of the International Society on Thrombosis and Haemostasis. Thromb Haemost 85:560
5. Gringeri A, Mannucci PM (2005) Italian guidelines for the diagnosis and treatment of patients with haemophilia and inhibitors. Haemophilia 11:611–619
6. Hay CR, Baglin TP, Collins PW et al (2000) The diagnosis and management of factor VIII

and IX inhibitors: a guideline from the UK Haemophilia Centre Doctors' Organization (UKHCDO). Br J Haematol 111:78–90

7. Negrier C, Goudemand J, Sultan Y, Bertrand M, Rothschild C, Lauroua P and the Members of the French FEIBA Study Group (1997) Multicenter retrospective study on the utilisation of Feiba in France in patients with factor VIII and factor IX inhibitors. Thromb Haemost 77:1113–1119
8. Tjonnfjord GE, Brinch L, Gedde-Dahl T, Brosstad FR (2004) Activated prothrombin complex concentrate (FEIBA) treatment during surgery in patients with inhibitors to FVIII/IX. Haemophilia 10:174–178
9. Shapiro AD, Gilchrist GS, Hoots WK et al (1998) Prospective randomised trial of two doses of rFVIIa (Novoseven) in haemophilia patients with inhibitors undergoing surgery. Thromb Haemost 80:773–778
10. Santagostino E, Morfini M, Rocino A et al (2001) Relationship between factor VII activity and clinical efficacy of recombinant factor VIIa given by continuous infusion to patients with factor VIII inhibitors. Thromb Haemost 86:954–958
11. Smith MP, Ludlam CA, Collins PW et al (2001) Elective surgery on factor VIII inhibitor patients using continuous infusion of recombinant activated factor VII: plasma factor VII activity of 10 IU/ml is associated with an increased incidence of bleeding. Thromb Haemost 86:949–953
12. Ludlam CA, Smith MP, Morfini M et al (2003) A prospective study of recombinant activated factor VII administered by continuous infusion to inhibitor patients undergoing elective major orthopaedic surgery: a pharmacokinetic and efficacy evaluation. Br J Haematol 120:808–813
13. Hoffman M, Monroe DM 3rd, Roberts HR (1998) Activated factor VII activates factor IX and X on the surface of activated platelets: thoughts on the mechanism of action of high-dose activated factor VII. Blood Coagul Fibrinolysis 9(Suppl 1):S61–65
14. Butenas S, Brummel KE, Bouchard BA, Mann KG (2003) How factor VIIa works in hemophilia. J Thromb Haemost 1:1158–1160
15. Nilsson IM, Jonsson S, Sundqvist SB et al (1981) A procedure for removing high titer antibodies by extracorporeal protein-A-sepharose adsorption in hemophilia: substitution therapy and surgery in a patient with hemophilia B and antibodies. Blood 58:38–44
16. Kroner BL (1999) Comparison of the international immune tolerance registry and the North American immune tolerance registry. Vox Sang 77(Suppl 1):33–37
17. Rodríguez-Merchán EC, Rocino A, Ewenstein B et al (2004) Consensus perspectives on surgery in haemophilia patients with inhibitors: summary statement. Haemophilia 10(Suppl 2):50–52
18. Solimeno LP, Perfetto OS, Pasta G, Santagostino E (2006) Total joint replacement in patients with inhibitors. Haemophilia 12(Suppl 3):113–116

Chapter 8
Postsurgical Pain

Horacio A. Caviglia, Pablo Nuova, Ana Laura Douglas Price and Miguel Moreno

Introduction

Internal medicine physicians sometimes find it difficult to handle postsurgical pain in patients with hemophilia. Pain mainly comes from two sources: painful stimuli of the surgical wound, and postural phenomena resulting from the deformities or arthropathies present.

Pain originating from the surgical wound must be treated effectively, preventing it from lasting too long and leading to chronic pain syndromes that are hard to resolve.

Postural pain is the pain the surgeon or the internist should be able to identify. Severe hemophiliacs undergoing elective surgery usually exhibit more than one affected joint. When the lower limb is involved, they often present a compensating hyperlordosis of the spine, flexion at the hip, knee flexion and/or valgus, external rotation at the tibia, ankle valgus, or equine foot. If the patient is a candidate for a knee replacement and presents with knee flexion, this may be accompanied by flexion of the hip and a compensating lumbar hyperlordosis.

If the patient is immobilized with the knee extended after the reconstructive procedure, he will not only suffer the pain caused by the surgery, but also have additional pain at the back of the knee due to tension of the posterior soft parts, which will manifest as posterior pain at the thigh and leg. The hip in flexion may also produce crural pain at the anterior surface of the thigh, originating from tension of the anterior soft parts of the hip. In addition, the patient may also suffer lumbar pain with sciatic irradiation, caused by hyperlordosis of the spine.

Therapeutic measures are simple: during early postsurgical periods, the knee should be left in the same position of flexion as before surgery, and a pillow placed under the lumbar spine. This avoids the pain described above, reduces the dose of analgesic necessary, and minimizes patient stress, making rehabilitation easier. On the second day, the therapist must start to work on progressive extension with a continuous passive movement splint (CPM), making daily progress with the range of movement. If there are no CPMs available, the therapist must start active and passive exercises in two daily sessions. By the seventh day, full extension of the knee must be accomplished [1-3].

H.A. Caviglia, L.P. Solimeno (eds.), *Orthopedic Surgery in Patients with Hemophilia*.

Intrasurgical Care

Even though most local anesthesic procedures are forbidden for these patients, due to their underlying pathology, new approaches for local anesthesia are now available. Ultrasound-guided block provides a safe way to block nerves while avoiding the risk of vascular puncture [4, 5].

Morphine analogues are the drugs of choice for intrasurgical treatment (morphine, meperidine, fentanyl, remifentanil), taking into account the type of surgery and its possible duration, in order to choose the most appropriate agent.

The non-steroidal anti-inflammatory drug (NSAID) acetaminophen (paracetamol) is used since it has a central mechanism of action and does not interference with coagulation.

Ketamine, in analgesic doses, clonidine and dexmedetomidine (due to their analgesic action on the posterior horn) appear to be excellent facilitators or potentiators of classic analgesics, thus allowing the use of lower doses, resulting in a synergism of potentiation, and enabling the patient to stay within the therapeutic range of the different agents.

Postsurgical Care

Within the first 48 h, an intravenous line is placed for administration of opiates, morphine being the one used most often. Continuous schedules (load-maintaining dose) with a rescue dose should be chosen, rather intermittent administration which does not maintain adequate levels of the drug in plasma over long periods of time.

The NSAIDs (etoricoxibe) and centrally acting analgesics (paracetamol) should be used with the opiates, using combined schedules that allow optimal exploitation of the benefits of both groups of drugs, while avoiding possible interactions.

After the first 48 h, the patient can be moved onto weak morphine analogues such as oxycodone, methadone, codeine, or dextropropoxphene for oral administration, or, if necessary, morphine itself in a sublingual form.

The postsurgical appearance of painful syndromes associated with neuropathy may require the administration of opiates of specific action such as methadone. Its use must be considered carefully for each particular case.

From the NSAID group, the patient should progress to using COX-2 inhibitors (etoricoxibe) and paracetamol (with regular oral administration and rescue), continuing with these in all therapies that last more than 72 h.

References

1. William ED, D Davis Glass (1990) Haematological diseases. In: Kadis LB, Benumof J, Katz J. Anesthesia and uncommon diseases. Philadelphia, Saunders, pp 378–436

2. Fudeta H, Hashimoto YK, Mori K (1976) Anesthesia in patients with hemophilia A and B. Jnp J Anesth 25:718
3. Simon E, Roux C, More J (1966) Drug combination in the treatment of pain in hemophiliacs. Bibl Haematologica 26:78
4. Baldi C, Bettinelli S, Grossi P et al (2007) Ultrasound guidance for locoregional anesthesia: a review. Minerva Anestesiol 11:587–593
5. Vanarase MY, Pandit H, Kimstra YW et al (2007) Pain relief after knee replacement in patients with a bleeding disorder. Haemophilia (4):395

Section III

Non-surgical Procedures

Chapter 9
Arthrocentesis

Roberto Bernal-Lagunas

Definition

Arthrocentesis is a therapeutic procedure that consists of joint aspiration in order to drain bleeding, or for drug administration in patients with hemophilia. The procedure can be performed under aseptic conditions in the office, or in the operating room. Patients do not require anesthesia.

Articular Drainage

Arthrocentesis [1–5] is indicated to extract the hematic contents of the joint in order to reduce pain, improve the general condition, and prevent articular cartilage damage due to the action of hemosiderin. The procedure is not indicated in every intra-articular episode, because it is not entirely harmless, and there is a risk of joint infection (septic arthritis).

Drainage is very easy due to capsular distension. The joint must be drained completely: Tachdjian recommends complete evacuation and washing if clots are present or there is any suspicion of septic arthritis [6].

It is advisable to perform arthrocentesis in the following situations:

- A bleeding, tense, and painful joint which shows no improvement 24 h after conservative treatment
- Joint pain that cannot be alleviated
- Evidence of neurovascular compromise of the limb
- Unusual increase in local temperature (septic arthritis)

A relative contraindication is the presence of inhibitor, and an absolute contraindication is local skin infection.

For post-procedure care, a splint and Jones dressing immobilization for 3 to 5 days helps to alleviate symptoms and prevent recurrence. Isometric exercises must be performed with the limb.

H.A. Caviglia, L.P. Solimeno (eds.), *Orthopedic Surgery in Patients with Hemophilia.*

Drug Administration

Intra-articular drug administration is a frequent procedure in hemophilic patients; it is best to permeate the joint before administering drugs, especially in cases of moderate or severe arthropathy (grade III or IV) when access to the joint is difficult because articular space is lost.

The most frequently administered drugs are:

- Anti-inflammatory: steroids (betamethasone)
- Chemical synovectomy: rifampicin [4, 7] and oxytetracycline chlorhydrate [8, 9]
- Radioactive synovectomy: gold198, yttrium90, rhenium86, dysprosium66, chromic phosphate32 [7, 10]
- Cartilage restorers : suprahial (sodium hyaluronate), Synvisc (hylan G-F 20)

Steroids are indicated in acute and chronic processes. They are used in acute processes, when repetitive hemarthrosis does not respond to conservative treatment, as they stop the inflammation and bleeding. In chronic cases (arthropathy grade IV), their action is analgesic and anti-inflammatory.

Chemical or radioactive synovectomy (synoviorthesis) is indicated in the treatment of chronic synovitis (arthropathy grade I and II). It produces subsynovial fibrosis at the point of drug contact, decreasing the frequency of bleeding episodes (these are frequent in the subsynovial tissue, which bleeds easily, resulting in persistent synovitis and hemarthrosis), in an attempt to avoid articular damage and allow recovery of articular function..

Cartilage restorers are indicated in grade III and IV arthropathy. The goal is to improve joint function and reduce progressive damage to the cartilage [12].

Technique [6, 10, 11]

Preparation

- The patient should have 20–30% coagulation levels. The patient with inhibitor requires special attention by a hematologist.
- The procedure can be carried out in the doctor's office or operating room.
- Anesthesia is generally not necessary.
- A sponge soaked with iodine is used to drape the region under aseptic conditions.

Equipment

- 20 ml syringe, with 16–18G needle, at least 38 mm long, for articulation drain and 20G for drug application.

Puncture Methods

The different approaches and puncture sites are shown in Figures 9.1–9.7. The hip is the most difficult joint to access and the procedure should be done in an operating room, under anesthesia and with fluoroscopy. Other joints are easier to access.

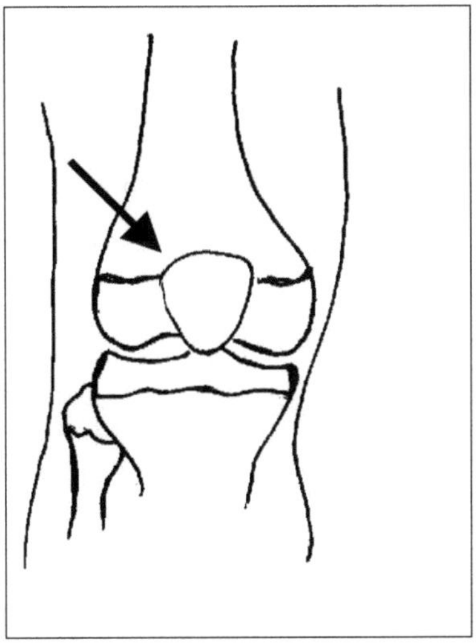

Fig. 9.1 The knee: it is recommended to approach near the superior pole of the patella

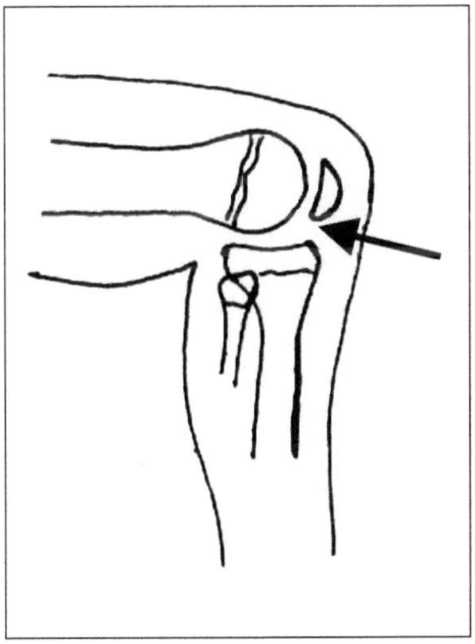

Fig. 9.2 The knee: anterolateral approach, similar to the anterior portal direction used in arthroscopy

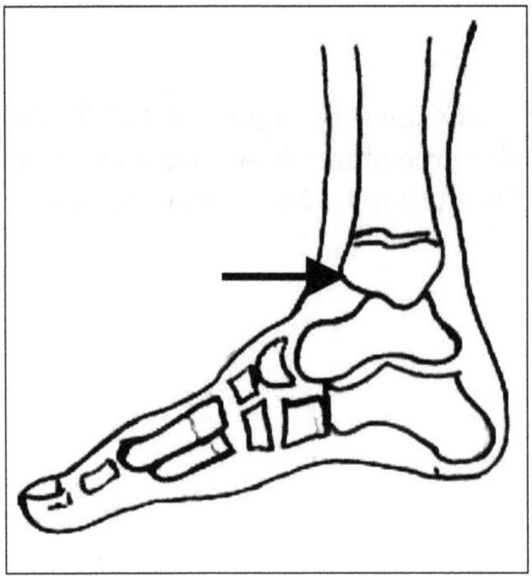

Fig. 9.3 The ankle: anterolateral approach

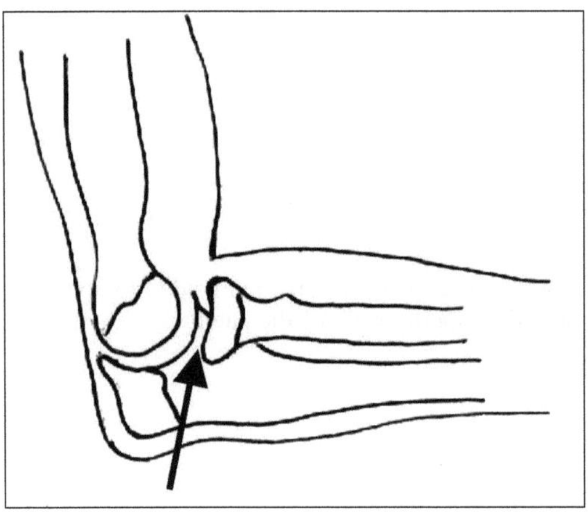

Fig. 9.4 The elbow: lateral approach to the radiohumeral articulation

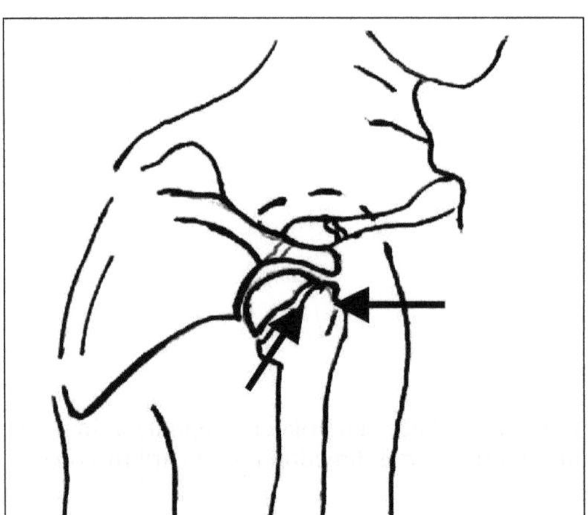

Fig. 9.5 The shoulder: anterior or lateral approach

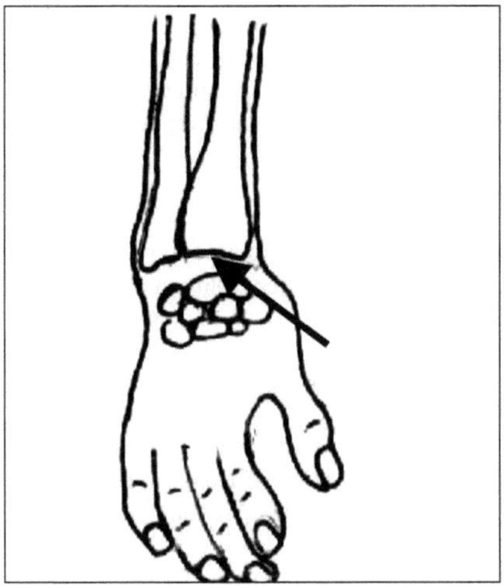

Fig. 9.6 The wrist: dorsal approach to the radioscaphoid joint

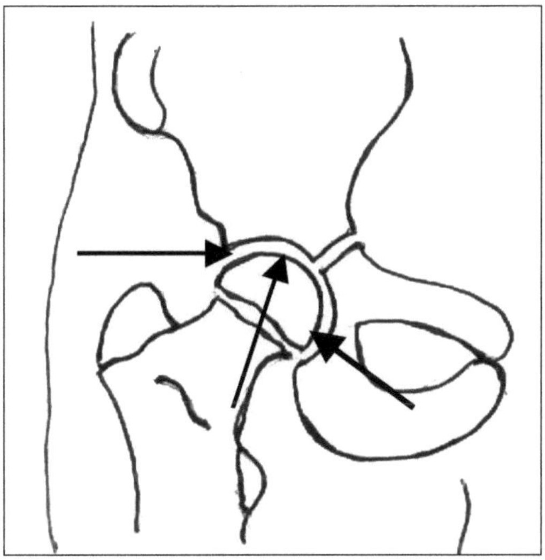

Fig. 9.7 The hip: entry can be made medially, anteriorly or laterally; it is recommended to use fluoroscopy to help

References

1. Crawford AH, Jacobsen FS (1992) Enfermedades hematológicas: Hemofilia. Tratado de ortopedia pediátrica (Canale ST). Primera edición. Español. MYB, pp 395–409
2. Gilbert MS (1997) Musculoskeletal complications of hemophilia: The joint. Treatment of hemophilia monographs. World Federation of Hemophilia 6
3. Gupta AD (2001) Treatment protocol in haemophilic arthropathy. Comprehensive hemophilia care in developing countries (With emphasis on musculoskeletal aspects). WFH. Ferozsons (Pvt) Ltd, pp 32–137
4. Rodríguez-Merchán EC (2000) Articular bleeding (hemarthrosis) in hemophilia. Treatment of hemophilia. Monographs. World Federation of Hemophilia 23

5. Roosendaal G, Lafeber F (2001) Genesis of musculoskeletal problems. Consequences for treatment in developing countries. Comprehensive hemophilia care in developing countries (With emphasis on musculoskeletal aspects). WFH. Ferozsons (Pvt) Ltd, pp 62–70
6. Tachdjian MO (1994) Ortopedia pediátrica. Hemofilia interamericana. Segunda edición. Español 1610–1630
7. Fernández-Palazzi F, Rivas S, Viso R et al (2000) Synovectomy with rifampicine in haemophilic haemarthrosis. Haemophilia 6:562–565
8. Fernández-Palazzi F, Caviglia H, Bernal LR, Tariq SM (2001) Physiotherapy resistant synovitis, treatment options in developing countries. Comprehensive hemophilia care in developing countries (With emphasis on musculoskeletal aspects). WFH. Ferozsons (Pvt), Ltd, pp 102–109
9. Fernández-Palazzi F, Caviglia H, Bernal LR (2001) Problemas ortopédicos del niño hemofílico. Rev Ortop Traumatol 2:144–150
10. Silva M, Luck JV Jr, Llinás A (2004) Chronic hemophilic synovitis: the role of radiosynovectomy. Treatment of hemophilia monographs. World Federation of Hemophilia 33
11. Staheli LT (2003) Ortopedia pediátrica. Técnicas: artrocentesis. Marbán SL Primera Edicion. Español, p 379
12. Tariq SM, Fernández-Palazzi F (2001) Haemarthrosis. Mangement in areas of limited resources. Comprehensive hemophilia care in developing countries (With emphasis on musculoskeletal aspects). Ferozsons (Pvt) Ltd, pp 110–114

Chapter 10
Intra-articular Hyaluronic Acid Therapy

Vincent K. Garg

Historical Aspects

In 1936, Karl Meyer and associates, while working with patients with rheumatoid arthritis at Columbia University, New York, isolated and characterized the active part of the synovial fluid of the swollen joints. They named the polysaccharide thus isolated hyaluronic acid (HA). HA is a linear polysaccharide that is composed of repeating disaccharide units of glucoronic acid and N-acetylglucosamine.

In the 1940s HA was isolated in almost all animal species, and in the 1950s it was shown to be associated with a number of diseases, including rheumatoid arthritis, osteoarthritis, certain malignancies, and skin diseases. In the 1960s and 1970s, the function of HA and its place in clinical practice became better defined. HA was first used as a visco-elastic product in surgical procedures on eyes. Later on, a Japanese product for osteoarthritis of the knee joint was introduced, after which several such products entered the market.

In 1997, the Food and Drug Administration (FDA) approved HA viscosupplementation therapy for the treatment of osteoarthritis.

Definition

Intra-articular injections of HA involve injections of hyaluronate into the joint in an attempt to improve the elasticity and viscosity of the synovial fluid and thereby reduce pain. HA is used in a series of injections into the joint at weekly intervals for 3–5 weeks. Studies suggest that the beneficial effects may last from 12 to 26 weeks.

Rationale of the Procedure

HA plays a fundamental role in the synovial joints, where it is present in both the cartilage matrix and the synovial fluid. It is synthesized by chondrocytes in

H.A. Caviglia, L.P. Solimeno (eds.), *Orthopedic Surgery in Patients with Hemophilia.*

the cartilage, and fibroblasts in the synovial lining. It plays a crucial role in determining the mechanical properties of articular cartilage. The high molecular weight and high concentration of HA in the joint provide a high visco-elastic solution that can act as a lubricant during slow movements, and as a shock absorber during rapid movements of the joints. Exogenous HA acts by its own presence, as well as by stimulation of endogenous HA production. Besides having mechanical benefits, HA has been found to be associated with a variety of anti-inflammatory effects in degenerative arthritis.

The synovial fluid from osteoarthritic joints has been found to have lower viscosity and elasticity than the synovial fluid of normal joints. This characteristic has led to the development of viscosupplementation therapy for degenerative arthropathy of the joints.

In a few available comparative studies with other products, HA appeared equivalent to methyl predisolone 40 mg (for 3 weeks) and to a single injection of triamcilonone 40 mg, as far as the pain-relieving effect was concerned. HA differs from other therapies in that it provides a sustained effect after treatment is discontinued [1-4].

Indications

Since the changes in hemophilic arthropathy are similar to those of degenerative arthropathy, one can safely use viscosupplementation therapy for hemophilic joints also. This therapy is useful for pain relief. However, it is not recommended as a first-line therapy for pain caused by degenerative arthropathy. An adequate trial with analgesics and physiotherapy should be done before opting for this therapy.

To sum up, viscosupplementation therapy is indicated only for moderate cases of degenerative arthropathy in patients who have failed to respond to non-invasive interventions and who have a reasonable degree of mobility.

Contraindications

- Inflammatory arthritis.
- Gross stiffness of the joint.
- Advanced hemophilic arthropathy (stage V of the Arnold and Hilgartner scale of hemophilic arthropathy).

Surgical Technique

Intra-articular injection of HA should be treated as a surgical procedure and not as one that can be performed in the doctor's office. The utmost care should be taken as far as asepsis is concerned.

1. The patient is made to lie in a supine position. Anti-hemophilic factor is infused so as to raise the factor level to almost 50%.
2. This is followed by a pre-operative antisepsis procedure.
3. The site of injection is then decided. The knee joint is commonly approached from either an anteromedial or anterolateral direction. For an anterolateral approach, the knee joint should be in an extended postion. If the surgeon wants to approach anteromedially, the knee joint needs to be flexed to 90°. In this position, the anterior portions of the medial and lateral joint lines can easily be palpated as dimples just medial or lateral to the lower pole of the patella. The medial joint line, which is easier to palpate, can be chosen as the site of injection. Alternatively, the joint can also be approached with the knee joint in a fully extended position. Most commonly, the superolateral edge of the patella is the site of injection, but other quadrants of the knee near the patellar edges can also be chosen. With this approach the needle is aimed under the patella.
4. Once a decision has been made regarding the site of injection, the area is anesthetized with a 2% solution of lidocaine, injected with a 26 gauge needle so as to raise a wheal of about 1–1.5 cm diameter.
5. HA comes in pre-filled syringes. With an 18 gauge needle, the joint space is approached through the anesthetized area of skin. If resistance is encountered, redirection of the needle may be needed. The injection is then administered.
6. A pressure bandage is applied.
7. In apprehensive patients, one may use tramadol or pentazocine injections intravenously just prior to the procedure.

If need be, viscosupplementation therapy can be repeated after 6–24 months.

Rehabilitation

The patient is allowed full weight-bearing soon after the procedure. The pressure bandage is removed after 24 h and the patient is encouraged to start doing active exercise against resistance as soon as possible.

References

1. Athanassiou-Metaxa M, Koussi A, Economou M et al (2002) Chemical synoviorthesis with rifampicine and hyaluronic acid in haemophilic children. Haemophilia 8(6):815–816
2. Fernández-Palazzi F, Viso R, Boadas A et al (2002) Intra-articular hyaluronic acid in the treatment of haemophilic chronic arthropathy. Haemophilia 8(3):375–381
3. Wallny T, Brackmann HH, Semper H et al (2000) Intra-articular hyaluronic acid in the treatment of haemophilic arthropathy of the knee. Clinical, radiological and sonographical assessment. Haemophilia 6(5):566–570
4. Fernández-Palazzi F (1998) Treatment of acute and chronic synovitis by non-surgical means. Haemophilia 4(4):518–523

1. The patient is made to lie in a supine position. Antihaemophilic factor is infused so as to raise the factor level to almost 50%.
2. This is followed by a pre-operative antisepsis procedure.
3. The site of injection is then decided. The knee joint is commonly approached from either an anteromedial or anterolateral direction. For an anterolateral approach, the knee joint should be in an extended position. If the patient [illegible]

[illegible]

[illegible]

ment of haemophilic arthropathy of the knee. Clinical, radiological, and ultrasound assessment. Haemophilia [illegible]

14. Fernandez-Palazzi F (1998) Treatment of acute and chronic synovitis by non-surgical means. Haemophilia 4(4):518-523

Chapter 11
Intra-articular Corticosteroid Therapy

Mahesh P. Shrivastava and Abhisek Bhattarai

Introduction

The hemophilias are inherited, lifelong, sex-linked bleeding disorders occurring predominantly in males [1]. People with hemophilia do not bleed faster than normal, but they can bleed for a longer time. Their blood does not have enough *clotting factor*, which is protein in blood that controls bleeding [2]. The incidence of hemophilia is rare. About 1 in 10,000 people are born with it. The most common type of hemophilia is factor VIII deficiency, also called hemophilia A or classic hemophilia. The second most common type is factor IX deficiency, also called hemophilia B or Christmas disease (named for Stephen Christmas, the first person diagnosed with factor IX deficiency). Hemophilia A is approximately five times more common than hemophilia B. Both types of hemophilia share the same symptoms and inheritance pattern — only blood tests can differentiate between the two [3]. It is very important to know which factor is defective so that the correct treatment can be given.

The severity of hemophilia is related to the degree of deficiency of the relevant clotting factor in the blood. Where there is less than 1% of the normal activity present, the condition is described as severe. Between 1% and 5% of normal activity is classed as moderate, and greater that 5–30% of normal activity is described as mild.

The most common symptom of hemophilia is bleeding, especially into the joints and muscles. Depending on the severity and mode of presentation, hemophilic arthropathy can be clinically categorized into acute, subacute and chronic hemophilic arthropathy [4].

In *acute hemarthrosis* the signs and symptoms develop rapidly (within hours) and the joints become warm, swollen, and painful. The overlying skin may become shiny, and the most commonly affected joint is the knee, followed by the elbow, ankle, hip, and shoulder.

Subacute hemarthrosis is a consequence of a few episodes of acute hemarthrosis. On palpation one can feel thickened synovium and boggy synovium. The condition is associated with restricted joint movement with less pain.

H.A. Caviglia, L.P. Solimeno (eds.), *Orthopedic Surgery in Patients with Hemophilia.*

Chronic hemarthosis is a consequence of acute and subacute hemarthosis which persists for more than 6 months and is characterized by persistent joint pain even at rest. At this stage there is gradual and progressive destruction of the joint. In the end the joint becomes totally destroyed and non-functional.

Role of Steroids

Intra-articular injection of steroid in hemophilia is a remarkably successful procedure that not only provides pain relief, but also improves quality of life and gives functional improvement of the affected joint. It also, to some extent, protects the joint from degenerative change. The success of intra-articular steroid therapy is predicted by the stage of disease and factor level in plasma.

Indications

Intra-articular corticosteroid therapy is widely used in rheumatoid arthritis or any other non-inflammatory degenerative joint disease. The use of intra-articular steroids in the treatment of hemophilic arthropathy has not been widely reported. Intra-articular steroid is used in those joints with grades II or III hemophilic arthropathic changes, where articular destruction is not yet so severe [5]. In these cases intra-articular steroid (long-acting steroid, usually dexamethasone) is used as a palliative treatment. Due to its anti-inflammatory action, it decreases the inflammation of the synovium, thereby decreasing pain caused by synovitis and arthritis.

Intra-articular steroid is also used in post-operatively chemical synoviorthesis to reduce pain, and in radioactive synoviorthesis to avoid radioactive burn of the needle tract or adjacent skin burn.

Contraindications

Corticosteroid injection should not be given in septic arthritis/septicemia; febrile patients; cases of serious allergy to previous injection; or any unknown cause of monoarthritis or neutropenia.

Evaluation of the Patient before Injection

A systematic approach to the evaluation of patient is necessary before injecting steroid into a joint because the joint may already be deformed and may need surgery. The patient may have multiple joint problems and may have high expectations from the overall outcome of the steroid therapy. Therefore, before injecting steroid into the joint, the whole procedure should be explained in detail, including its complications and the prognosis after injection.

It is essential to take a full patient history, do an adequate physical examination (how many joints involved, degree of severity, joint destruction, movement, muscle wasting, muscle mass, and neuromuscular coordination and joint perception), note previous medication, and find information about previous history of any injection if present, any other chronic disease, or whether the patient has had complications during previous injection, and history of factor transfusion.

The patients should also be warned of uncommon side-effects: exacerbation of pain for 24–48 h, septic arthritis, tissue atrophy, depigmentation, anaphylaxis, avascular necrosis, cartilage damage, and soft-tissue calcification.

As a general rule it is strongly recommended that no one joint should be injected more than four times in a year and there should be an interval of 6 weeks between injections.

Relevant investigations include X-ray of the affected joint (to be aware of the radiological changes in the involved joint, e.g., joint destruction, narrowing of the joint space, and joint deformity), and the factor level in plasma to prevent post-injection bleeding (the factor level must be above 40% before injecting steroid) as well as bleeding and clotting profile. Before injecting steroid, one must clearly know the preventive measures to control bleeding after injection, and the indication for surgery.

Principles of Injection Techniques

The procedure is carried out in a sterile environment. All the steps mentioned below need to be followed strictly to maintain relatively aseptic conditions.

- The exact spot of the needle insertion is marked.
- The hands are thoroughly washed and sterile gloves and gowns are used.
- The skin is cleansed with antiseptic solutions.
- The skin is anesthetized either with local anesthetic or refrigerant alcohol spray.
- A clean needle with an empty syringe is inserted into the joint and aspiration of the joint carried out.
- The needle is left in place, the syringe is detached, and another syringe containing the drug is placed onto the end of the needle.
- The syringe plunger is pulled back to ensure there is no arterial or venous injury.
- The drug should be injected into a joint without encountering any resistance.
- The syringe and needle are removed and the injection site is covered with a sterile dressing pad.
- Finally, the joint is rested for 24 h (48 h for a weight-bearing joint), and any possible side-effects thoroughly dealt with.

Route and Position

In hemophilic arthropathy, the most commonly affected joints are the knees, ankles, and elbows. The shoulders and the hips can also be involved. The general principles for intra-articular corticosteroid therapy are the same whichever joint is involved, but the approaches and the positions of the patients while giving intra-articular steroid therapy differ from one joint to another as described below [6].

The Shoulder

The shoulder can be approached by a superior, posterior, anterosuperior, or antero-inferior route.

Anterosuperior Route

The patient lies in a supine position with the shoulder held in external rotation. The entry point is 1 cm inferior to the acromioclavicular joint, and the direction of the needle is postero-inferior until it reaches the bone.

Antero-inferior Route

The patient is supine with the shoulder held in external rotation and 20–30° abduction. The needle is directed superolaterally.

Posterior Route

The patient may sit or be in a prone position with the arm abducted to 20°. The entry point is the line of intersection between a vertical line drawn 2 cm medial to the lateral margin of the acromion and a horizontal line 2 cm below the inferolateral edge of the acromion. The needle is perpendicular to the skin and directed posteriorly until it touches the humeral head.

Superior Route

The patient is in a sitting position with the arm abducted to 45°. The entry point is the angle formed by the posterior edge of the clavicle and medial border of the acromion.

The Elbow

The patient is in a supine position with the arm across the abdomen and forearm in a neutral position. The needle is inserted at the center of the angle formed by the olecranon, radial head, and the lateral epicondyle.

The Ankle

Entry of the needle is through the anterior route. The patient position is supine, and the ankle position is neutral. The needle is inserted in the depression between the tibialis anterior and the tendon of the extensor digitorum longus.

The Knee

The patient position is supine with knee extension. The route of injection is lateral parapatellar and lateral suprapatellar, and the injection is directly given in the suprapatellar pouch and lateral corner of the patella.

The Hip

For the hip, the patient position is supine and the injection site is identified with the help of an image intensifier. The entry point is directly over the femoral head, which is just lateral to the femoral vessel and three finger breadths below the mid-inguinal point. The route is suprolateral and inferomedial.

Choice of Drug and Procedure

Before injecting steroid, appropriate factor replacement is necessary to ensure the factor level is at least 40%. The procedure should be carried out in the theater with all antiseptic precautions and all the facilities for the management of post-injection bleeding or any other complication that may arise.

The area of injection should be carefully cleansed and sterilized and the operator should use sterile gowns and gloves. Young children and anxious adults may require sedation.

The needle size will depend upon the size of the joint. For a simple joint injection, a 16 or 18 gauge needle is sufficient, and a 12 or 14 gauge needle may be necessary if evacuation of blood or viscous synovial fluid from the joint is needed before injection.

Dexamethasone, a long-acting steroid, is the drug of choice for intra-articular injection. The steroid should be diluted in 2% local anesthetic solution. Both solutions should be kept in the same disposable syringe. An injection should be given three times, with a 3-week interval between each injection, to complete one cycle. According to the response obtained (given by the patient and radiological change observed by the clinician), 6 months after the last injection, a new cycle of three injections may be performed.

The usual dose is 2 ml of corticosteroid (dexamethasone — sodium phosphate and sodium acetate of dexamethasone) diluted in 2–10 ml of 2% lidocaine hydrochloride. The dose of medicine should be selected according to the size of the joint.

Management after Injection

After injecting the steroid into a joint, local ice application is helpful to reduce post-injection bleeding. Application of Robert Jones-type bandage, rest, and support to the joint with a splint may have beneficial results. If the patient does not complain of any pain and bleeding for 24 h, then the applied splint is removed and physiotherapy started. A regular exercise protocol should be used. Robert Jones-type bandage should be applied for 4–7 days.

Effect

The clinical outcome can last for months, or maybe a year, depending on the severity of disease, the number of injections, the severity of joint involvement, and the presence or absence of HIV. If pain re-appears and the range of movement decreases, the procedure can be repeated after 6 months. The radiological changes observed before and after the procedure may remain unchanged and deterioration may be due to the natural history of the disease. It may not be associated with the number of injections, amount of steroid, or number of cycles performed.

Conclusion

Prevention of chronic synovitis is the key to management of hemophilic arthropathy. There are various treatment options for hemophilic synovitis and hemophilic arthropathy, such as prophylaxis, aspiration, oral steroids, synoviorthesis (chemical, radioactive), or synovectomy (open or arthroscopic). Intra-articular steroid can also be used safely. This is an alternative palliative treatment focused particularly on pain relief, to arrest functional impairment before an aggressive surgical procedure is required.

References

1. World Federation of Hemophilia (1996) Facts for Health Care Professional. Haemophilia, p 2
2. World Federation of Hemophilia (2004) What is Hemophilia, p 1
3. National Hemophilia Foundation (1998) Caring for your Child with Hemophilia, p 2
4. Gupta AD (2001) Treatment Protocol in Haemophilic Arthropathy-Comprehensive Haemophilia Care in Developing Countries, p 133
5. Fernandez-Palazzi F (1998) Treatment of acute and chronic synovitis by non-surgical means. Haemophilia 4:519
6. Rodriguez-Merchan EC, Goddard NJ (2001) The Technique of SynoviorthesisHaemophilia, 7(2):11–15

Chapter 12
Rifampicin Synoviorthesis of the Ankle Joint

Shubhranshu S. Mohanty

Introduction

Hemophilia, a hereditary blood clotting disorder, characterized by joint bleeds (either spontaneous or injury-induced), is known to cause arthropathy in affected males. The only preventive treatment available to protect from joint bleeds is replacement of the relevant clotting factor that is deficient. After several bleeding episodes, persistent synovitis with swelling of a joint develops in patients with hemophilia, despite adequate therapy. This condition seems to be inflammatory rather than hemorrhagic. Chronic synovitis persists in moderate and severe hemophilia, despite improved and increased availability of clotting factors [1]. Patients with synovitis are again prone to develop recurrent bleeds and joint damage, which is quite disabling.

Rifampicin synoviorthesis is a procedure where rifampicin is injected into a joint [2]. The procedure is based on rifampicin's proteolytic and anti-fibrinolytic properties, so it achieves synovial sclerosis and fibrosis [2]. This should control the recurrent episodes of bleeding and prevent progressive destruction of articular cartilage by chemical ablation of synovium. Radioactive material such as ^{90}yttrium is also helpful in chemical ablation of the synovium.

Definition of the Problem

Chronic synovitis is a common problem associated with teenage hemophilia. About 60–70% of all hemophiliacs are affected by this condition at present. It develops as a reaction to the intra-articular hemosiderin deposits, and is a problem for which no solution has been developed to date. Hemosiderin deposits trigger an intense synovial inflammatory reaction [3].

Hypertrophic synovitis occupies extra space and is likely to be injured causing additional bleeding. This process begins again and is responsible for the chronic synovitis in the joints of hemophiliac patients that is seen most commonly in the knee, followed by the shoulder and ankle. The hypertrophic synovitis is characterized by villus formation and markedly increased synoviocytes,

H.A. Caviglia, L.P. Solimeno (eds.), *Orthopedic Surgery in Patients with Hemophilia.*

vascularity, and chronic inflammatory cells. Due to limited capacity of the synoviocytes to absorb iron, the excess clot formed is unlikely to be removed completely by the fibrinolytic system, and the remaining clot leads to the development of fibrous adhesions. Failure to treat the synovitis may cause progressive pathological changes in the synovium and progression of the joint disease.

Clinically, a patient with ankle synovitis may have a distended joint; it may not be painful, and the range of movements may be restricted because of muscle atrophy. Untreated patients may develop problems like capsular and ligamentous laxity, leading to rapid joint deformity. On palpation, synovial thickening, effusion, deformities, and restriction of dorsiflexion may be observed (Fig. 12.1).

Radiologically, soft tissue thickening may be seen. Synovitis is usually limited to epiphyseal osteoporosis, mild joint space narrowing, and subchondral irregularity (Fig. 12.2). Special investigations like magnetic resonance imaging (MRI) (Fig. 12.3) and ultrasonography are of help to delineate the extent of synovial thickening, soft tissue damage, and intra-articular changes. A red blood cell (RBC)-labeled bone scan would also assess the vascularity of the synovium.

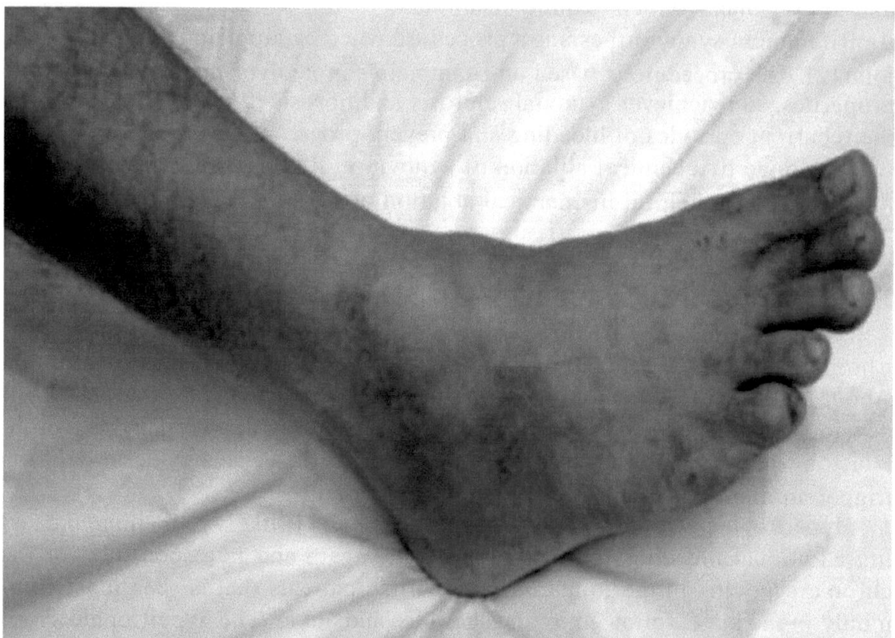

Fig. 12.1 Clinical picture of hemophilic synovitis of the right ankle

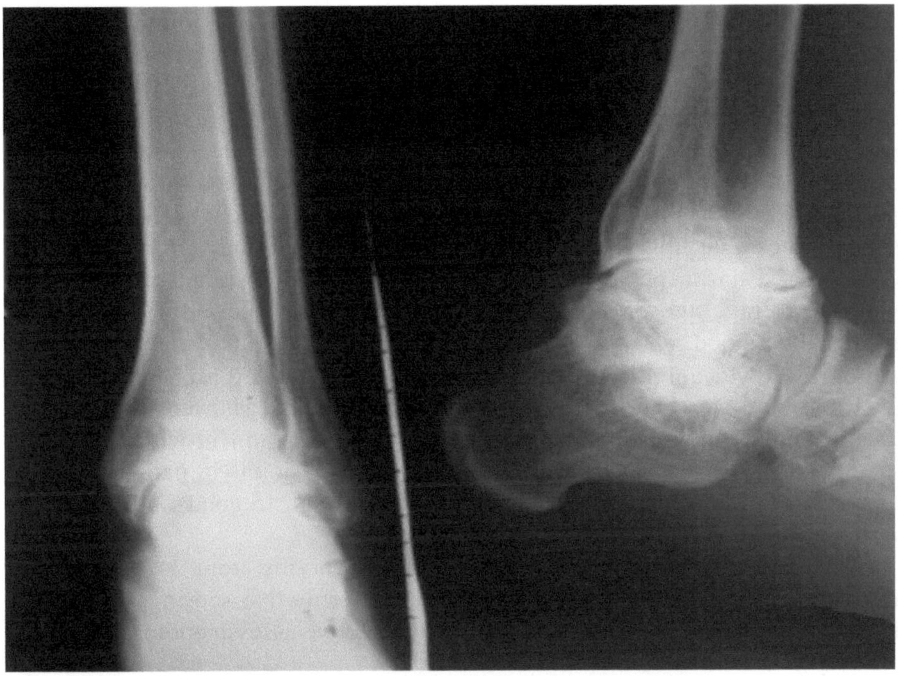

Fig. 12.2 Radiological picture of hemophilic synovitis of the right ankle

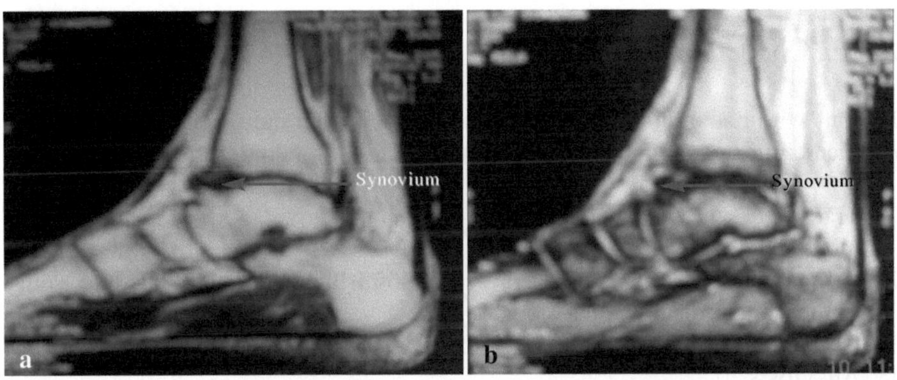

Fig. 12.3 a T_1 and **b** T_2-weighted MRI picture of hemophilic arthropathy of the right ankle

Literature Review

Rifampicin synoviorthesis has been empirically used for the treatment of hemophilic synovitis. Three Latin American centers have conducted clinical trials on this subject and are of the opinion that it is best indicated in younger patients (<15 years) and small joints (ankles and elbows) [3]. The Hemophilia Center of

Sao Paulo (Brazil) followed up 3 years of injection of 21 knee joints, two ankles and one elbow in patients with an average age of 19 years. Results show an excellent or good result (with or without pain, no hemarthrosis) in 71.1% of cases. The orthopedic department of Caracas (Venezuela) studied 19 joints in patients with an average age of 19 years. A 4-year follow-up showed 58% were excellent (no pain, no hemarthrosis) and 28% good (no hemarthrosis, but pain persisted). Similar results were obtained in a 10-year follow-up of radioactive synoviorthesis at this center [4]. One prospective study from Argentina (Fernández-Palazzi, personal communication) studied a patient sample of 19 with an average age of 9 years. Two-year follow-up showed 79% excellent results, 16% good, and 5% poor. Moreover, similar results were evident with radioactive ^{90}yttrium injection in a 25-month follow-up at this center.

Rodríguez-Merchán had a group of 20 patients and showed that effective chemical ablation with rifampicin was equivalent to treatment with radioactive materials [2]. Fernandez-Palazzi et al [4] studied 39 joints in patients with an average age of 18 years. They had 21 excellent results, 15 good, and 3 fair/poor results.

Though all of these studies had a follow-up varying from 2–7 years, their results are based on symptomatic improvement only. No scoring system was used, nor were the results supported by any objective assessment to confirm the efficacy of treatment.

Procedure

Patient Selection

Patients with hemophilic arthropathy are selected from outpatient departments. A detailed clinical examination is performed to classify them into four grades [3]:

I Transient synovitis with no post-traumatic sequelae (>3 episodes in 6 months)
II Permanent synovitis (increased size of joint involved, synovial thickening, limited range of movements)
III Chronic arthropathy with axial deformities and muscle atrophy
IV Ankylosis

Indications

- All grade I and II hemophilic arthropathy
- Patients with progressive bleeds (>3 episodes in 6 months) into the joint

Absolute Contraindications

- Acute hemarthroses.
- Unhealthy skin condition over a joint, e.g., furuncle, ulcer, scarred skin.

Relative Contraindications

- Children under 5 years of age.
- Fixed deformities.
- Uncooperative/anxious patients.
- Patients with inhibitors.

Clinical and Laboratory Tests

- Assessment is performed according to:
  - World Federation of Hemophilia (WFH) scoring system [5]
  - Disability evaluation score [6].
- Routine investigations like full blood count, HIV, X-ray of the joint are performed. Pettersson's criteria [7] are followed to give a radiological classification.
- Special investigations like factor assay, inhibitor assay, ultrasonography of the ankle to assess fluid in the synovium, RBC-labeled scan to study the synovial circulation, and MRI of the joint are performed to measure the thickness of synovium anterior and posterior to the talus, hemarthrosis, articular cartilage destruction, subarticular erosion, and osteophyte formation.

Consent Form for the Procedure

Written consent is taken from the patient or the parents after explaining the method in detail in their own language, and discussing possible complications such as acute hemorrhage, infection etc.

Factor Correction

Coagulation factor correction up to 20% is done before each injection.

Procedure of Joint Injection under Aseptic Conditions

Position

The patient should be in a supine position with the knee flexed to 90° and the foot flat on the table, so that the ankle joint remains in slight equinus.

Location

The needle is inserted about 2.5 cm. proximal and 1.3 cm medial to the tip of lateral malleolus. This will be just lateral to the peroneus tertius tendon [8] (Fig. 12.4).

The procedure is carried out as follows:

1. Aspiration of articular contents; sample sent for factor and inhibitor assay.
2. Injection of rifampicin (150 mg) in 2.5 ml water (Fig. 12.5).
3. Cold therapy applied to the joint for 20 min (Fig. 12.6).
4. Compression dressing applied for 24 h (Fig. 12.7).
5. Rehabilitation programme for 6 days.

The procedure is repeated every week for 6 weeks. If the patient had partial relief the procedure is repeated after 6 months.

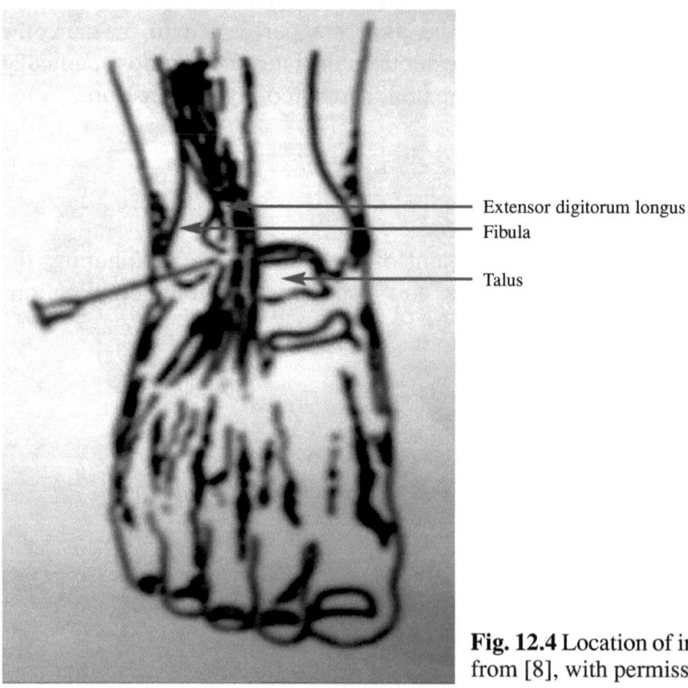

Fig. 12.4 Location of injection. Reproduced from [8], with permission from Elsevier

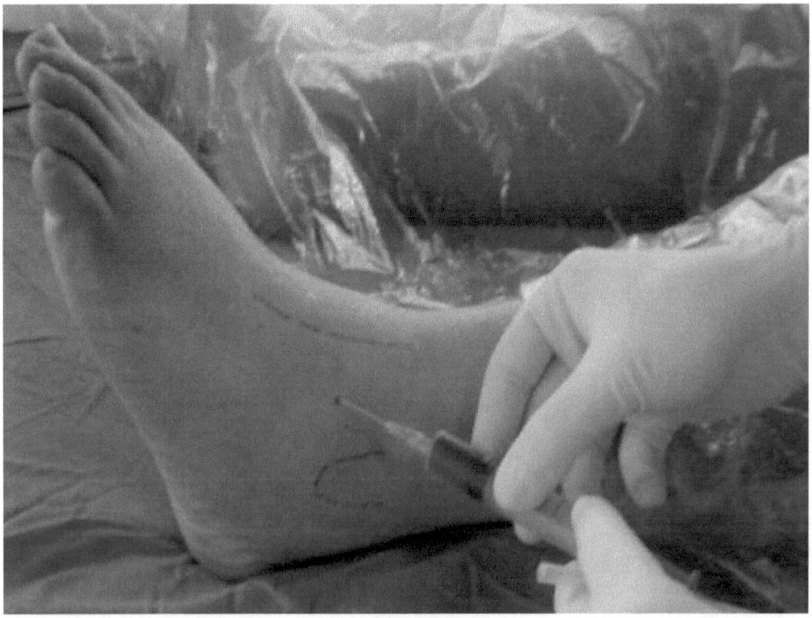

Fig. 12.5 Injection of rifampicin into the left ankle

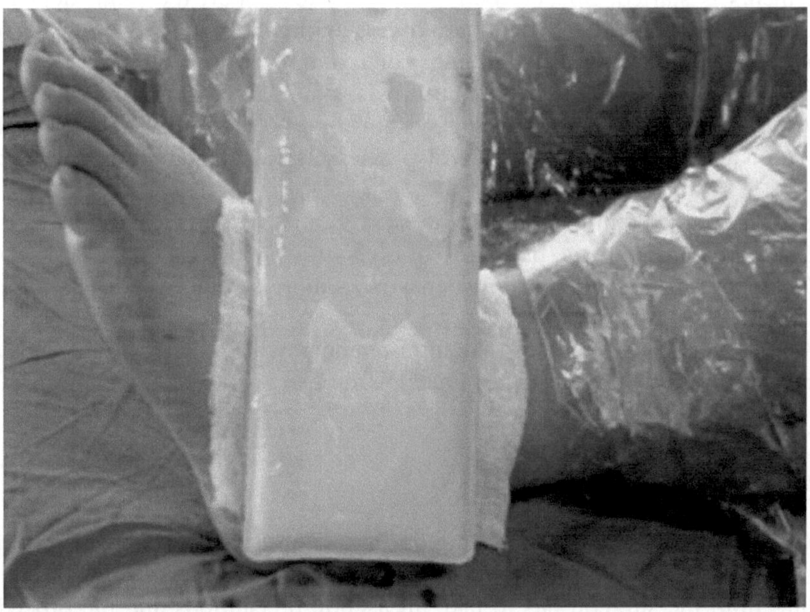

Fig. 12.6 Cold compression over a gauze piece

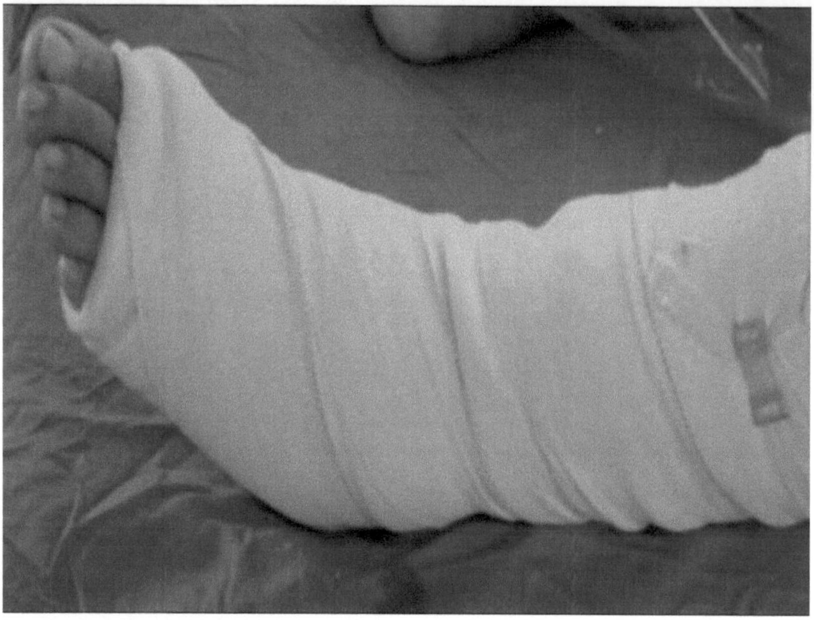

Fig. 12.7 Compression dressing

Rehabilitation Schedule

The joint is mobilized after 24 h. An assisted range of both passive and active movements is started. Special splints are used to support the joint, depending upon the individual case. Patients are assessed clinically before each injection. Then they are followed every 3 months for 1 year, every 6 months for 2 years to check for pain, any evidence of hemarthrosis, synovial thickening, and the range of movements. The different scoring systems like WFH score, disability evaluation score and Pettersson scores are also assessed. Results are graded as [3]:

- *Excellent*: no hemarthrosis, no pain.
- *Good*: no hemarthrosis, pain present (synovitis persisted).
- *Poor*: both pain and hemarthrosis persisted/more advanced arthropathy.

All the special investigations like ultrasonography, RBC-labeled scan and MRI are repeated 3 months after the last injection to objectively assess the progress.

Complications

- *Acute hemorrhage*: acute bleeding during the procedure is expected as injection is a form of external trauma (Fig. 8).
- *Infection*: the surgeon has to take all aseptic precautions and the procedure should preferably be carried out in a sterile operation theater set-up.

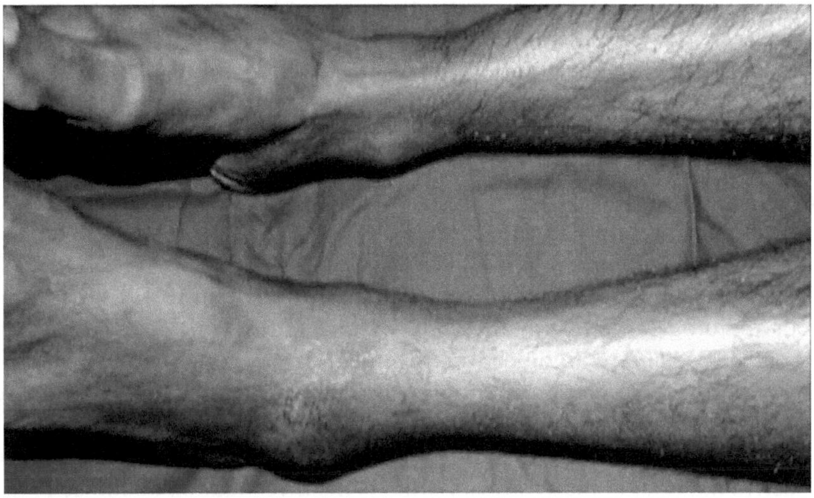

Fig. 12.8 Acute bleed in the left ankle after intra-articular rifampicin injection

Our Experience

Our samples of 37 patients included 13 ankle joints, which were injected between January 1999 and November 2001. Two joints were of grade I and II of grade II. The average age of patients was 23.5 years (range 11–45 years). Ten patients had severe hemophilia and three moderate. Patients most commonly had hemophilia A (10 patients) and three had hemophilia B. The average follow-up period was 4.6 years (range 3.5–6.4 years). The average Disability Limitation Score before injection was 60.8. There was thickening of the synovium shown by ultrasound and MRI. The maximum synovial thickness was measured. The vascularity of the synovium was increased as evidenced by RBC-labeled bone scan.

The clinical assessment showed excellent results in nine (69.2%) joints. Good results were seen in three and poor in one. One ankle joint developed acute bleeding during the procedure, which improved with factor correction and conservative measures. The average Disability Limitation Score improved from 60.8 to 45.6. The Pettersson radiological scoring improved from an average of 8.66 to 6.1. There was considerable reduction in the vascularity of the synovium as evidenced by the bone scan, and the average reduction in synovial thickness was 1.6 mm.

Discussion

Rifampicin synoviorthesis is an excellent therapeutic alternative for hemophilic synovitis to prevent further articular damage. The Latin American clinical trials show that it is best indicated in younger patients (<15 years) and small joints (ankles and elbows) [3]. Our patients often present late due to lack of awareness of patients in our series.

Moreover, these centers show 71–86% excellent/good results in a 2–4-year follow-up. We had similar results in 92% of cases, with an average follow-up of 4.6 years. Similar results were obtained in a 10-year follow-up of radioactive synoviorthesis at this center [4]. However, we have very limited experience of radioactive synovectomy.

The current literature does not reveal any objective assessment demonstrating the effect of rifampicin at the site of injection. Our study is the first of its kind to reveal the local effect of intra-articular rifampicin. It was demonstrated in four radiological investigations, i.e., X-ray, ultrasound, RBC-labeled bone scan, and MRI. The radiological improvement of the joint is coincidental with clinical improvement. Petterson criteria are instrumental in delineating the scoring system. Hemophilia is associated with increased vascularity of the synovium due to hypertrophy, and the effect of synovial ablation is reduction of uptake of radioactive material in the synovium. MRI is the investigation of choice to measure the synovial thickness, and it has assessed the efficacy by measuring the reduction in thickness. However, ours is a short follow-up of only 4.6 years, and long-term objective assessment is awaited.

We did not see any serious side-effects. Acute bleeds during the procedure are expected as injection is a form of external trauma. As intra-articular injection in a minor procedure, it is considered cost-effective to infuse 20% factor correction. However, the acute bleed should be managed in the routine manner.

One of the long-term effects of rifampicin could be antibody development to this antibiotic. No literature shows this complication. However, we have a study in progress to detect antibodies in all these patients during their follow-up.

Acknowledgements

I would acknowledge the help of Dr. (Mrs.) N.A. Kshirsagar, Dean, Dr. V.J. Laheri, Head of Orthopaedics, Dr. Dipika Mohanty, Ex-Director, Dr. K. Ghosh, Director of IIH, Dr. J.S. Kale, Occupational Therapy, Dr. F. Jijina, Haematology, Dr. D. Patkar, MRI for carrying out the procedures published in this article.

References

1. Rodríguez-Merchán EC (1997) Pathogenesis, early diagnosis and prophylaxis for chronic haemophilic synovitis. Clin Orthop 343:6–11
2. Pietrogrande V (1987) XIV International Congress of World Federation of Haemophilia, Costa Rica. Personal communication
3. Caviglia H, Galatro G, Duhalde C, Perez-Bianco R (1998) Haemophilic synovitis: is rifampicin an alternative? Haemophilia 4:514–517
4. Fernández-Palazzi F, de Bosch NB, de Vargas AF (1984) Radioactive synovectomy in haemophilic haemarthrosis. Follow up of fifty cases. Scand J Haematology 33:291–300

5. Hoffmann P, Ahlberg A, Duthie RB et al (1981) Orthopaedics and haemophilia: the state of the art. Haemostasis (Suppl 10):126
6. Kale JS (2000) Disability assessment for haemophiliacs. Indian J Occ Ther 32(3):9–12
7. Pettersson H, Ahlberg A, Nillson IM (1980) A radiological classification on haemophilic arthropathy. Clin Orthop 149:153–159
8. Canale ST (2003) Campbell's operative orthopaedics, 10th Ed., Vol.1, Mosby, Philadelphia, p 689

Chapter 13
Radioactive Synoviorthesis of the Knee

Horacio A. Caviglia, Victoria Soroa, Gustavo Galatro and Noemi Moretti

Introduction

There is a clear relationship between recurrent joint bleeding, synovitis, and arthropathy in patients with hemophilia. Synovitis is inflammation of the specialized connective tissue lining of a joint cavity. The golden moment in treatment is when no associated arthropathy is present, because synovitis and muscular hypotrophy are reversible; in contrast arthropathy is not a reversible process [1,2].

Definition

Radioactive synoviorthesis is radionuclide therapy of joint synovitis by intra-articular injection of ^{90}Y silicate/citrate, chromic phosphate – ^{32}P *or* ^{186}Re sulphide.

Radiopharmaceuticals

The properties of the radiopharmaceuticals that can be used [3, 4, 5] are summarized in Table 13.1 and the lists below.

^{32}P:

- Is a pure beta particle emitter with a maximum energy of 1.71 MeV.
- Has a mean energy of maximum beta penetration in tissue of 7.9 MeV.
- Has a mean beta penetration of 2.2 mm with no gamma emission.
- Has a physical half-life of 14.3 days.

^{186}Re:

- Is a beta particle with a maximum energy of 0.98 MeV, and a 9% abundant gamma emission with a photopeak of 0.137 MeV.

H.A. Caviglia, L.P. Solimeno (eds.), *Orthopedic Surgery in Patients with Hemophilia.*

Table 13.1 Radiopharmaceuticals that can be used

Radionuclide	Maximum beta energy (MeV)	Gamma emission, % (KeV)	Tissue range (mm)		Half-life (days)	Activity (MBq)
			Maximum	Mean		
^{90}Yttrium	2.26		11.0	3.6	2.7	185–250
^{186}Rhenium	0.98	9 (137)	3.7	1.2	3.7	37–185
^{188}Rhenium	2.1	15 (155)	11.0	3.8	0.7	148–703
^{32}Phosphorus	1.71		7.9	2.6	14.3	11–74

- Has a mean energy of 0.349 MeV.
- Has an average penetration range of 1.2 mm.
- Has a physical half-life of 3.7 days.

^{188}Re:
- Is a beta particle with a maximum energy of 2.1 MeV, and a 15% abundant gamma emission with a photopeak of 0.155 MeV.
- Has a mean energy of 0.349 MeV.
- Has an average penetration range of 3.8 mm.
- Has a physical half-life of 0.7 days.

^{90}Y:
- Is a beta particle with a maximum energy of 2.26 MeV.
- Has a mean energy of 0.935 MeV.
- Has an average soft tissue range of 3.6 mm.
- Has a physical half-life of 2.7 days.

Recommended Activity

Table 13.2 shows recommended activity for the knee and elbow.

Table 13.2 Recommended activity (MBq)

Joints	^{90}Yttrium	^{188}Rhenium	^{32}Phosphorus	^{186}Rhenium
Knee	185 (285)	518	37	185
Elbow	111	300	22	111

- Children 2 to 6 years old: use one-third the activity for an adult.
- Children 6 to 10 years old: use half the activity for an adult.
- Children 10 to 16 years old: use three-quarters the activity for an adult.

Grade of Hemophilic Arthropathy

The classification developed by Fernández-Palazzi and Caviglia is very useful to clarify the indications for treatment (Table 13.3) [6].

Table 13.3 Grading of haemophilic arthropathy

Grade	Description
I	Transitory synovitis post-bleeding without sequelae
II	Joint remains enlarged; synovial thickening and some muscle wasting
III	Same as grade 2 plus restricted range of movement (contractures) and axial deformities
IV	Great diminution in rate of movement or fibrous or bony ankylosis

Indications

Radioactive synoviorthesis is indicated in patients in grade I and II, and exceptionally in some early cases in grade III. In grade I cases, synoviorthesis is indicated as a preventive treatment if there are more than two episodes of hemarthrosis in 6 months [6].

Inclusion criteria

- Patients with hemophilic arthropathy grades I and II.
- Grade I: preventive when there are more than two episodes of bleeding within 6 months.
- All grade II.
- Early grade III patients (optional).

Exclusion Criteria

Absolute Contraindications

- Grade III patients with advanced osteoarthritis.
- All grade IV patients.
- Age: less than two years.
- Lesion or infection on the skin in the joint area.
- Presence of acute episode of bleeding at the time of injection.
- Ruptured popliteal cyst (knee).
- Pregnancy.
- Breastfeeding.

Relative Contraindications

- Extensive joint instability with bone destruction.
- Evidence of significant cartilage loss within the joint.

Pre-operative Evaluation

- Extensive documentation of patient history using a standard set of questions which include: age, diagnosis (hemophilia A or B), severity of hemophilia, previous anti-hemophilia factor (AHF) therapy, number of episodes of hemarthroses, pain (visual analogue scale in 10 steps).
- Clinical examination: joint swelling (circumference of joint), range of motion, and walking ability.

The hematologist should perform a pre-operative corrective test with factor VIII and IX to define the most adequate doses and to detect whether any inhibitor is present. The latter case implies an alternative strategy in the replacement therapy (for example, recombinant factor VIIa).

The time interval between joint puncture and radiosynoviorthesis should be 2 weeks, and that between arthroscopy or joint surgery and radiosynovectomy should be 6 weeks.

The minimum interval between repeated treatments in the same joint is 6 months.

Radiology

Radiographs of the joints to be treated should be obtained in anteroposterior and lateral view, in order to asses the degree of hemophilic arthropathy and compromise of the cartilage surface of the joint at the time of diagnosis.

Magnetic Resonance Imaging (MRI)

The MRI is the best method to evaluate the damage of the joint cartilage and so prevent migration of the radioisotopic material in the blood to subchondral bone.

Ultrasound

Ultrasound is used to evaluate synovial structure and thickness and exclude ruptured Baker's cyst. In the presence of a ruptured Baker's cyst, radiosynoviorthesis is contraindicated.

Bone Scintigraphy

Scintigraphy may be used to asses soft tissues and the severity of active inflammation of the affected joints (three-phase ^{99m}Tc MDP/HDP/HEDP (methylene diphosphonate/hydroxymethane diphosphonate/hydroxyethylidene diphosphonate) bone scintigraphy).

Procedure

The patient must informed of possible complications:

- Risks associated with joint puncture: local hemorrhage, bruising, infection, and extravasation.
- Risk of post-injection pyrexia or radiopharmaceutical allergy.
- Risk of exposure to beta-emitting radiation including radiation necrosis and future malignancy.
- The facilities required will depend on national legislation for the administration of pure beta-emitting therapeutic agents.
- The administration of radiocolloids for radiosynovectomy should be undertaken in an approved facility, equipped for sterile injection procedures, by appropriately trained medical staff with supporting scientists and nurses. A room with laminar flow is not necessary.
- Pre-operative replacement therapy: raise AHF to 30% above coagulation level.
- Local skin anaesthesia is advisable. In young patients and uncooperative patients, sedation or general anesthesia may be necessary.
- Joint puncture for radiosynovectomy carries the same risk as any joint puncture and should follow the rules of strict asepsis.
- Puncture of all joints other than the knee should be performed under fluoroscopic (X-ray) screening or ultrasound guidance.
- The knee can be routinely injected without imaging guidance once intra-articular needle placement has been ensured by aspiration of joint fluid (Fig. 13.1).
- Aspiration of the joint if necessary (Fig. 13.2)
- Inject the radiopharmaceutical into the joint using a special syringe (Fig. 13.3).
- After injection of radiopharmaceutical, flush the needle with 1 ml saline. This prevents the rare complication of a cutaneous burn if the radioactive material leaks out of the joint.
- Manipulate the joint through a full range of motion to distribute the radioactive particles throughout the joint space. Correct deposition and homogeneous distribution of the radiopharmaceutical agent in the joint space is fundamental.
- Carry out a post-therapy scan with a gamma camera to confirm and document the distribution of radiopharmaceuticals in the joint, using gamma emission or ‘Bremsstrahlung’.
- Immobilize the injected joint by splinting for 2 or 3 days.

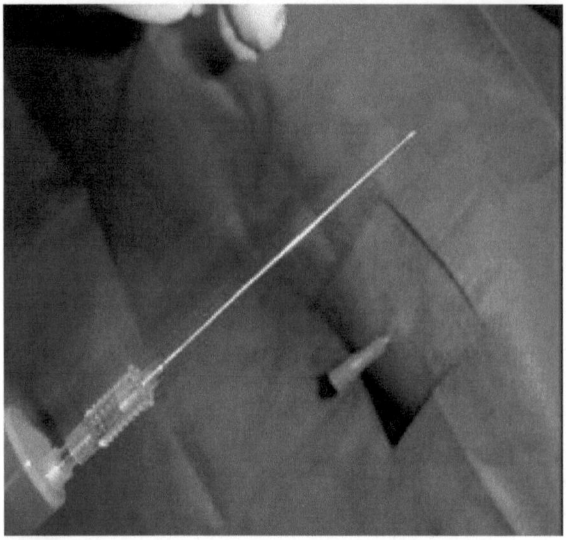

Fig. 13.1 Puncture of the knee without imaging guidance

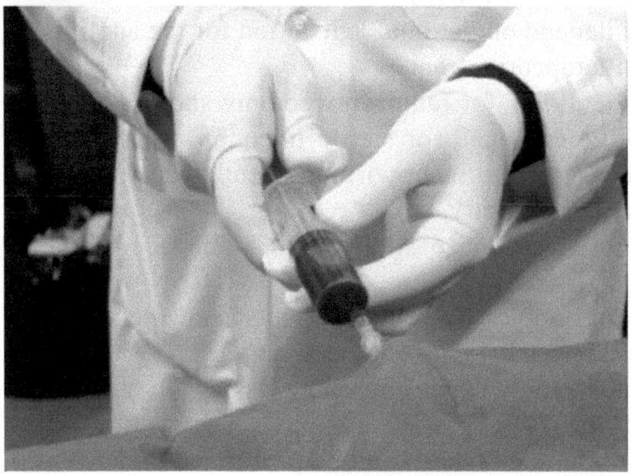

Fig. 13.2 Aspiration of the joint contents

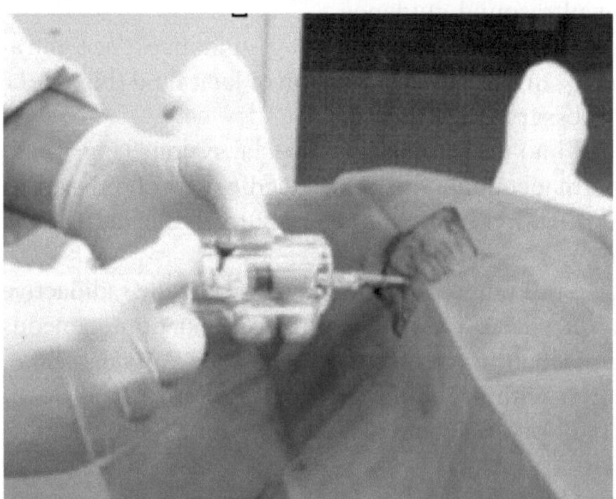

Fig. 13.3 Injection of ^{32}P

- Post-therapy whole-body scan should then be carried out for determination of the leakage rate 2–3 days after treatment.
- After removal of the splint, full weight-bearing is allowed. Patients are encouraged to regain a full range of motion in the knee and the elbow. Vigorous athletic activities are prohibited for one month.
- Active physical therapy is recommended.

Radiosynoviorthesis is a safe, cheap and cost-effective procedure for patients with hemophilic synovitis. It is an effective procedure that decreases the frequency of recurrent intra-articular bleeding related to joint synovitis. It can also be used in patients with inhibitors with minimal risk of complications.

References

1. Caviglia HA, Fernández-Palazzi F, Maffei E et al (1997) Chemical synoviorthesis for hemophilic synovitis. Clin Orthop 343:30–36
2. Rodríguez-Merchán EC, Luck JV, Silva M, Quintana M (2003) Synoviorthesis in haemophilia. In: Rodríguez-Merchán ed. The haemophilics joints. New perspectives. Blackwell Publishing, Oxford, pp 73–79
3. Ingrand J (1973) Charactheristics of radioisotopes for intra-articular therapy. Ann Rheum Dis 32:3–9
4. Deutsch E, Brodack JW, Deutsch KF (1993) Radiation sinovectomy revisted. Eur J Nuclear Med 20:1113–1127
5. Coya Vina J, Ferrer M, Martin Curto LM (2003) Radioactive isotopes for radiosynoviorthesis. In: Rodríguez Merchan ed. The haemophilics joints. New perspectives. Blackwell Publishing, Oxford, pp 68–72
6. Fernández-Palazzi F, Caviglia HA (2000) On the safety synoviorthesis in haemophilia. In: Rodríguez-Merchán EC, Goddard NJ, Lee CA (eds). Musculoskeletal aspects of haemophilia. Oxford, Blackwell Science, pp 50–55

Section IV
Upper Limb

Chapter 14
Arthroscopic Treatment of Hemophilic Arthropathy of the Shoulder

Gianluigi Pasta, Olivia Samantha Perfetto and Luigi P. Solimeno

Introduction

The shoulder has never been considered a target joint in hemophiliac patients, although many adult hemophiliacs suffer from shoulder symptoms [1–3].

Repeated articular bleeding leads to hypertrophic and hypervascularized synovia. Almost simultaneously, intra-articular bleeding produces proteolytic enzymes, cytokines, and oxygen metabolites, which lead to direct damage of articular cartilage. Synovial and articular degenerative processes influence each other, contributing to end-stage hemophilic arthropathy. The clinical picture of hemarthrosis is characterized by pain, swelling, and limited abduction. Rotator cuff tears, and consequent positive impingement signs, are a common component of hemophilic arthropathy of the shoulder, although swelling and disabling pain are the surgical indication for shoulder arthroscopy [1–3].

Diagnosis

Standard X-ray generally leads to correct evaluation of articular involvement and allows the use of a staging system [4], but we generally use arch view X-ray as well. Joint incongruity and superior migration of the humeral head are the best radiographic indicators of a cuff tear. Magnetic resonance imaging (MRI) is necessary for correct detection of rotator cuff tears and synovial hypertrophy.

Treatment

Conservative treatment should be considered first. Prophylactic treatment and a rehabilitation program are recommended to reduce the frequency of hemarthrosis and preserve articular function.

Repeated bleeding that does not respond to conservative treatment calls for arthroscopic synovectomy.

H.A. Caviglia, L.P. Solimeno (eds.), *Orthopedic Surgery in Patients with Hemophilia.*

Surgical Technique

Factor levels are maintained at 100% for the operative procedure, and at approximately 80% for post-operative days 1 to 5.

The patient is placed in the lateral decubitus position, and 10–15 lb of traction are applied using skin traction.

Once the patient has been positioned, prepared, and draped, the bony anatomical landmarks and proposed portal sites are identified and outlined with a skin-marking pen. The bony sites marked are the anterior, lateral, and posterior corners or borders of the acromion, the spine of the scapula, the distal clavicle and acromioclavicular joint, and the coracoid process. In order to evaluate the glenohumeral and subacromial joints, the arthroscopic procedure is performed through anterior, posterior, and superior portals.

A 4 mm, 30° arthroscope is used. The posterior portal is the primary entry route for shoulder arthroscopy, but for a complete diagnostic examination of the shoulder an anterior portal is essential. We generally establish the anterior portal using the retrograde method with a Wissinger rod. The superior and anterior portions of the joint are reached with surgical instruments placed through the anterior portal and the arthroscope in the posterior portal. Normally, the synovectomy is performed using a radiofrequency device and/or motorized synovial resector.

We sometimes add 1 ampule of epinephrine to the 3 l arthroscopy bag to keep blood from clouding the arthroscopic view.

Post-operative Treatment

The arm is placed in a sling and passive motion exercises are begun on the day after a synovectomy. The sling is discarded as soon as comfort permits. Active assisted range-of-motion exercises and isometric strengthening exercises for the deltoid and the rotator cuff are begun within the first week. Light resistance exercises using elastic tubing are started in the second week.

Results

The pain and frequency of hemarthroses lessens considerably, with a consequent improvement in the range of motion. Any complications are recorded.

Conclusion

In our experience, arthroscopic synovectomy of the shoulder reduces hemarthroses, with an unchanged or slightly augmented articular function. Pain reduction is considered satisfactory in all patients. Our findings coincide with those of the current international literature on radiographic evidence of cessation of articular degeneration [5].

References

1. Gilbert MS, Klepps S, Cleeman E et al (2002) The shoulder: a neglected joint. Int Monitor Haemophilia 10:3–5
2. Hogh J, Ludlam CA, Macnicol MF (1987) Hemophilic arthropathy of the upper limb. Clin Orthop 218:225–231
3. MacDonald PB, Locht RC, Lindsay D, Levi C (1990) Haemophilic arthropathy of the shoulder. J Bone Joint Surg Br 72:470–471
4. Pettersson H, Ahlberg A, Nilsson IM (1980) A radiological classification of hemophilic arthropathy. Clin Orthop 149:153–159
5. Wiedel JD (2002) Arthroscopic synovectomy: state of the art. Haemophilia 8(3):372–374

Chapter 15

Radial Head Excision for Patients with Hemophilic Arthropathy of the Elbow

Mauricio Silva and James V. Luck Jr.

Introduction

The elbow is the second most frequently affected joint in hemophilia. Chronic hemophilic synovitis of the elbow usually leads to enlargement of the radial head and severe arthropathy (Fig. 15.1). A derangement of the proximal radio-ulnar joint secondary to hypertrophy and marginal irregularities of the radial head is the major source of pain, recurrent bleeding, and restricted forearm rotation commonly seen in patients with hemophilic arthropathy of the elbow. Limitations in forearm rotation often result in significant disability. For example, loss of supination of the dominant extremity interferes with eating, handling money, and personal hygiene. Excision of the radial head has been successfully used to improve the symptoms associated with advance hemophilic arthropathy of the elbow.

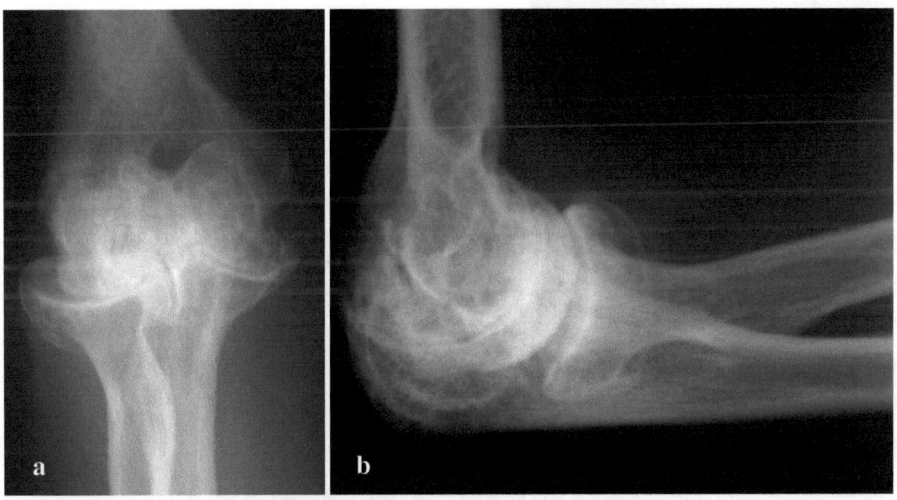

Fig. 15.1 Anteroposterior (**a**) and lateral radiographs (**b**) of an elbow with advanced hemophilic arthropathy. Note the loss of articular cartilage at both the radio-humeral and ulno-humeral articulations, the enlargement of the radial head, and the irregularities of the radio-ulnar facet. Reprinted from [4], with permission from The Journal of Bone and Joint Surgery, Inc.

H.A. Caviglia, L.P. Solimeno (eds.), *Orthopedic Surgery in Patients with Hemophilia.*

Indications

In general, the ideal candidate for this procedure is a hemophiliac patient with a history of chronic synovitis of the elbow that has resulted in enlargement of the radial head, pain, and disabling limitation in forearm pronation and supination, but who still has a relatively adequate cartilage interval at the ulno-humeral joint and a complete flexion–extension arc of motion (Fig. 15.2). In most cases, however, some degree of hemophilic arthropathy is already observed at the ulno-humeral joint, with associated flexion–extension arc limitations and capsular contractions. In these cases, patient expectations need to be discussed at length, clearly explaining that although forearm rotation is expected to improve, minimal or no improvements in flexion–extension should be anticipated.

Diagnostic Studies

A detailed history and physical examination should be obtained. The typical clinical picture of a patient with a significantly enlarged radial head is that of a hemophiliac patient, between the third and fourth decade of life, with a history of chronic synovitis of the elbow in early years, who complains of pain that is

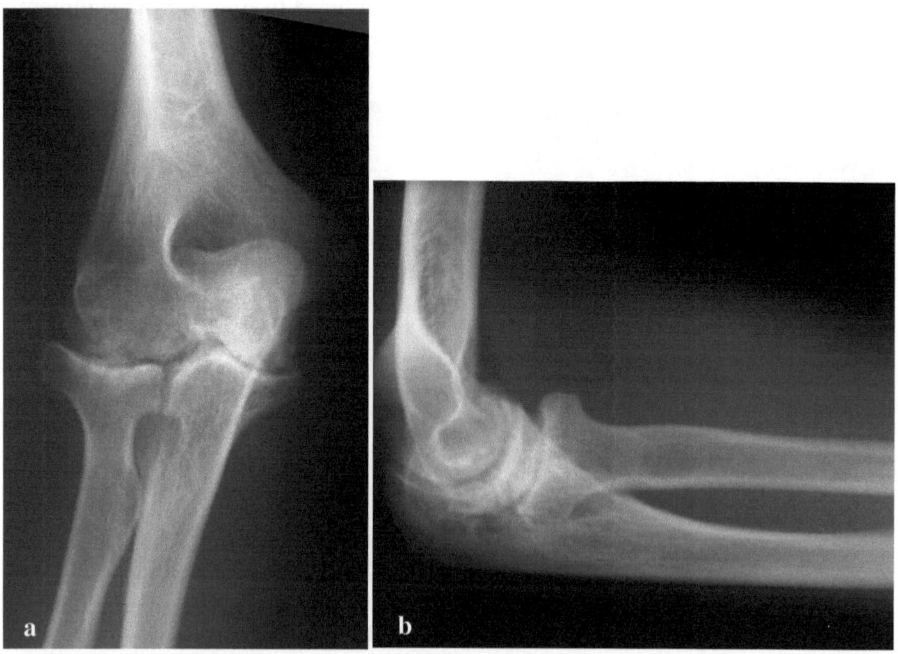

Fig. 15.2 Anteroposterior (**a**) and lateral (**b**) radiographs of a patient with hemophilic arthropathy. There is evidence of an enlarged radial head, with irregularities at the radio-ulnar facet, but with a relatively preserved cartilage interval of the ulno-humeral articulation

usually located at the posterolateral aspect of the elbow, and who has developed a chronic, progressive, and disabling limitation of forearm rotation. A history of frequent, recent recurrent bleeding can be also observed. It is important to differentiate this patient from the hemophiliac patient that presents with recurrent bleeding, pain, and disabling functional limitations that are only temporary and that improve once the bleeding is controlled. In a patient with a significantly enlarged radial head, the limitations for forearm rotation persist even in the absence of bleeding.

In a patient with an enlarged radial head and restricted motion, hemarthrosis history, its frequency, and the type of treatment received should be obtained, since the presence of active synovitis could indicate the additional need for synovectomy. The presence of pain, and its location, should be recorded. In general, pain due to impingement of a hypertrophic radial head against the ulnar facet is located posterolaterally and is aggravated by supination. The elbow flexion and forearm rotation arcs of motion should be measured and recorded. Anterior and posterior capsular releases can be considered in patients with flexion and extension contractures, although, in our experience, these procedures have resulted in minimal improvement in the flexion–extension arc. The pre-operative status of the radial and ulnar nerves should be specifically examined. Although low, there is a potential risk of radial nerve injury during the surgical procedure. Occasionally, patients will experience an ulnar neuropathy as a result of chronic synovitis impinging on the ulnar groove.

Appropriate anteroposterior, lateral, and oblique radiographs of the affected elbow, obtained prior to the procedure, usually provide all the necessary information for pre-operative planning. The status of the radio-humeral, ulno-humeral, and proximal radio-ulnar joints should be carefully assessed. The size and contour of the radial head should be examined, as well as the presence of loose bone fragments. Careful attention should be given to analysis of the morphology of the humeral trochlea. Deepening of the trochlear groove can be observed in patients with severe hemophilic arthropathy of the elbow, usually resulting in ulno-humeral impingement and a reduced flexion arc. If this is the case, the flexion arc might be improved, at least partially, by resection of the origin of the impingement, usually part of the coronoid process.

Procedure

Excision of the radial head is accomplished by a transverse osteotomy of the radial neck, performed just below the level of the ulnar facet (Fig. 15.3). An effort should be made to preserve at least part of the annular ligament in order to improve the stability of the remaining proximal radius. Once the radial head is excised, extensive synovectomy can be performed by the same surgical approach. Capsular releases and additional ulnar resections (coronoid, olecranon), aimed to improve contracture deformities and the flexion arc, can also be carried out during the same surgical procedure.

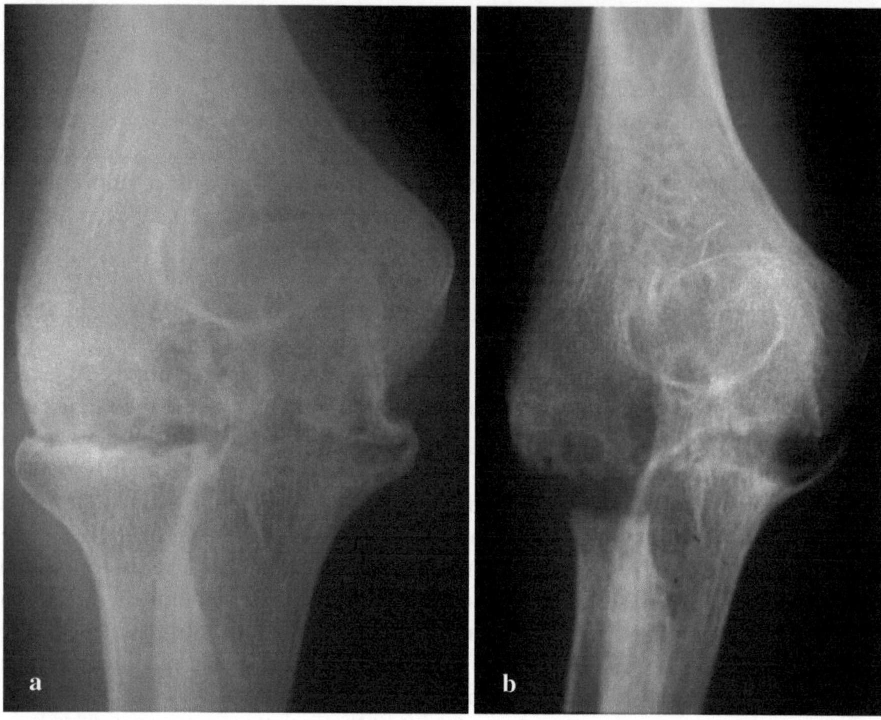

Fig. 15.3 Pre-operative (**a**) and post-operative (**b**) radiographs of a hemophiliac patient that underwent a radial head excision. Note the level of the resection just distal to the radio-ulnar facet. Reprinted from [4], with permission from The Journal of Bone and Joint Surgery, Inc.

Surgical Technique

For the purpose of radial head excision, the patient is placed in the supine position on a regular operating table. The affected upper extremity is placed across the patient's chest, using a regular arm-rest oriented parallel to the operating table to support the elbow. Pre-operative prophylactic antibiotics are administered intravenously. After a tourniquet sleeve is applied to the arm with appropriate padding, the arm is prepped and draped following sterile techniques. The upper extremity is then exsanguinated and the tourniquet is raised to an appropriate pressure.

A standard Kocher approach is used for this purpose. The skin incision begins proximal to the lateral epicondyle of the humerus and is extended distally and posteriorly, in an oblique manner, over the fascia of the anconeus and extensor carpi ulnaris muscles. Usually, the incision is about 6 cm in length. The interval between these two muscles is identified and incised, carrying the dissection down to the joint capsule. The deep radial nerve is protected by the extensor carpi ulnaris and extensor digitorum communis muscle mass. Care must be taken to avoid retraction that would put pressure on the radial nerve. A subperiosteal release of the epicondylar insertion of the anconeus and part of the common extensor origin is usually needed to obtain adequate exposure of the joint capsule. A longitudinal incision is made in the capsule, exposing the radio-humeral joint. The remaining common extensor origin can be reflected from the lateral epicondyle and distal humerus, giving exposure to the posterior aspect of the ulnohumeral joint for débridement and synovectomy, if necessary.

Positioning of small Homman's retractors facilitates exposure of the proximal radius (Fig. 15.4). As indicated before, the level of resection of the radial head is just below the ulnar facet. A transverse osteotomy of the radial neck is performed at this level, using an osteotome or an oscillating saw. An effort should be made to preserve the integrity of the annular ligament, in order to improve the stability of the remaining proximal radius. Once the radial head is excised, extensive synovectomy can be performed by the same surgical approach. Through a separate incision, ulnar nerve entrapment can be relieved by medial synovectomy and release of the ulnar groove with or without transposition.

Once the goal of the operation has been achieved, the tourniquet is released. Careful hemostasis should be performed before closing the surgical incision, especially if synovectomy has been performed. Bone bleeding is controlled with the application of bone wax to the exposed osteotomy surface. In most cases a drain is placed. The joint capsule is closed using an absorbable suture. The skin is closed with intradermal, non-absorbable sutures. A compression dressing and a long arm plaster splint are applied, with the forearm in maximum supination for the first four days.

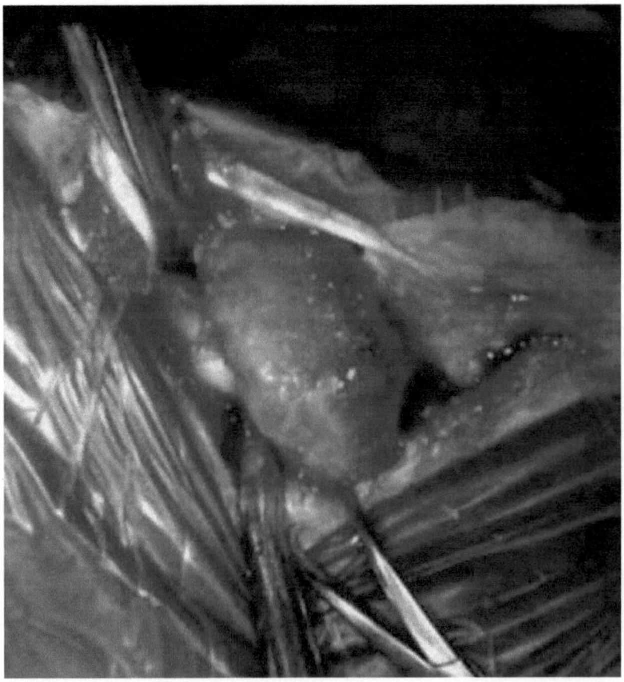

Fig. 15.4 Small Homan's retractors facilitating exposure of the radial head

Rehabilitation

On the fourth post-operative day, the splint is removed, the wound is checked, and physical therapy is initiated. The principal goal of the physical therapy program is to maintain the forearm rotation that was gained intra-operatively. The secondary goal is to, at the very least, restore the pre-operative flexion arc. Continuous passive motion devices may be used as an adjunct to physical therapy. In general, our patients undergo physical therapy twice a day while in hospital. After discharge from the hospital, the patient receives physical therapy three times a week for at least 8 weeks.

Results of Radial Head Excision

The excision of the radial head has been shown to provide sustained pain relief, reduction in the frequency of bleeding, and improvement in forearm pronation and supination in patients with advance hemophilic arthropathy of the elbow [1–4]. However, minimal or no improvements in flexion–extension range should be expected after the excision of the radial head [1, 4]. Although very few complications have been described after this procedure, the possibility of radial nerve palsy should be considered [4]. In the few reports available, no infections have been described after radial head excision.

Conclusion

Excision of the radial head is a simple, safe, and effective procedure that should be considered in hemophiliac patients with advance hemophilic arthropathy of the elbow associated with disabling limitations in forearm rotation.

References

1. Luck JV, Kasper CK (1989) Surgical management of advanced hemophilic arthropathy. An overview of 20 years' experience. Clin Orthop 242:60–82
2. Lofqvist T, Nilsson IM, Petersson C (1996) Orthopaedic surgery in hemophilia. 20 Years' experience in Sweden. Clin Orthop 232–241
3. Nagelberg S, Gilbert MS, Luck JV et al (1985) Radial head resection and partial elbow synovectomy for hemophilic arthropathy. Orthop Trans 9:420
4. Silva M, Luck JV (2007) Result of radial head excision and synovectomy in patients with hemophilia. J Bone Joint Surg Am 89:2156–2162

Chapter 16

Tendon Lengthening in Volkmann's Ischemic Contractures in Hemophilia

Hernan Blanchetiere, Ana Laura Douglas Price and Enrique Pener

Indications

- Generally in patients that show a contracture in the flexion of the finger flexor apparatus, but also have a good perception, positioning, and sensibility of the hand [1].
- Volkmann's ischemic contractures, flexion contractures in cerebral palsy [2].

Definition of the Procedure

The procedure is based on enlargement of the flexor apparatus of the wrist and fingers, using a procedure at the muscle–tendon junction in the forearm. Multiple ruled and programmed tendon incisions are made in each muscle plane, according to the necessity in each particular case [3].

Diagnosis

The patient must be studied in relation to his level of function and sensitivity, muscle contractures, and movement control. Functional tests for different parts of the body can be carried out routinely in less than 10 s. Sensitivity evaluation is made in the palm of the hand by testing discrimination between two points that must each be smaller than a centimeter.

The mobility of each finger and articular segment must be explored individually, to eliminate intrinsic articular rigidity phenomena.

X-rays are useful as complementary studies, to evaluate the condition of the joint and analyze previous trauma. Electromygraphy is necessary to document the presence of neurological injury.

H.A. Caviglia, L.P. Solimeno (eds.), *Orthopedic Surgery in Patients with Hemophilia.*

Surgical Technique

The patient is placed in the dorsal decubitus position under general anesthesia, using a table to support the limb that is undergoing surgery, and a hemostatic sleeve is placed on the proximal third of the arm.

A longitudinal incision is made in the midline of the anterior face of the forearm at one-third medial level, and the subcutaneous cellular matrix and deep aponeuroses in the same line as the cutaneous incision are exposed.

The cutaneous flap is freed and separators with teeth are placed. The superficial muscle is exposed, the anterior cubital muscle visualized, and the cubital vascular and nervous network identified and protected. The same procedure is carried out at the level of vessel and radial nerves in the radial edge of the flexor carpi radialis longus (Fig. 16.1) [4].

Two incisions are made, approximately 1.5 cm apart at the tendon–muscle junction, without altering the underlying muscle matrix of the flexor carpi radialis longus muscle and the anterior cubital muscle. The proximal incision is transverse, and the distal one oblique. The flexor carpi radialis longus and the finger flexors are each enlarged with a transverse incision (Fig. 16.2).

Hyperextension of the wrist and fingers is carried out, separating the tendon structures affected and conserving the continuity of underlying muscular fibers.

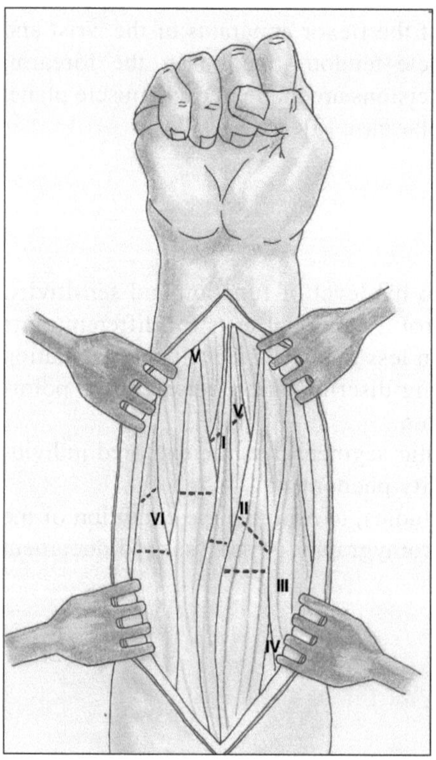

Fig. 16.1 Approach and muscles exposed; *I*: flexor carpi radialis brevis; *II*; flexor carpi radialis longus; *III*: brachio-radialis; *IV*: pronator teres; *V*: flexor digitorum superficialis; *VI*: flexor carpi ulnaris

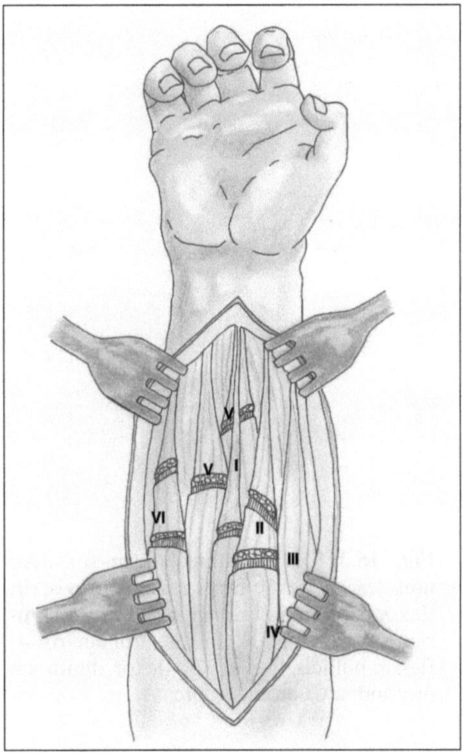

Fig. 16.2 Enlarged muscles at superficial level; *I*: flexor carpi radialis brevis; *II*; flexor carpi radialis longus; *III*: brachioradialis; *IV*: pronator teres; *V*: flexor digitorum superficialis; *VI*: flexor carpi ulnaris

Separators are positioned (Fig. 16.3), and the brachioradialis muscle and radial vessels are moved to the radial side, and the flexor carpi radialis longus to the cubital side next to the middle nerve previously identified, and the flexor digitorum superficialis.

The flexor pollicis longus and the flexor digitorum profundus are enlarged through two incisions in their tendon parts, as described for the superficial muscles.

An evaluation of the forearm supination is made and, if a pronation contracture is found, an enlargement of the pronator teres is made by two oblique incisions separated by 1.5 cm in their tendon fiber, without injuring the underlying muscle matrix. Forced supination takes place, allowing slipping with consequent muscle extension (Fig. 16.4).

The hemostatic sleeve is taken off and careful hemostasis carried out. The deep aponeurosis is not closed, a drain is placed and the subcutaneous matrix and skin are closed separately.

A plaster splint is made to immobilize the elbow in a 90° position, with the forearm in supination, wrist in extension of 50° and the fingers and thumb in neutral position.

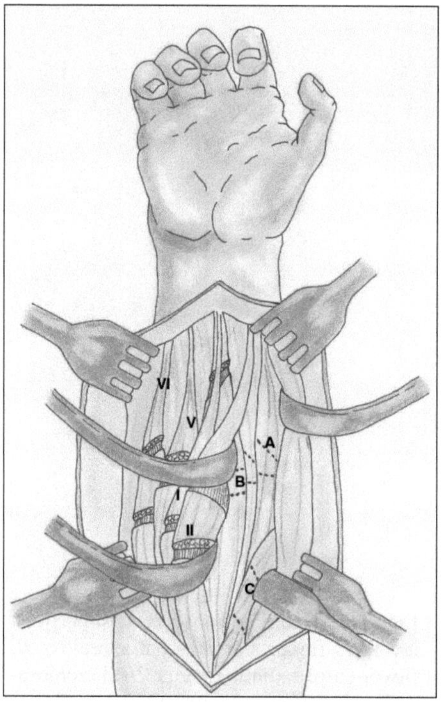

Fig. 16.3 Exposition technique for deep muscles; *I*: flexor carpi radialis brevis; *II*; flexor carpi radialis longus; *V*: flexor digitorum superficialis; *VI*: flexor carpi ulnaris; *A*: flexor pollicis longus; *B*: flexor digitorum profundis; *C*: pronator teres

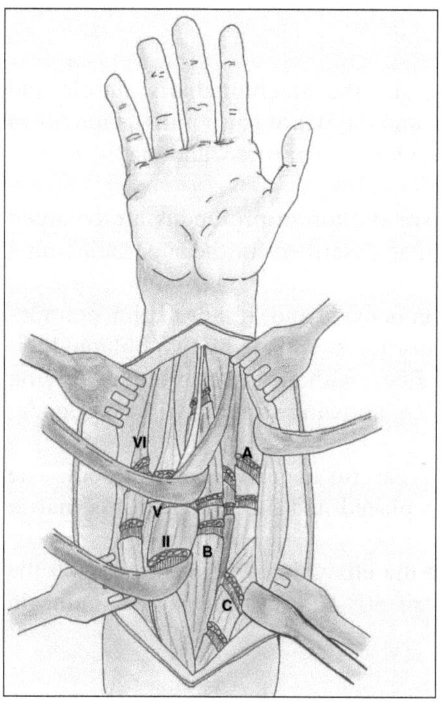

Fig. 16.4 Enlarged muscles at deep level; *II*: flexor carpi radialis longus; *V*: flexor digitorum superficialis; *VI*: flexor carpi ulnaris; *A*: flexor pollicis longus; *B*: flexor digitorum profundis; *C*: pronator teres

Rehabilitation

After four weeks of immobilization, exercises for articular movement and muscle strength begin. The splint is postioned to maintain the extension lengths reached [5].

References

1. Ilyas AM, Wisbeck JM, Shaffer GW, Thoder JJ (2005) Upper extremity compartment syndrome secondary to acquired factor VIII inhibitor. A case report. J Bone Joint Surg Am 87(7):1606–1608
2. Volkmann R (2005) Ischaemic muscle paralyses and contractures. J Hand Surg [Br] 30(2):233–234
3. Stevanovic M, Sharpe F (2006) Management of established Volkmann's contracture of the forearm in children. Hand Clin 22(1):99–111
4. Teng AL, Huang JI, Wilber RG, Wilber JH (2005) Treatment of compartment syndrome: transverse fasciotomy as an adjunct to longitudinal dermatofasciotomy: an in vitro study. J Orthop Trauma 19(7):442–447
5. Ultee J, Hovius SE (2005) Functional results after treatment of Volkmann's ischemic contracture: a long-term followup study. Clin Orthop 431:42–49

Section V

Lower Limb

Chapter 17
Hip Osteotomy in Hemophilia

Thomas A. Wallny and Clayton N. Kraft

Introduction

In comparison to other large joints, the hip is less frequently afflicted by intra-articular bleeding, probably due to the localization of the synovial lining, thereby being less prone to mechanical injury [1]. While intra-articular bleeding in childhood typically induces morphological changes as observed in Perthes, disease [2, 3], knee and ankle arthropathy of the hemophiliac adult is frequently associated with a valgus deformity of the hip [1, 4]. The reason for this may be that in earlier years the typical treatment regime (for hemophiliacs) was immobilization, resulting in severe disturbance of muscular development, combined with varus deformity of the knee [4].

The physiological configuration of the lower extremities is based on a correct anatomical axis, stable ligaments, and a precise muscular interaction between agonists and antagonists. In hemophilic arthropathies, deformities of the knee and hip joint are frequently observed, probably associated with mechanical overloading of the joint due to muscular malfunction and secondary loss of the ideal biomechanical axis. This pathological mechanism is supported by increasing ligament insufficiency, resulting in joint instability, which ultimately facilitates the hemophiliac's tendency to bleed into the joint. Apart from severe pain and a disabled joint, premature osteoarthritis is the result. Correction of the deformity may therefore play a pivotal role in decreasing the incidence of spontaneous bleeding episodes [4, 5].

Besides this, the typical malalignment in hemophiliac arthropathy of the hip is a coxa valga with minor acetabular dysplasia. The uncovered lateral aspect of the articular surface of the femoral head leads to high stresses at the weight-bearing portion of the articular surfaces of the hip.

Indication

The primary goals of all joint-retaining surgical procedures are to relieve pain and improve function. It must be pointed out that total hip arthroplasty may be

H.A. Caviglia, L.P. Solimeno (eds.), *Orthopedic Surgery in Patients with Hemophilia.*

delayed but not with certainty prevented by hip osteotomy. Only patients with radiographically verified deformities who are suffering from motion-induced groin pain and in whom conservative treatment has not helped should be considered for surgery. The aim of this reconstructive hip procedure is to achieve as close to normal proximal femoral angulation as possible, without compromising congruity of the joint. In view of the fact that the primary problem lies in the malalignment of the joint, a valgus neck-shaft angle of more than 135° is frequently found. As one is dealing with hemophilic arthropathy, arthrotic radiographic changes are frequently more pronounced than one would usually tolerate for the non-bleeder hip joint.

The basic biomechanical idea behind varus intertrochanteric femoral osteotomies is to elevate the greater trochanter and move it laterally, while moving the abductor and psoas muscles medially, thereby improving joint congruency and decreasing muscle forces around the hip. A medial displacement of 10 mm should be achieved to keep the ipsilateral knee aligned under the femoral head and to maintain the correct mechanical axis of the leg. With patients frequently also suffering from knee and ankle-joint malalignments, the indication as well as the surgical procedure can be challenging.

Pre-operative Diagnosis and Planning

Routine anteroposterior (AP) and frog leg views of the hip are taken, as well as standing AP X-rays of the lower limb to assess limb alignment. Note that a greater valgus neck-shaft angle will be feigned by rotation of the femoral neck. For this reason it is essential that intra-operative analysis with an image intensifier is performed in internal rotation and abduction of the hip, so as to determine the true rotation and valgus angle of the femoral neck to the shaft. Placement of the seating chisel is determined by the formula 180° minus the angle of the blade plate (90°) minus the angle of correction. If a correction of, for instance, 20° is planned, this would mean inserting the blade at 70° to the shaft axis.

Surgical Technique [6]

The patient is placed on the operating table in a supine position. Through a lateral incision, the trochanteric region as well as the proximal femoral shaft are exposed. The lateral vastus muscle is detached in L-form and by means of Hohmann-retractors the lateral proximal femoral shaft is sufficiently exposed to accommodate the osteosynthetic material.

1. A Kirschner wire is inserted anterior to the femoral neck and in line with its longitudinal axis. A second Kirschner wire is inserted through the greater trochanter into the femoral neck to check the antetorsion of the femoral neck. A third wire is inserted on the level with the lesser trochanter (Fig. 17.1).

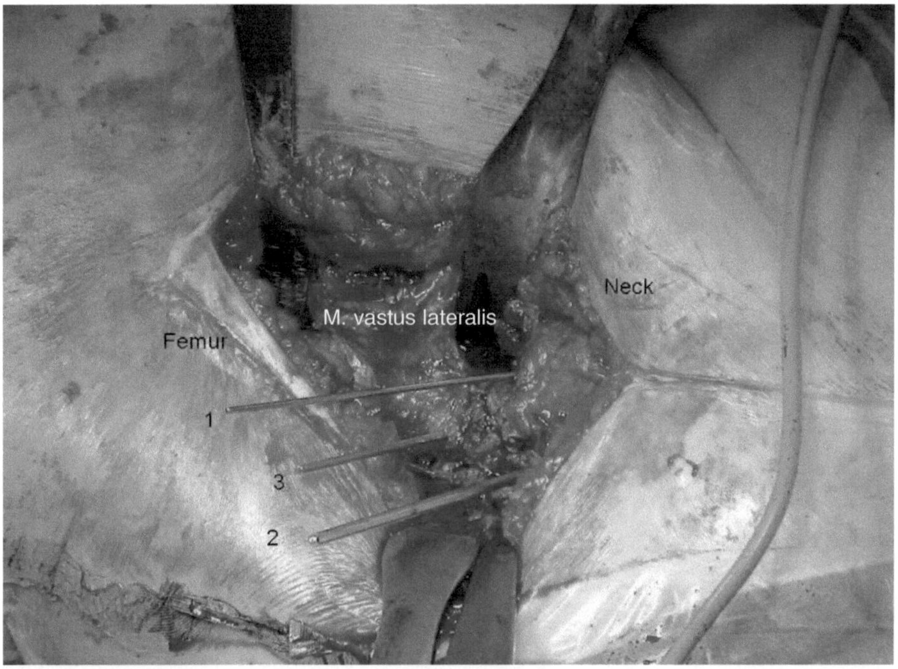

Fig. 17.1 Using fluoroscopy, Kirschner wires are inserted anterior to the femoral neck (*1*), through the greater trochanter into the femoral neck (*2*), and on the level of the lesser trochanter (*3*) as guide wires

These positions should be checked by anteroposterior and lateral fluoroscopy; these wires serve as guides for insertion of the blade plate.

2. The seating chisel is inserted on a level with the innominate tubercle. In hard cortical bone, before inserting the chisel, several drill holes should be placed in the lateral femoral cortex to avoid splintering.
3. Using the removable aiming device, the seating chisel is inserted at the angle appropriate to obtain the desired amount of varus position at the osteotomy; the chisel is driven into the bone a distance equal to the length of the blade part of the plate (Fig. 17.2). Without removing the seating chisel, a Hohmann retractor is placed posterior to the trochanteric area to protect the soft tissue.
4 The desired osteotomy wedge is outlined on the anterior and the lateral cortex using the second wire as a guide. With an oscillating saw, the femur is divided parallel with and at least 2 cm distal to the seating chisel (Fig. 17.3). It is very important that the osteotomy is made at least 2 cm from the seating chisel, because otherwise the blade may pull out of the bone when compression is applied. It is also essential that the proximal cut runs absolutely parallel to the chisel. Using the seating chisel as a lever, the osteotomy is opened and the proximal fragment tilted into a varus position. Then a cut is made

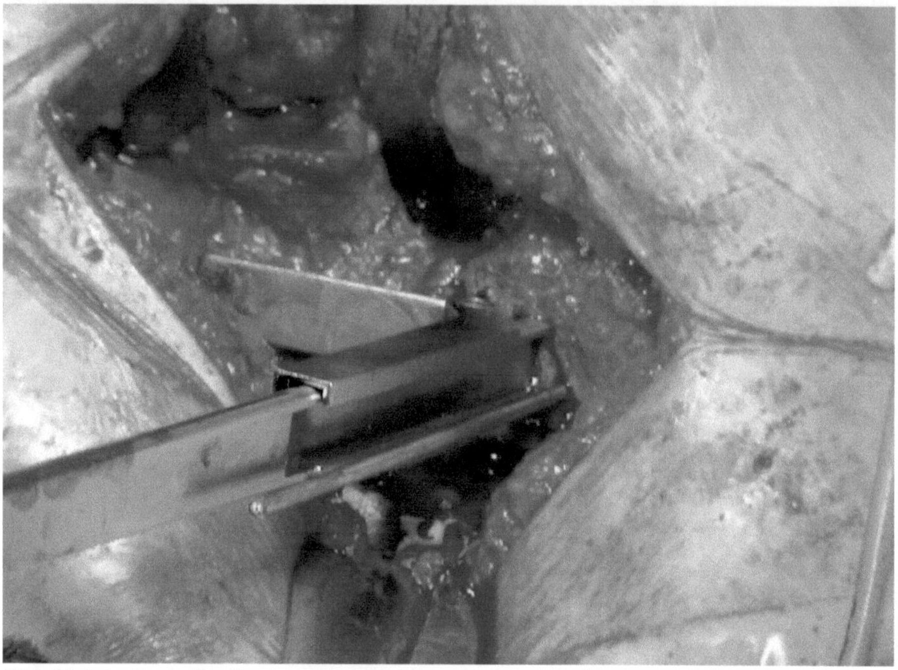

Fig. 17.2 Again under fluoroscopic control, a seating chisel is inserted through the greater trochanter into the neck of femur with the removable aiming device along the axis of the femur

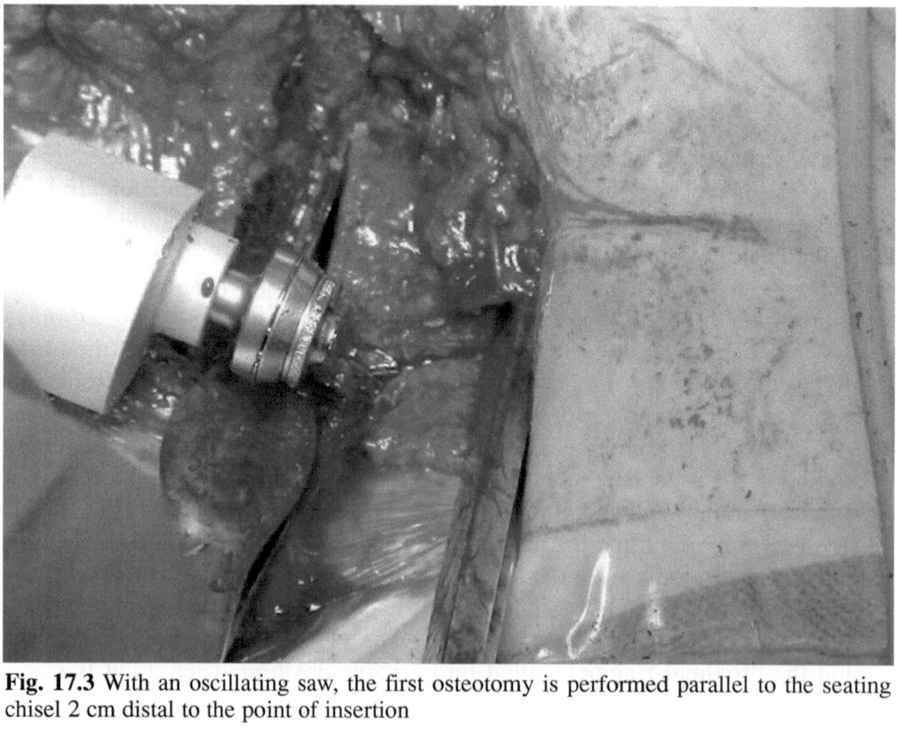

Fig. 17.3 With an oscillating saw, the first osteotomy is performed parallel to the seating chisel 2 cm distal to the point of insertion

across the proximal end of the distal fragment at a right angle to the long axis of the femoral shaft (Fig. 17.4) and a small wedge of bone based medially is removed. The distal cut must be perpendicular to the axis of the shaft fragment if rotational correction is desired. All correcting wedges are taken from the proximal fragment to avoid loss of apposition when the distal fragment is rotated. If the chisel was placed correctly and the osteotomies performed as above, the bone wedge that is then removed should have the exact angle of correction

5. The seating chisel is removed with the extractor, and the blade part of the plate is inserted into the prepared tunnel (Fig. 17.5, note the two Kirschner wires to control rotation). The osteotomy is fixed as recommended by the AO-ASIF (Arbeitsgemeinschaft für Osteosynthesefragen/Association for the Study of Internal Fixation Group) [7], with an ASIF-condylar blade plate and cortical screws. The fragments are correctly aligned, and the plate held against the femoral shaft with a self-retaining bone clamp (Fig. 17.6). The hip is flexed and extended, and the rotational alignment carefully checked. If necessary, the compression device is hooked into the distal hole of the plate and fixed to the femoral shaft. The device is tightened with the wrench and compression applied to the osteotomy. As much compression as can be applied manually when the cortical bone is heavy and strong is used. Again the rotational alignment is carefully checked. Holes are drilled in the femur,

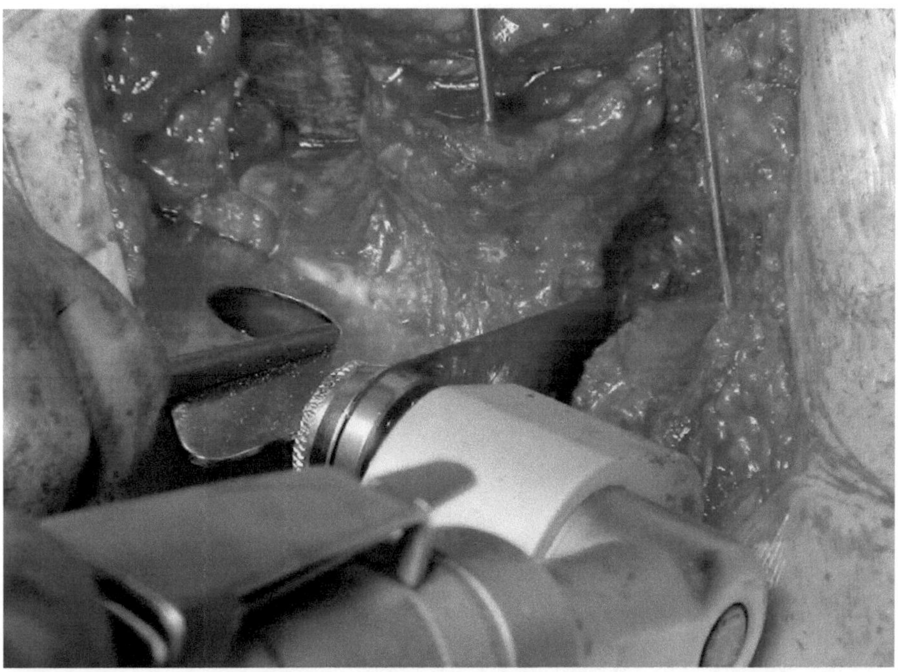

Fig. 17.4 The second osteotomy is then performed perpendicular to the femoral axis

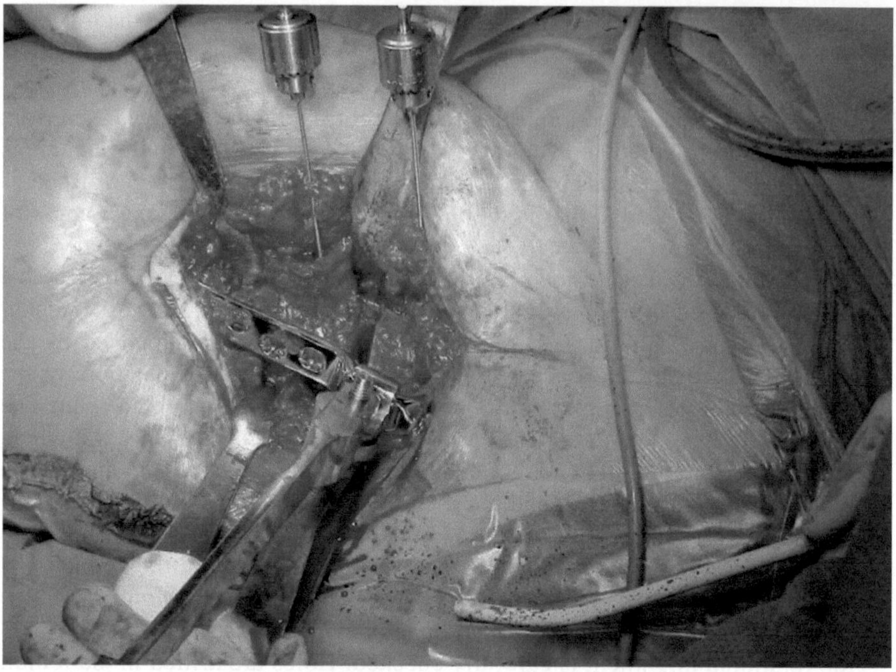

Fig. 17.5 The seating chisel is removed and in the prepared tunnel the blade of the condylar plate is pushed into the greater trochanter and neck of femur

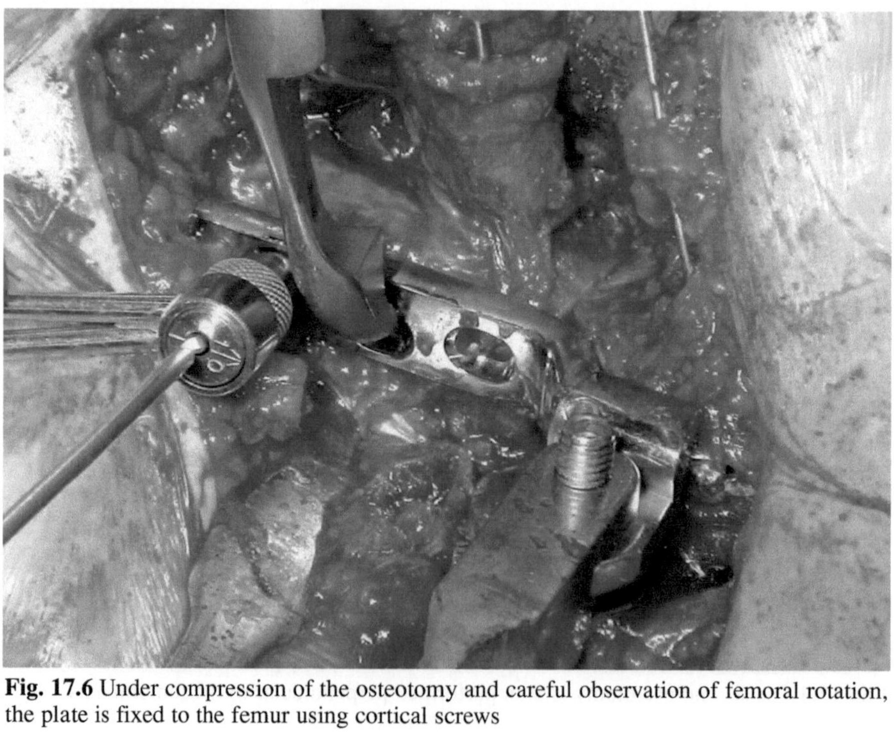

Fig. 17.6 Under compression of the osteotomy and careful observation of femoral rotation, the plate is fixed to the femur using cortical screws

and the plate is fixed to the femur. The tension of the iliopsoas and adductor muscles is checked. If necessary, relaxation can be obtained by tenotomy. Towards the end of the operation, anteroposterior and lateral fluoroscopic control of the correct position of the osteosynthetic material as well as the achieved correction must be performed and documented. Plastic tubes are inserted for suction drainage and the wound is closed.

Post-operative Care

Post-operative care consists of early functional treatment the day after surgery. When the patient is able to raise the limb from the bed with the knee extended, walking should be started with partial weight-bearing (10 kg) of the treated leg over a period of 10–12 weeks, using crutches. Full weight-bearing after complete consolidation of the osteotomy gap is achieved on average 12 weeks after surgery. In an uneventful healing phase, control radiography should also be performed one day and 6 and 12 weeks after surgery.

Pitfalls

1. Correction of the valgus neck-shaft angle should increase and not decrease the weight-bearing area of the femoral head.
2. Extensive avascular necrosis of the femoral head and collapse of the femoral head are contraindications.
3. Rotation contractures of 25°or more, and flexion of 50° or less are contraindications.
4. An adduction deformity must be treated by tenotomy of the adductor muscles.
5. Stable internal fixation is a prerequisite for union of the osteotomy. Displacement should be limited to 50% of the diameter of the shaft. An incidence of non-union as high as 20% has been reported.

Personal Data [8]

Eleven hips affected by hemarthropathy in nine patients suffering from a severe hemophilia A were treated with an intertrochanteric varus osteotomy. The average follow-up period was 15.4 years. The pre-operative clinical score of the Advisory Committee of the World Federation of Hemophilia (WFH) was 5.3 points (range 4 to 7) and the Pettersson score 6.4 points (range 2 to 10).

Average varus correction was 22°, and post-operative derotational angle was found to be 15°.

The average WFH score at follow-up had increased to 3.6 points. Seven hips showed clinical improvement, and two hips showed a post-operative deterioration, while two further hips remained unchanged. The Pettersson score increased to an average of 7.7 points. Here the radiographs of six patients indicated postoperative deterioration, three remained unaltered, and two showed improvement. In one of our patients, ensuing total hip replacement (THR) became necessary 25 years after osteotomy.

Osteotomy Versus Total Hip Replacement

In hemophiliac patients, more often than not, a number of joints are afflicted. Degenerative processes may have significantly progressed despite a comparatively young age, and it is therefore hypothetical whether the alternative arthroplasty may avoid further surgery. Nonetheless, it is imperative to consider the status of the ipsilateral knee when planning an osteotomy of the hip [9]. In severe arthrotic degeneration, early joint replacement is recommended. Despite its many advantages, this is not an ideal solution for the frequently relatively young hemophiliac patient, primarily due to a limited life span of the alloplastic material. A higher revision rate than in non-hemophiliacs has been reported [10–12]. As yet it remains to be shown whether early hip replacement in young hemophiliac patients [13] leads to such an increase in quality of life that the long-term complications, particularly implant loosening, are justified. The basic idea of correcting the biomechanical axis is to postpone or possibly even avoid prosthetic joint replacement. The patients we reported on above were predominantly treated at a time when total hip replacement was only in the process of establishing itself as a management option for the young hemophiliac patient. The fact these patients benefited from corrective osteotomy over an astonishingly long period of time demonstrates that this management option for the treatment of hemophilic arthropathy of the hip can be contemplated.

We cannot conclusively answer whether intertrochanteric varus osteotomy for hemophilic arthropathy of the hip is always a feasible alternative to joint arthroplasty. The decision for or against this procedure must be individually assessed, and the patient must be well informed of the advantages and disadvantages of both procedures. There seems to be an individual, but also hemophiliac-associated, tendency that patients profit from the osteotomy, though admittedly with reduced degree of activity. Complete physiological restoration of the joint after osteotomy is not possible. Ensuing intensive muscle training plays a significant role in the long-term success of the surgical procedure.

References

1. Rodríguez-Merchán EC (1996) Effects of hemophilia on articulations of children and adults. Clin Orthop 328:7–13
2. Pettersson H, Wingstrand H, Thambert C et al (1990) Legg-Calve-Perthes disease in hemophilia: Incidence and etiologic considerations. J Pediatr Orthop 10:28–32
3. Wallny T, Brackmann HH, Seuser A et al (2003) Haemophilic arthropathy of the hip in children – prognosis and long-term follow-up. Haemophilia 9:197–201

4. Hofmann P, Rössler H, Brackmann HH (1977) Orthopedic problems in hemophilia. Pathophysiology and results of operations. Z Orthop 115:342–355
5. Smith MA, Urquhart DR, Savidge GF (1981) The surgical management of varus daformity in haemophilic arthropathy of the knee. J Bone Joint Surg Br 63:261–265
6. Müller ME (1973) In: Tronzo RG (ed) Surgery of the hip joint. Lea & Fabiger, Philadelphia
7. Müller ME, Allgöwer M, Schneider R, Willenegger H (1991) Manual of internal fixation. 3rd ed. Springer, New York
8. Wallny T, Brackmann HH, Hess L et al (2002) Long-term follow-up after varus osteotomy for haemophilic arthropathy of the hip. Haemophilia 8:149–152
9. Poss R (1984) The role of osteotomy in the treatment of osteoarthritis of the hip. J Bone and Joint Surg Am 66:144–151
10. Nelson IW, Sivamurugan S, Latham PD et al (1992) Total hip arthroplasty for hemophilic arthropathy. Clin Orthop 276:210–213
11. Kelley SS, Lachiewicz PF, Gilbert MS et al (1995) Hip arthroplasty in hemophilic arthropathy. J Bone Joint Surg Am 77:828–834
12. Lofqvist T, Sanzen L, Petersson C, Nilsson IM (1996) Total hip replacement in patients with hemophilia. Acta Orthop Scand 67:321–324
13. Luck JV, Kasper CK (1989) Surgical management of advanced hemophilic arthropathy. Clin Orthop 242:60–82

Chapter 18
Total Hip Arthroplasty in Patients with Hemophilia

Remzi Tözün and Nadir Şener

The most common clinical manifestation of hemophilia is arthropathy secondary to repeated intra-articular bleeding and chronic synovitis. In patients with hemophilia, 80–85% of the bleeds occur into the joints [1, 2]. The articular bleeding can cause synovial hypertrophy, and a vicious circle of chronic synovitis develops with rebleeding. The blood in the joint makes the synovial tissue become catabolically active, and inhibits synthesis of the cartilage matrix. The blood has also a direct harmful effect on cartilage irrespective of the synovial changes [3]. The articular problems in patients with hemophilia begin in the early years of life. If untreated, this condition is followed by degenerative changes, and a stiff or painful joint will result. Hemophilic arthropathy is a disabling condition that may cause chronic pain and immobilization, and impair the quality of life of the hemophiliac patient. Prophylactic therapy can slow the natural course of hemophilic arthropathy. However, due to its excessive cost, prophylaxis is only possible in a small proportion of patients with hemophilia.

The most commonly affected joints in patients with hemophilia are the knees, followed by the elbows and ankles, with the shoulders and hips affected to a much lesser extent [2]. Spontaneous bleeding in the hip joint is uncommon. Thus, end-stage hemophilic arthropathy requiring arthroplasty is infrequent in the hip. Although there have been several reports of the results of total knee arthroplasty for hemophilic arthropathy, there have been few papers concerning the results of total hip arthroplasty (THA) in hemophiliac patients. Therefore, we aimed to discuss the technique and results of THA in patients with hemophilia, with a review of the literature.

The indication for THA in patients with hemophilia is severe, disabling pain with activity and at rest. We prefer cementless prostehesis designs with ceramic-on-ceramic surfaces, because hemophiliac patients who need joint replacement surgery are usually young. Our factor substitution protocol is according to the method of Löfqvist et al [4]. The surgical technique is the same as for standard arthroplasty using the lateral approach in the lateral decubitus position (Figs. 18.1 and 18.2). Minimally invasive surgery and hypotensive anesthesia techniques are helpful to control excessive bleeding. Electrocauterization of all small bleeding points is inevitable. Post-operative rehabilitation in the hemophiliac patient who

H.A. Caviglia, L.P. Solimeno (eds.), *Orthopedic Surgery in Patients with Hemophilia.*

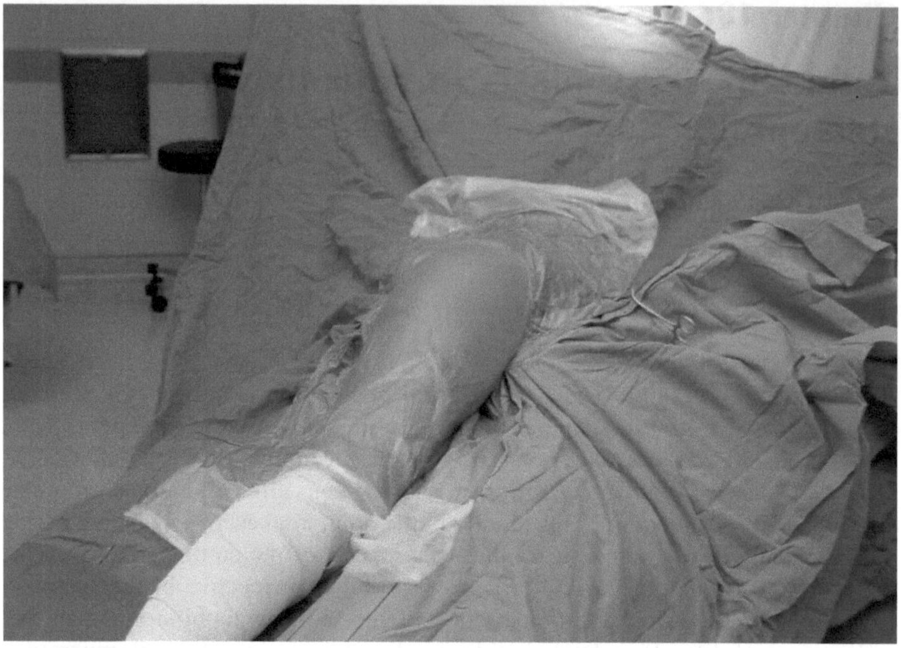

Fig. 18.1 Position of patient on the operating table

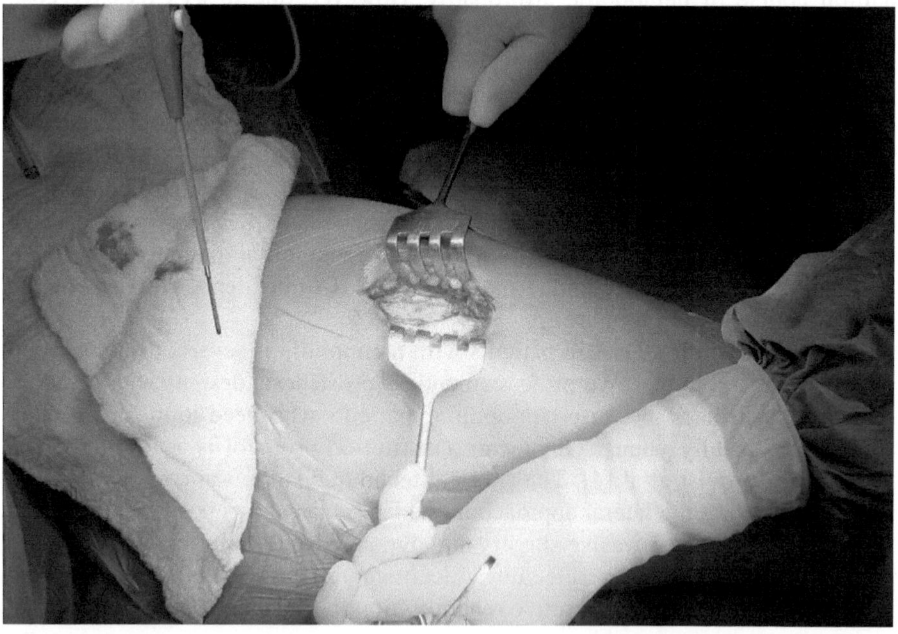

Fig. 18.2 Intra-operative view of the minimally invasive incision

has undegone THA does not differ from that for standard arthroplasty. We allow full weight-bearing with Canadian crutches on the first post-operative day, if the primary stability of the prosthesis is acceptable.

One of the first series of THA procedures in patients with hemophilia was published by Luck and Kasper in 1989 [5]. They reported that the first prosthetic arthroplasty of the hip in a patient with hemophilia in the United States was a cup arthroplasty performed by J. Vernon Luck in 1968. Between 1968 and 1982, three more cup arthroplasties and 10 primary cemented THAs were performed at their institution [5]. Eight arthroplasties out of 13 required revision. They reported their long-term experience with various types of hip prosthesis. In this group of patients the procedure can only be rated as fair, with a revision rate of about 60% over 20 years [5].

Nelson et al reviewed 21 patients with 22 THAs with insertion of a Charnley prosthesis [6]. The median age of these patients was 48.1 years. At a median of 7.6 years after the operation, their total rate of mechanical failure was 36%. These results are much worse than for cemented components in patients in the same age range without hemophilia [7]. The authors discussed that the hemorrhagic diathesis may contribute to early loosening of the prosthesis by predisposing to microhemorrhages at the bone–cement interface when the factor levels fall over time. At the end of their report they concluded that THA is an appropriate operation for disabling hemophilic arthropathy [6].

In 1995, Kelly et al presented a multicenter retrospective study of 27 patients with 34 THAs [8]. The mean age of the patients was 38 years, and the mean duration of follow-up was 8 years, with a minimum of 2 years for all patients. There were 26 THAs performed with cement, and six without; and one bipolar arthroplasty performed with cement and one hybrid THA. Six of the 28 cemented femoral components and six of the 26 cemented acetabular components were revised because of aseptic loosening. None of the cementless prostheses loosened. The authors reported they started to choose cementless components for all primary and revision arthroplasties in patients with hemophilia after the poor results they had with cemented components. They ascribed the high rate of failure of cemented components to a suboptimum technique, rather than to microhemorrages at the bone–cement interface as theorized by Nelson et al. [6, 8].

Löfqvist et al performed 13 Charnley cemented prosthesis procedures in 11 patients during 1973 and 1988, and reviewed them in 1996 [4]. The mean age was 46 years, and the mean duration of follow-up was 7 years. Four hips were revised at a mean of 10 years. Two hips necessitated revision due to aseptic loosening and the other two revisions were due to infection, both in HIV-positive patients. The authors emphasized the high frequency of aseptic loosening after THA as well as the predisposition of the HIV-positive patients to infection. Despite their modest results, they concluded that THA is of value in some hemophiliacs.

In 1998, Heeg et al reported the long-term results of three total hip and nine total knee arthroplasties [9]. The mean follow-up was 6.9 years. There was no infection in this series. The functional improvement was perfect, with an average increase in the hip score from 36 to 85 points. They concluded that hip and knee arthroplasty is a good option in symptomatic hemophiliac patients with disabling arthropathy, in order to obtain pain relief and functional improvement.

Two years later, in a Japanese article, Takedani et al published the medium-term follow-up results of arthroplasty for hemophilic arthropathy with 26 total knee and 9 total hip arthroplasties [10]. The authors reported good results in terms of pain relief but only marginal improvement in the range of motion.

In 2003, Rodríguez-Merchán et al reported 23 THAs in 22 hemophiliac patients [11]. The mean age of the patients was 32 years and the mean duration of the follow-up was 10.5 years. Eleven hips had cementless fixations and 12 had cemented fixations. Nineteen patients were alive at the follow-up. Two patients underwent revisions for aseptic loosening, and there were no infections.

A serious problem affecting the survival of hemophiliac patients is the high prevalence of HIV seropositivity and the eventual development of AIDS. Between 33% and 92% of patients with hemophilia A, and between 14% and 52% of those with hemophilia B, carry the HIV antibody [11]. In two studies of THA for hemophilic arthropathy, approximately 50% of the patients were known to be seropositive for HIV, and the overall mortality rate at median 7-year follow-up was 20–30% [5, 7]. Hicks et al reviewed the outcome of 102 arthroplasties in 73 HIV-positive patients from different centers [12]. The mean age of patients at surgery was 39 years, and the median follow-up was 5 years. There were 27 arthroplasties of the hip, 74 of the knee and one of the elbow. They found an overall rate of infection of 7.2% regardless of HIV status, and 11.7% in HIV-positive patients. Patients with low CD4 counts were more likely to develop deep sepsis. In contrast to these findings, Powell et al recently reported that knee and hip arthroplasty infection rates in patients with hemophilia were not increased, and HIV infection is not a contraindication to knee or hip arthroplasty in the appropriate clinical setting [13].

Another serious problem is hemophiliac patients with a high titer of inhibitors who require elective orthopedic surgery. With the availability of activated prothrombin complex concentrate and activated recombinant factor VII (rFVIIa), patients with inhibitors can undergo such surgical operations and expect a high rate of success [11].

In conclusion, the results of THA in hemophiliac patients are inferior to those obtained in osteroarthritis, and the incidence of aseptic loosening is higher. Patients with advanced hemophilic arthropathy have a remarkably stiff-legged gait due to severe ankylosis of the knee and ankle. This gait pattern is one reason for the loosening [4]. Furthermore there is a high rate of prosthetic infection in patients with hemophilia. HIV-positive patients also seem to have an increased infection rate. Despite the medical and surgical complexities and high rate of complications, THA should be considered in the treatment of hemophilic arthropathy in patients who have severe pain and disability (Figs. 18.3 and 18.4). THA in patients with hemophilia should only be performed by experienced surgeons in special referral centers. The patients should be prepared by a multidisciplinary team. Pre-operative medical preparation of the patients is as important as surgical preparation.

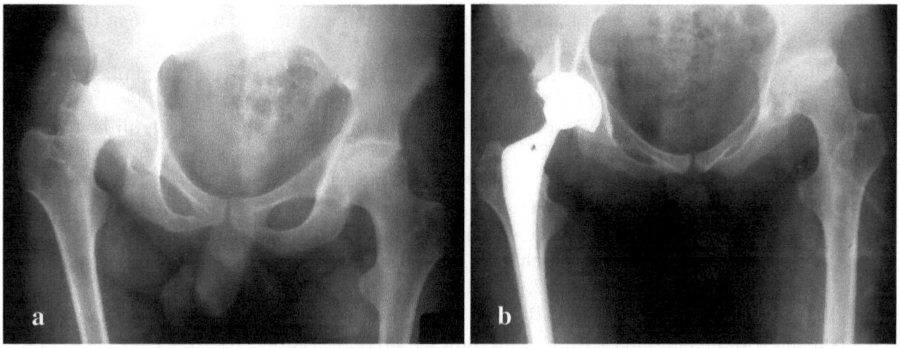

Fig. 18.3 A 31-year-old hemophiliac patient with severe hemophilic arthropathy of the left hip. **a** Radiograph before operation. **b** Post-operative radiograph after cementless THA at 13 months

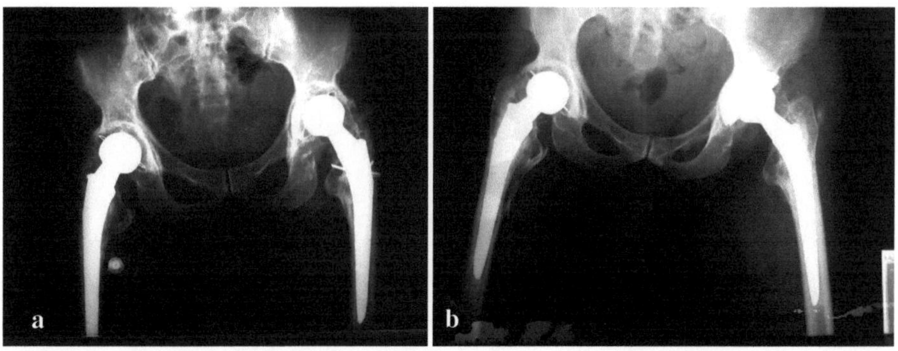

Fig. 18.4 a Radiograph showing cemented acetabular component loosening in a hemophiliac patient. **b** Revised acetabular component replaced with a cementless one; the femoral component was well fixed

References

1. Arnold WD, Hilgartner MW (1997) Hemophilic arthropathy: current concepts of pathogenesis and management. J Bone Joint Surg Am 59:287–305
2. Rodríguez-Merchán EC (2003) Orthopedic surgery for persons with hemophilia: general principles. In: Rodríguez-Merchán EC (eds) The Haemophilic Joints: New Perspectives. Blackwell Publishing Ltd, Oxford, 3–11
3. Caviglia H, Galatro G, Vatani N et al (2003) Osteophytes, subchondral cysts and intraoseous cysts of the haemophilic joints. In: Rodríguez-Merchán EC (eds) The Haemophilic Joints: New Perspectives. Blackwell Publishing Ltd, Oxford, 181–186
4. Löfqvist T, Sanzen L, Petersson C, Nilsson IM (1996) Total hip replacement in patients with hemophilia. Acta Orthop Scand 67:321–324
5. Luck JV, Kasper CK (1989) Surgical management of advanced hemophilic arthropathy: an overview of 20 years' experience. Clin Orthop 242:60–82
6. Nelson IW, Sivamurugan S, Latham PD et al (1992) Total hip arthroplasty for hemophilic arthropathy. Clin Orthop 276:210–213

7. Collis DK (1984) Cemented total hip replacement in patients who are less than fifty years old. J Bone Joint Surg Am 66:353–359
8. Kelley SS, Lachiewicz PF, Gilbert MS et al (1995) Hip arthroplasty in hemophilic arthropathy. J Bone Joint Surg Am 77:828–834
9. Heeg M, Meyer K, Smid WM et al (1998) Total hip and knee arthroplasty in hemophilic patients. Haemophilia 4:747–751
10. Takedani H, Mikami S, Abe Y et al (2000) Total hip and knee arthroplasty for arthropathy in a haemophiliac. Rinsho Ketsueki 41:97–102
11. Rodríguez-Merchán EC, Riera JA, Wiedel JD (2003) Total hip replacement in the hemophilic patient. In: Rodríguez-Merchán EC (eds) The Haemophilic Joints: New Perspectives. Blackwell Publishing Ltd, Oxford, 111–115
12. Hicks JL, Ribbans WJ, Buzzard B et al (2001) Infected joint replacements in HIV-positive patients with hemophilia. J Bone Joint Surg Br 83:1050–1054
13. Powel DL, Whitener CJ, Dye CE et al (2005) Haemophilia 11(3):233–239

Chapter 19
Pitfalls in Total Hip Replacement

Horacio A. Caviglia and Luigi P. Solimeno

Introduction

Total hip replacement in hemophilia requires an appropriate indication, preoperative planning, a well-carried-out procedure, and rehabilitation to obtain a good long term-result. In clinical series, it is a procedure that has demonstrated a higher rate of failure than for non-hemophiliac patients [1–8].

The indications for total hip replacement in hemophilia are summarized by the following clinical situations:

1. Medial hip fractures without ipsilateral hip and knee arthropathy.
2. Primary arthrosis of the hip in patients with hemophilia without hemophilic arthropathy of the ipsilateral hip and the knee joint.
3. Secondary arthrosis of the hip in patients with hemophilia and arthropathy of the ipsilateral knee without active synovitis of the joint.
4. Secondary arthrosis of the hip in patients with hemophilia and arthropathy of the ipsilateral knee with active synovitis of the joint.

Next we will analyze these clinical situations; these present anatomical differences and therefore the procedure for hip replacement is different for each one. However, it is firstly necessary to explain the precautionary measures that be should taken for all these groups, as a result of the patients' hematological illness.

Patient Positioning

When placing the patient in position on the operating room table, the following guidelines should be observed:

- Do not place the patient in forced positions; make the necessary adjustments to position the patient in light of the deformities presented. This diminishes post-operative pain and the presence of hemarthrosis and hematomas.

H.A. Caviglia, L.P. Solimeno (eds.), *Orthopedic Surgery in Patients with Hemophilia.*

- Padding should be well placed in all regions, in order to avoid lesions such as decubitus or post-operative neurapraxias, especially in patients with marked muscular hypotrophy.

Surgical Approach

Carry out the procedure you consider most appropriate according to the clinical case and what you are more accustomed to using.

Mobilization of the Extremity to be Operated

Mobilization of the extremity to be operated should be maneuvered with utmost care, during both preparation and surgery, especially when the patient presents ipsilateral knee arthropathy, since they will be affected by regional osteoporosis, and supracondylar fractures are easily caused.

Control of Intra-operative Bleeding

Hemostasis should be meticulously controlled throughout the whole procedure. If a hypotensive anesthesia is used, blood pressure should be normalized before concluding the closure, to control hemostasis.

Selection of the Implant

The clinical results show better progress with non-cemented implants. Therefore, avoid using a cemented prosthesis if possible.

The Cementing Process

If a cemented replacement is used, remember that bleeding should be well controlled during cementing of the components, to achieve an appropriate bone–cement interface (Figs. 19.1 and 19.2). For this it is necessary to:

- Maintain an appropriate plasma level of coagulation factor concentrates, by infusing the necessary concentrate.
- Use an anesthetic technique of controlled hypotension during the cementing process.
- Have an effective washing system and aspiration to carry out the cementing.
- Dry the intramedullary channel with a gauze moistened with a 1% adrenaline solution before cementing.

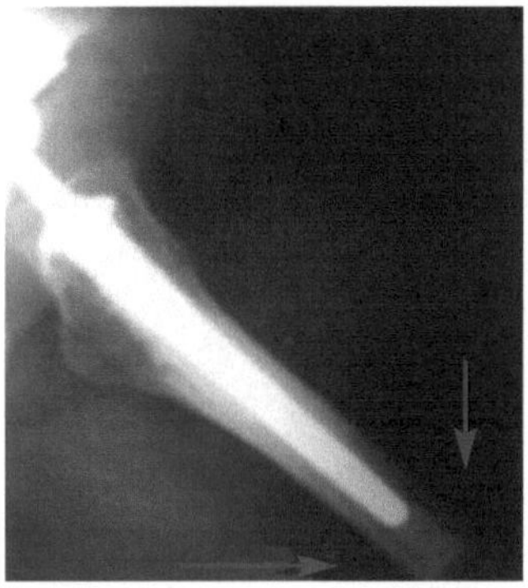

Fig. 19.1 Bone–cement interface defect

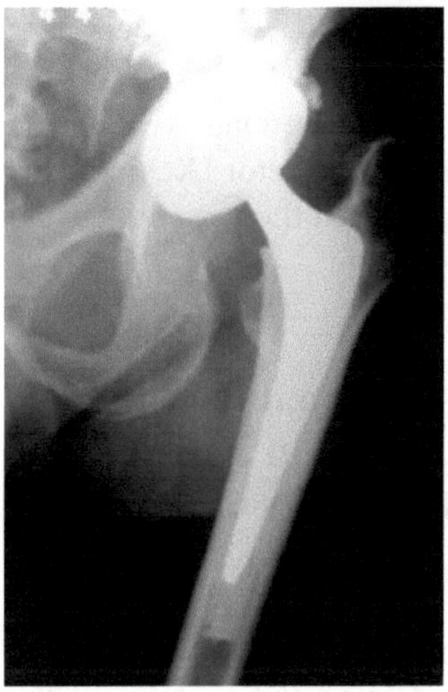

Fig. 19.2 Appropriate bone–cement interface

- Use a femoral intramedullary plug.
- Mix the cement in a vacuum, if possible.
- Apply the cement with a syringe to ensure optimal pressurization.

Use of Bone Graft

If the patient requires the placement of an autologous bone graft, it should not be taken from the iliac crest or any other areas. This is because, there can be post-operative bleeding in the donor area, with corresponding hematoma or risk of developing a pseudotumor. Therefore always use the patient's femoral head as a graft. If the bone graft is not sufficient to solve the bony defect, or in revision surgery, use bone substitutes, or frozen bone either from a bank source or lyophilized according to the type of bone deficiency present.

Wound Closure

Before beginning wound closures, spray the surfaces with fibrin line (Tissucol) in order to encourage hemostasis.

Use of Post-operative Suction Drainage

Post-operative drainage is used for 6–12 h; there is an exception when we need to control the debit. When the suction drain is taken out, the patient should be covered by factor substitute therapy.

Antithrombotic Prophylaxis

Antithrombotic prophylaxis is used in two clinical situations. One is when the patient has hemophilia type B and receives non-recombinant factor IX, since this contains a thrombin activator. The second indication is when the patient has had a previous thrombosis.

Medial Hip Fractures without Ipsilateral Arthropathy of the Hip and Knee, and Primary Arthrosis of the Hip in Patients with Hemophilia without Hemophiliac Arthropathy of the Ipsilateral Hip and the Knee Joint

In hemophiliac patients with medial hip fractures, and in primary arthrosis without hemophiliac arthropathy of the ipsilateral hip and knee, the anatomy is the same as for patients without hemophilia. For this reason, the total hip replacement is technically similar.

Secondary Arthrosis of the Hip in Patients with Hemophilia and Arthropathy of the Ipsilateral Knee without Active Synovitis of the Joint

Patients who suffer from hemophilic arthropathy of the ipsilateral hip and knee usually present the following characteristics:

- Coxa valga: this is associated with the hemophilic arthropathy of the hip and the knee; it is very frequent and can develop a secondary arthrosis.
- Proximal femoral hypoplasia: the whole proximal femoral head is hypoplasic with a small medullary channel.
- Increase in the femoral antecurvatum (Figs. 19.3 and 19.4).

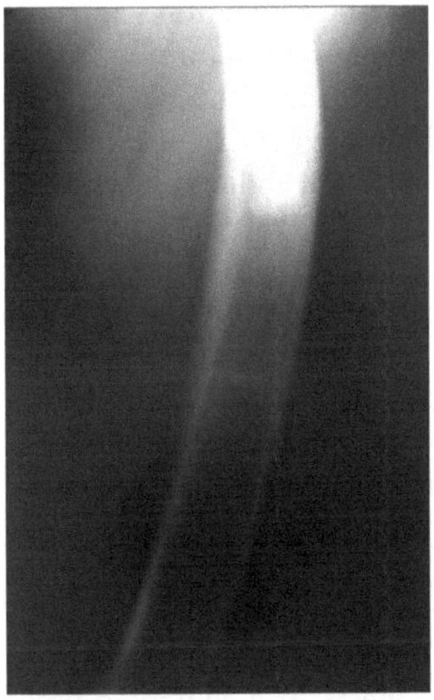

Fig. 19.3 Femoral antecurvatum

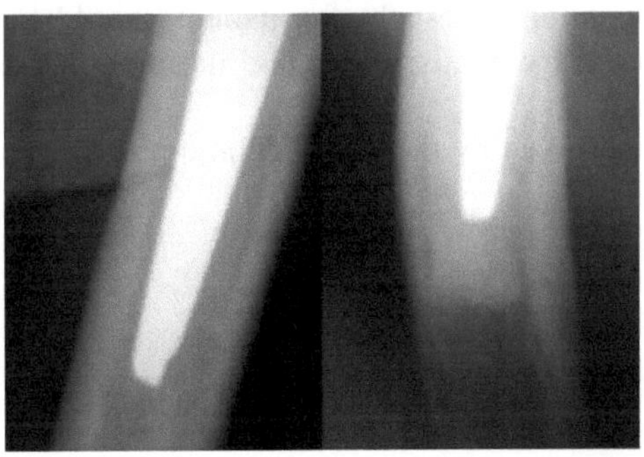

Fig. 19.4 Relationship between the femoral antecurvatum and the size of the implant

- Contracture in hip adduction that usually develops a secondary genus valgus.
- A difference in leg length.

All these characteristics should be investigated and taken into consideration in the pre-operative planning and you should rely on all the necessary elements for the surgical procedure.

- In the presence of a dysplasic acetabulum, the nature of its reduced dimensions requires the use of small acetabulums or necessitates the use of bone graft to replace the deficit of bone stock. Generally, in young patients it is therefore best to use a non-cemented acetabulum. The surface-to-surface component most frequently used is a head of chrome-cobalt with a polyethylene insert. In these cases the thickness of the polyethylene should always be greater than 8 mm. To avoid polyethylene wear, a ceramic head with polyethylene–ceramic or ceramic–ceramic interface should be implanted. The head should be a minimum of 28 mm to avoid its fracture.

- In cases where a non-cemented acetabulum is used (Fig. 19.5), a ceramic interface should be avoided in order to avoid impingement of the components. The acetabulum should be placed in 45 ± 5° of abduction, with an anteversion of 10 ± 5°.
- On occasions, the coxa valgus will require prosthesis with appropriate offset to avoid post-operative Trendelenburg and instability of the hip and an ensuing tendency to dislocation.
- Femoral hypoplasia: the whole proximal femoral head is hypoplasic, with a small medullary channel. In many cases it is necessary to use a prosthesis for dysplasia. It should be carried out with appropriate pre-operative planning. The size of the implant should be controlled in relation to the femoral antecurvatum, to avoid further complication. In the case of using a non-cemented prosthesis, it is essential to ensure that the model of prosthesis can be adapted to the femoral anatomy. If you cannot be absolutely sure of this, you should opt for the application of a cemented prosthesis. If a cemented prosthesis is used, the cement should be pressurized.
- The adduction contracture of the hip may require an adductor tenotomy when the hip cannot be taken to the abduction. As such, the patient should be informed of the presence of the secondary genus valgus and its implication for the final outcome of the procedure.
- The difference in leg length can be resolved by the usual techniques.

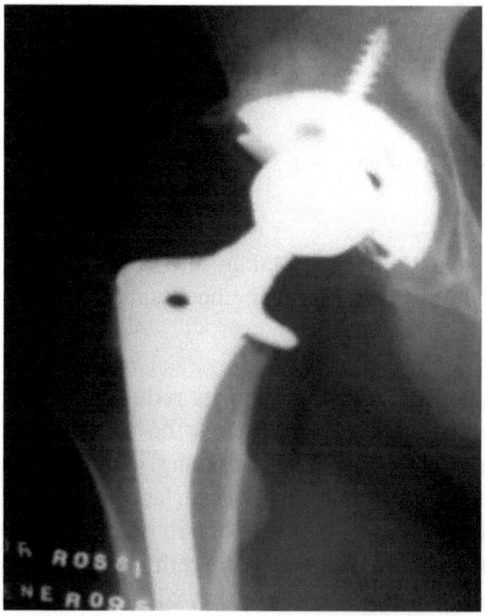

Fig. 19.5 Non-cemented prosthesis

Secondary Arthrosis of the Hip in Patients with Hemophilia and Arthropathy of the Ipsilateral Knee with Active Synovitis of the Joint

The characteristic of these cases is that the active synovitis produces a loss of acetabular and femoral bone stock accompanied by marked synovitis (Fig. 19.6).

All the synovitis should be removed, to avoid secondary hemarthrosis in the joint replacement.

The deficit in acetabular bone stock is usually greater and the hip has a higher tendency for dislocation. The femoral head shows more serious destruction (Fig. 19.7) that usually continues down to the femoral neck, and the bone stock is not sufficient to cover that of femoral bone loss. Therefore, for the resolution of the acetabular defect (Fig. 19.8), a bone supply from the bone bank, or bone substitute such as coralline hydroxyapatite will be necessary.

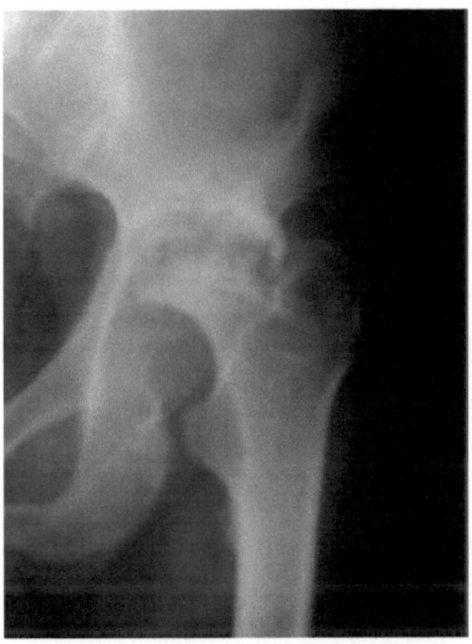

Fig. 19.6 Arthropathy with active synovitis

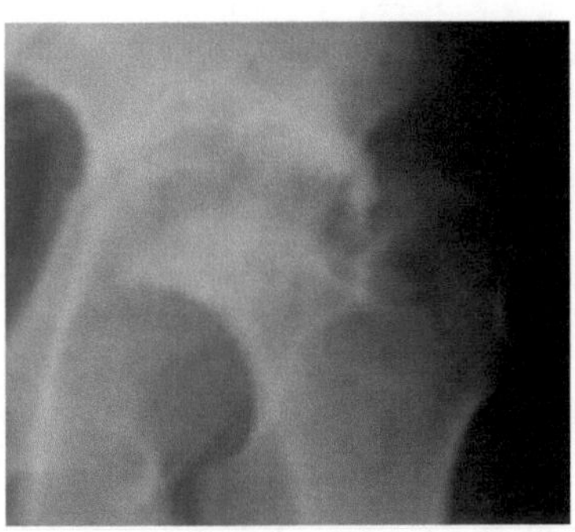

Fig. 19.7 The femoral head destruction and acetabular defect

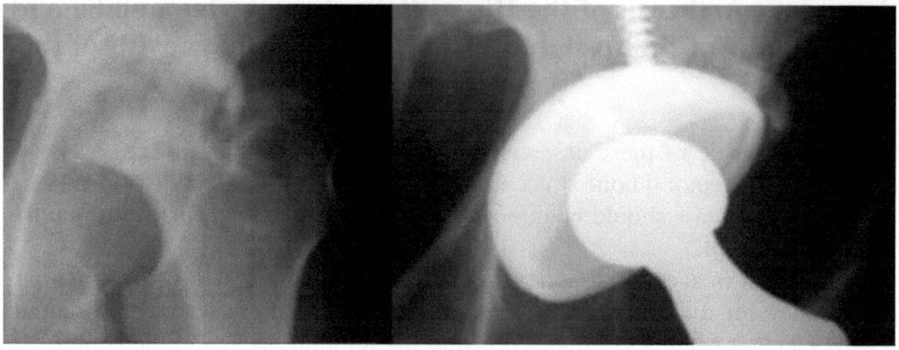

Fig. 19.8 Resolution of the acetabular defect

In this chapter we have tried to summarize what the most frequent errors in the application of this procedure are, as well as the precautions the surgeon needs to take in order to avoid the complications that may arise in carrying out such procedure.

References

1. Collis DK (1984) Cemented total hip replacement in patients who are less than fifty years old. J Bone Joint Surg Am 66:353–359
2. Heeg M, Meyer K, Smid WM et al (1998) Total hip and knee arthroplasty in hemophilic patients. Haemophilia 4:747–751
3. Kelley SS, Lachiewicz PF, Gilbert MS et al (1995) Hip arthroplasty in hemophilic arthropathy. J Bone Joint Surg Am 77:828–834
4. Löfqvist T, Sanzen L, Petersson C, Nilsson IM (1996) Total hip replacement in patients with hemophilia. Acta Orthop Scand 67:321–324
5. Luck JV, Kasper CK (1989) Surgical management of advanced hemophilic arthropathy: an overview of 20 years' experience. Clin Orthop 242:60–82
6. Nelson IW, Sivamurugan S, Latham PD et al (1992) Total hip arthroplasty for hemophilic arthropathy. Clin Orthop 276:210–213
7. Rodriguez-Merchan EC, Riera JA, Wiedel JD (2003) Total hip replacement in the hemophilic patient. In: Rodríguez-Merchán EC (ed.) The haemophilic joints: new perspectives. Blackwell Publishing Ltd, Oxford, pp 111–115
8. Takedani H, Mikami S, Abe Y et al (2000) Total hip and knee arthroplasty for arthropathy in a haemophiliac. Rinsho Ketsueki 41:97–102

Chapter 20
Management of the Hemophilic Knee

Emérito Carlos Rodríguez-Merchán

Introduction

It is well known that in hemophilia the knees tend to bleed from an age as early as 2–5 years. The synovium is only able to reabsorb a small amount of intra-articular blood; if there is an excessive amount, the synovium will hypertrophy to compensate, so that eventually the affected joint will show an increase in size of the synovium: so-called hypertrophic chronic hemophilic synovitis (Fig. 20.1) The hypertrophic synovium is richly vascularized, so that small injuries will easily make the joint rebleed. The final result will be the classic vicious cycle of hemarthrosis–synovitis–hemarthrosis [1, 2]. In this article I will review the most important therapeutic approaches for the hemophilic knee.

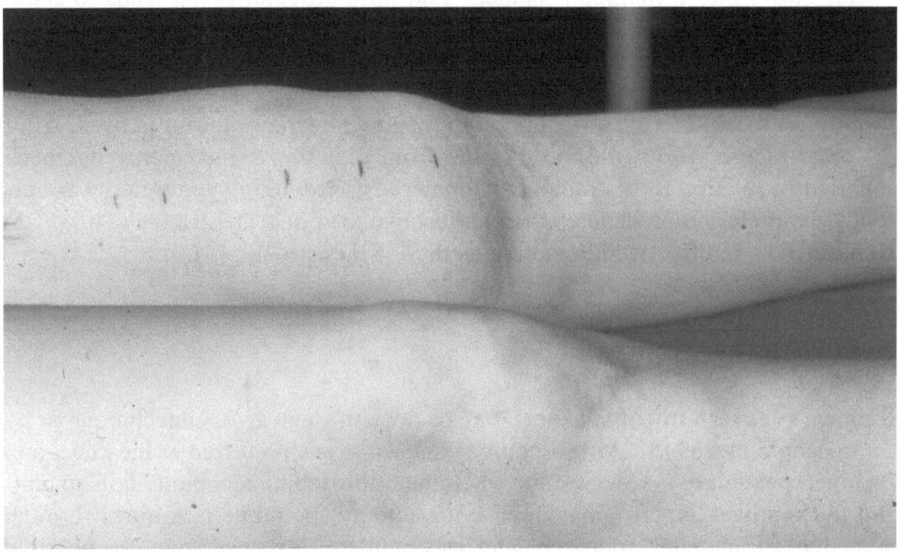

Fig. 20.1 Clinical view of an intense hemophilic synovitis in an adolescent. Note the contralateral side for comparison

H.A. Caviglia, L.P. Solimeno (eds.), *Orthopedic Surgery in Patients with Hemophilia.*

Hemarthrosis (Arthrocentesis)

An arthrocentesis of the knee is a unique and effective procedure that can be carried out many times at the outpatient clinic or in the patient's home [1, 2]. Articular puncture should be used for the evacuation of knee hemarthroses in hemophilia.

Synoviorthesis

Radiation synovectomy consists of destruction of synovial tissue by intra-articular injection of a radioactive agent. Radioactive substances have been used for the treatment of chronic hemophilic synovitis of the knee for many years. Radiation causes fibrosis within the subsynovial connective tissue of the joint capsule and synovium. It also affects the complex vascular system, in that some vessels become obstructed; however, articular cartilage is not affected by radiation. Radioactive substances, therefore, have a radionecrotic effect [1–3]. The indication for a synoviorthesis (medical synovectomy) is chronic hemophilic synovitis causing recurrent hemarthroses that are unresponsive to hematological treatment. Synoviorthesis is the intra-articular injection of a specific material to diminish the degree of synovial hypertrophy, thereby decreasing the number and frequency of hemarthroses. There are two basic types of synoviorthesis: chemical synoviorthesis and radiation synoviorthesis. On average, the efficacy of the procedure ranges from 76% to 80%, and it can be performed at any age. The procedure slows the cartilaginous damage that intra-articular blood tends to cause in the long term.

Synoviorthesis can be repeated up to three times with 3-month intervals if radioactive materials are used (yttrium-90, phosphorus-32, and rhenium-186), or weekly up to 10–15 times if rifampicin (chemical synovectomy) is used. After 30 years of use worldwide, no damage from radiation synovectomy has been reported in relation to the radioactive materials. Radiation synovectomy is currently the preferred procedure when radioactive materials are available; however, rifampicin is an effective alternative method if they are not [4].

Synovectomy

Surgical synovectomy of the knee, may be done through an open technique or by arthroscopic means [5]. Arthroscopic synovectomy is preferred at the knee, and the open procedure is reserved for when the arthroscopic technique fails to control the synovial hypertrophy. Open synovectomy should be performed through a medial parapatellar approach, and as complete a synovectomy as possible should be carried out (Fig. 20.2). It is well known that it is impossible to perform a complete synovectomy by a medial parapatellar approach; however, a complete synovectomy is not mandatory in hemophiliac patients because it has

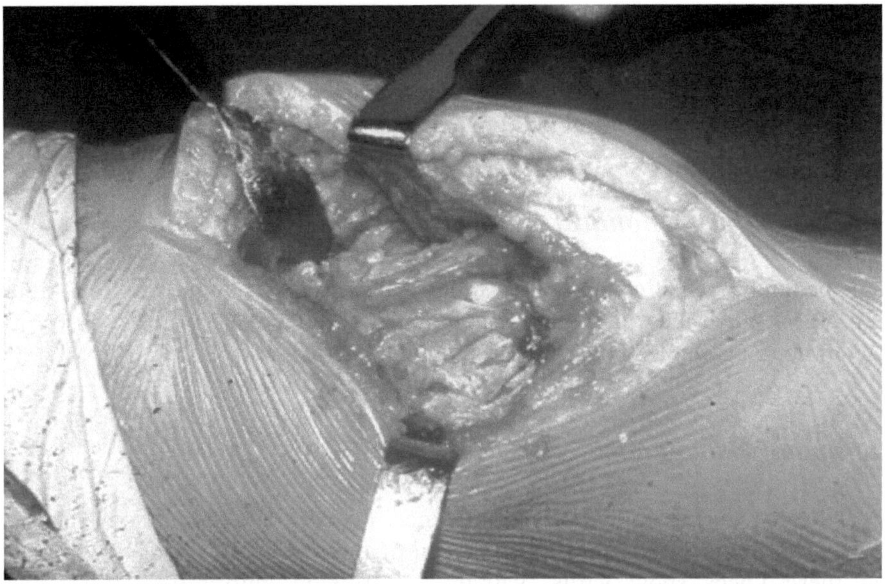

Fig. 20.2 Intra-operative view of knee synovitis during an open surgical synovectomy

been shown that a wide partial synovectomy is enough to decrease the amount of bleeding synovium sufficiently to decrease the number of articular bleeds. Suction drainage must be used for 24–48 h after surgery, and patients should be discharged with a home exercise regime.

Arthroscopic synovectomy should be done through three portals (anterolateral, anteromedial, and lateral or medial suprapatellar portals). In other words, at least three portals are needed to perform a "complete" synovectomy. As complete a synovectomy as possible should be performed with the use of a motorized resector. After surgical synovectomy (by any method), the knee should be immobilized in a Robert Jones dressing for 3 days, and active movement encouraged. Holmium:YAG laser would appear to be superior to conventional arthroscopic synovectomy, which utilizes mechanical devices, because laser seems to improve the quality of local hemostasis and the speed of post-operative recovery.

Rehabilitation

The importance of pre-operative and post-operative rehabilitation of the knee joint in hemophilia must be emphasized. Children must utilize the resources available and seek early consultation with their center's rehabilitation physician and/or physiotherapist. Rehabilitation using the techniques available has been shown to speed recovery, reduce pain, and prevent contractures. Physiotherapy is important in knee rehabilitation following surgical procedures, and the physiotherapist must work closely with the orthopedic surgeon.

Severe Hemophilic Arthropathy

A number of orthopedic procedures can be carried out on the hemophilic knee when a severe degree of arthropathy is reached [1, 2, 6].

Curettage of Subchondral Bone Cysts

Some hemophiliac patients present large subchondral cysts on the proximal tibia (Fig. 20.3). When these cysts are symptomatic, curettage and filling with fibrin glue and/or cancellous bone graft are recommended [1, 2].

Alignment Osteotomies

Occasionally, during childhood, adolescence, or early adulthood, some hemophilic knee joints suffer from an alteration of their normal axis. It is common that these knees show varus, valgus, and flexion deformities. When the malaligned joint is painful, the patient will need an alignment osteotomy [7]. The most commont osteotomies performed on the knee of hemopiliac patients are: proximal tibial valgus osteotomy, supracondylar femoral varus osteotomy, and knee extension osteotomy.

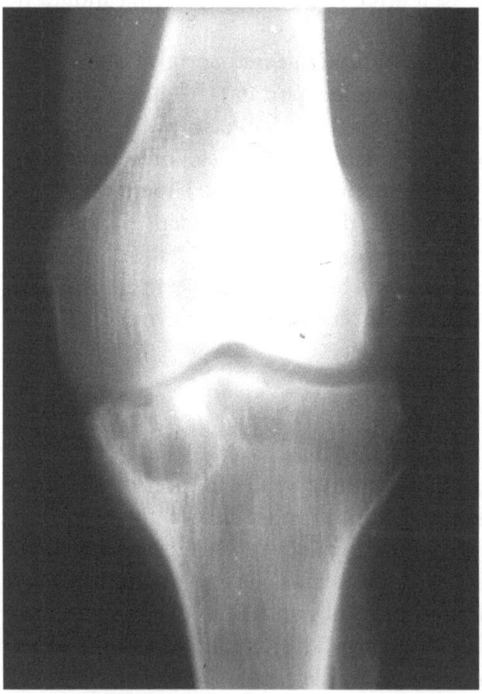

Fig. 20.3 Subchondral cyst in a haemophilic knee (anteroposterior view)

In all of these procedures the rationale is to produce a fracture at an appropriate place, in order to re-align the joint to a normal axis. After the osteotomy it is necessary to ensure adequate bone fixation by any kind of internal fixation device. It is interesting to note that I have sometimes corrected a flexion contracture of the knee at the same time as a spontaneous supracondylar fracture of the femur. When axial malalignment occurs in a joint with severe hemophilic arthropathy, a total joint arthroplasty would be commonly indicated, and hence both problems can be solved at the same time.

Joint Débridement

Joint débridement is commonly performed on young patients suffering from severe hemophilic arthropathy, where the orthopedic surgeon in charge considers the patient too young for total joint replacement to be indicated. Débridement is a procedure that can alleviate articular pain and bleeding for a number of years, and that delays the need for a total joint arthroplasty [1, 2]. Joint débridement consists of opening the joint in order to remove the existing osteophytes, resect the synovium, and carry out curettage of the articular cartilage of the femoral condyles, tibial plateaus, and patella. Some authors do not believe débridement is effective, and therefore when facing severe arthropathy in a young patient they will immediately recommend a total joint replacement. It should be emphasised that if débridement fails a joint arthroplasty can be performed by the same approach. Some authors perform joint débridement by arthroscopic means with quite similar results to those with open surgery. On many occasions synovectomy and débridement are performed together, because hemophilic synovitis and early arthropathy commonly co-exist. Again, postoperative rehabilitation is paramount to avoid loss of range of movement, and therefore it should be associated with adequate hematological control in order to avoid rebleeding.

Total Knee Arthroplasty

Between the second and fourth decades, many hemophiliac patients develop severe articular destruction. For the knee the best solution is a total knee arthroplasty. The role of total knee replacement in individuals with hemophilia is very important [1, 2]. Hemophiliac patients infected by human immunodeficiency virus (HIV) are at risk of bacterial and opportunistic infection because of worsening immunodepression. In these patients, the risk of infection after orthopedic surgery is of considerable concern. Arthroplasty appears to have seven times the risk of infection of other procedures [8].

Total knee replacement for advanced hemophilic arthropathy has good or excellent results in about 85% of cases (Fig. 20.4). The principal risk is late infection, which can occur regardless of HIV status. However, this risk appears

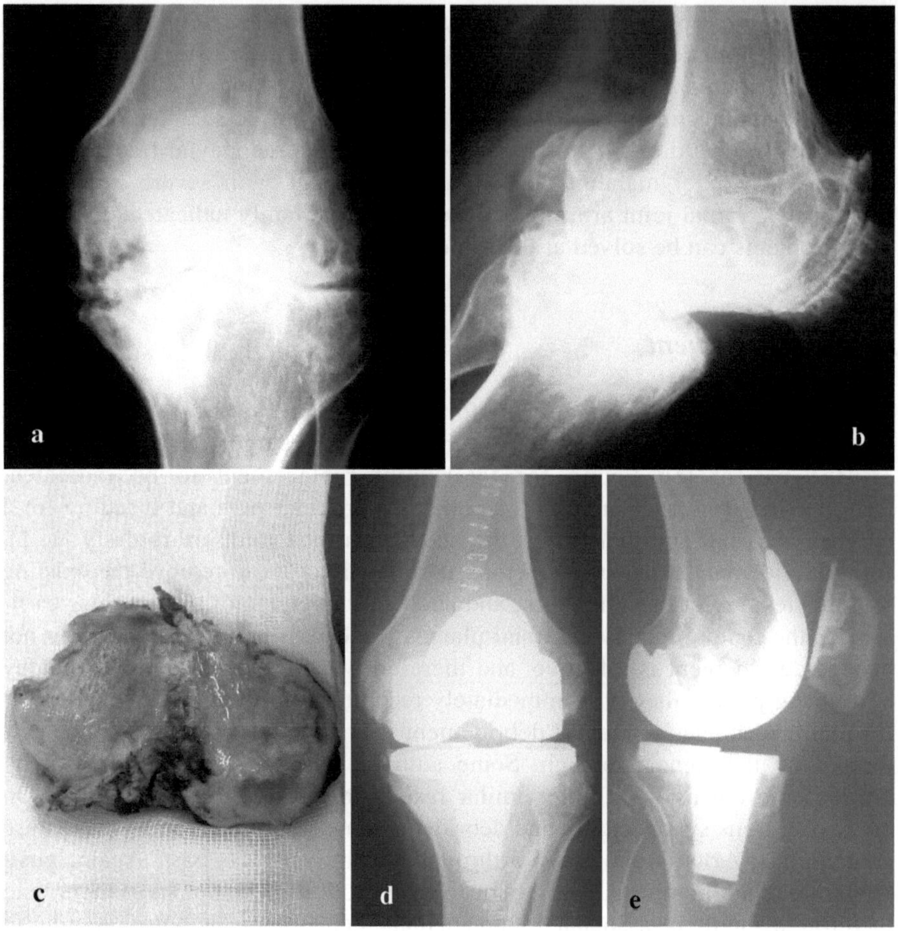

Fig. 20.4 Total knee arthroplasty for severe haemophilic arthropathy: **a** anteroposterior pre-operative radiograph, **b** lateral pre-operative view, **c** intra-operative view of the resected proximal tibia, **d** post-operative anteroposterior view, **e** lateral post-operative radiograph

to be increased patients with a CD4 count under 200/ml. It should not be inferred that a total knee replacement should be avoided in an HIV-positive hemophilia patient today, but it is important that the orthopedic surgeon, treatment team, and patient weigh the risks and benefits carefully.

Knee Flexion Contractures

The management of articular contracture in a patient with hemophilia represents a major challenge. The problems that arise are complex, and require a range of knowledge from an understanding of basic biological events to fine details of surgical technique. The treatments available are physiotherapy, orthotic and corrective devices, and surgical procedures. End-stage arthropathy of the knee is the most frequent cause of severe pain and disability in hemophiliac patients. Some have such severe arthropathy that a total joint arthroplasty is required [1, 2].

Physiotherapy and Orthotic and Corrective Devices

The aim of physiotherapy is to maintain muscle power and a good range of joint movement. The problems of hemophiliac patients are unique and complex, and the assignment of a special physiotherapist to their care is an invaluable aid. Several specific devices have been used to overcome hemophilic contractures.

Serial Casting

The most basic of these is the serial application of plaster of Paris casts, which are changed approximately weekly as the deformity is gradually overcome. Serial casting can be complicated by skin necrosis, joint cartilage compression, and joint subluxation.

Reversed Dynamic Slings and Inflatable Splints

More recently, serial casting has been supplemented by the use of reversed dynamic slings and inflatable splints (Flowtron machine, Huntleigh Medical, Luton, England). Reversed dynamic slings require admission to hospital and close supervision, whereas Flowtron is easy to use and suitable for home treatment. These non-invasive methods are generally only successful in mild contractures, or are used as adjuncts after radical soft-tissue release, to gradually stretch the tight neurovascular structures. The amount of corrective force that may be applied with casts, splints, and braces is limited by the inability of skin to tolerate direct pressure. Additionally these methods can cause articular subluxation.

Extension/De-subluxation Hinge (EDH) Devices

An extension-only hinge device between cylinder casts on the thigh and calf can be used for the treatment of severe knee flexion contractures.

Surgical Procedures

Late or severe cases may require surgical correction in the form of soft-tissue procedures, osteotomies, or mechanical distraction using external fixators.

Soft-Tissue Procedures

Soft-tissue procedures (hamstring release at the knee) are often insufficient to gain full correction. In this situation, the chronically contracted vessels and nerves prevent full correction.

Osteotomies

Supracondylar extension osteotomy of the femur creates a secondary deformity (angulation and shortening) instead of correcting the deformity, and may lead to abnormal joint-loading forces in the ambulatory patient.

Mechanical Distraction using External Fixators

Russian investigators have developed external fixators that produce gradual joint distraction to allow ambulatory treatment. These fixators represent a more efficient way to apply forces to the skeletal deformity. The advantages of this technique include versatility and minimized risk of neurovascular complications. Problems encountered included a rebound phenomenon after frame removal, with loss of the temporarily increased total arc of motion.

Experimental evidence suggests that low-load prolonged stretch is preferred to high-load brief intermittent stretch in elongation of collagen. There are still two unanswered questions: why does the muscle stretch and how can the rebound phenomena be minimized? Continued combined clinical and basic research will hopefully provide answers to these questions. The results obtained with mechanical distraction external fixators warrant its wider application.

Patients with Inhibitors

The development of an inhibitor against factor VIII or factor IX is the most common and most serious complication of replacement therapy in patients with hemophilia A or B, resulting from the exclusive use of virus-inactivated, plasma-derived concentrates or recombinant products. When present, the inhibitor inactivates the biological activity of infused factor (F) VIII or IX, making the patient refractory to treatment. Between 10% and 30% of patients with severe hemophilia A, and 2–5% of patients with severe hemophilia B or mild/moderate hemophilia A, develop an inhibitor against factor VIII or IX after treatment with either plasma-derived or recombinant products. Inhibitor detection using the Bethesda assay, measured in Bethesda units (BU), is part of the regular follow-up for all hemophiliac patients treated with such products. After development of the inhibitor, the inhibitor titer decreases if no FVIII- or FIX-containing products are used for a long period, so the inhibitor may become undetectable. However, the inhibitor usually reappears after a new challenge with FVIII- or FIX-containing products (anamnestic response).

Two approaches for the management of patients with inhibitors have been proposed. Immune tolerance induction using high-dose FVIII or FIX daily or twice daily for a period of a few months to several years may completely eliminate the inhibitor, allowing the patient to be effectively treated with FVIII or FIX once again. However, immune tolerance induction fails in around 20% of cases, and is not recommended for all patients due to the high probability of failure or adverse events. Furthermore, this procedure is very costly. The other possibility is to treat bleeding episodes with prothrombin complex concentrates (PCCs), activated prothrombin complex concentrates (aPCCs ; Autoplex, Feiba), or, more recently, with recombinant activated factor VIIa (rFVIIa; NovoSeven). In case of failure of aPCC or rFVIIa in life-threatening or limb-threatening bleeds or as first-line treatment for major bleeds, high-dose human or porcine FVIII or human FIX may be efficacious if the inhibitor is low or is lowered using plasmapheresis or protein A immunoadsorption. However, the anamnestic rise of the inhibitor will render treatment with FVIII or FIX ineffective within a few days, making the patient resistant to rescue with FVIII or FIX for months or even years.

Recombinant FVIIa has made major elective orthopedic surgery possible in patients with high-titer inhibitors. Most of these procedures would not have been possible without rFVIIa, as it would have been difficult to overcome the inhibitor even with high doses of human or porcine FVIII or FIX. The reported experience with aPCC, for example, is minimal despite aPCCs being available for more than 20 years. rFVIIa is a novel and real alternative for major elective orthopedic surgery in inhibitor patients. The standard regimen is 90 µg/kg body weight every 2 h for the first 48 h, with increasing intervals between doses after this first post-operative period. Lower doses are much less efficient, and administration by continuous infusion is not yet approved for rFVIIa, as a few bleeds and one episode of disseminated intravascular coagulation have been reported with continuous infusion of rFVIIa.

Previous reports have shown that current hematological advances allow hemophiliac patients with inhibitors to undergo surgery with a greater expectation of success, leading to an improved quality of life [9–11]. Thorough analysis of each case by a multidisciplinary team will help to identify further inhibitor patients in whom surgery can be performed both safely and effectively (Fig. 20.5). Both factor VIII inhibitor bypassing agent (FEIBA) and rFVIIa have been used satisfactorily by the author of this chapter to control hemostasis during and after surgery in patients with inhibitors.

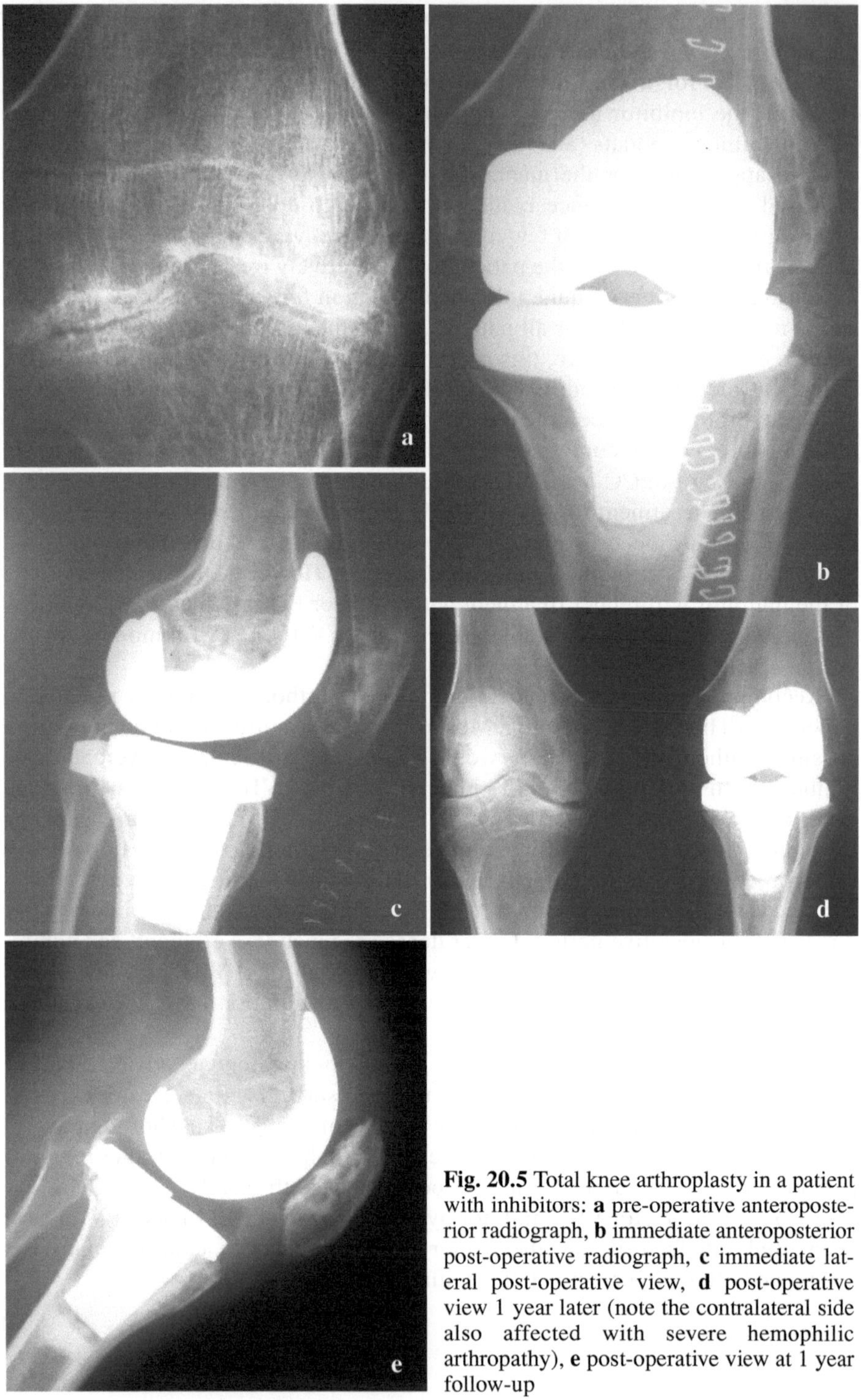

Fig. 20.5 Total knee arthroplasty in a patient with inhibitors: **a** pre-operative anteroposterior radiograph, **b** immediate anteroposterior post-operative radiograph, **c** immediate lateral post-operative view, **d** post-operative view 1 year later (note the contralateral side also affected with severe hemophilic arthropathy), **e** post-operative view at 1 year follow-up

Risk of Infection in HIV-Positive Patients

Spontaneous Septic Arthritis (Arthrotomy)

Immunodepressed patients may suffer spontaneous septic arthritis of the knee that can sometimes mimic hemarthrosis. Pyrexia and culture of the intra-articular fluid will help us to reach diagnosis. Intravenous antibiotics can often solve the problem, but on other occasions it may be necessary to perform surgical drainage and lavage of the joint by an arthrotomy.

Post-operative Infection

Taking into account that a majority of the population of adults with hemophilia is HIV-positive, their immunological status is likely to be deficient when surgery is considered. Furthermore, most of these patients are positive for hepatitic C. In fact, when undertaking any surgery on hemophiliac patients the risk of post-operative infection is higher than in the normal population, because of their immunodepression. However, some controversy exists on this point since, while some authors have reported a much higher post-operative infection risk in patients with a CD4 count lower than 200/ml, others have not found such a high level of infection. In any case, there is no doubt that immunosupression somehow increases the risk of post-operative infection, particularly when performing joint arthroplasties, and the patient should be informed of this increased risk. Nevertheless, modern treatments against immunodeficiency can make it possible for hemophiliac patients to undergo orthopedic surgery with a relatively satisfactory immunological status.

Conclusion

Contemporary knowledge appears to demonstrate that radiation synoviorthesis is a very effective procedure that decreases both the frequency and intensity of recurrent intra-articular bleeds related to knee synovitis. The procedure should be performed as soon as possible to minimize the degree of articular cartilage damage. It can also be used in patients with inhibitors, with minimal risk of complications. No damage has been reported in relation to the use of radioactive materials. Radiation synovectomy is currently the preferred procedure when radioactive materials are available; however, chemical synoviorthesis is an effective alternative method if they are not. Radioactive synoviorthesis is the best choice for patients with persistent synovitis. Personal experience and the general recommendation is that when three early consecutive synoviorthesis procedures (repeated every three months) fail to halt synovitis, a surgical synovectomy should be immediately considered. For advanced hemophilic arthropathy of the knee, the best solution is a total knee replacement [12–17]. Other surgical and non-surgical procedures are less commonly needed for the hemophilic knee.

Continuous prophylaxis could halt or slow the development of the orthopedic complications of hemophilia that we still see today. However, this has not been achieved so far, even in developed countries; therefore, orthopedic surgeons are still needed to carry out many different surgical procedures in the knee. HIV infection has meant that immunodepressed persons in developed countries sometimes require an arthrotomy for treatment of spontaneous septic arthritis; moreover, they have a high risk of post-operative infection after any surgical procedure, particularly a joint arthroplasty. Current hematological advances allow hemophiliac patients with inhibitors to undergo surgery with a greater expectation of success.

References

1. Rodríguez-Merchán EC, Goddard NJ, Lee CA (2000) Musculoskeletal Aspects of Haemophilia. Blackwell Science Ltd, Oxford, UK
2. Rodríguez-Merchán EC (2003) The Haemophilic Joints: New Perspectives. Blackwell Science Ltd, Oxford
3. Rivard GE, Girard M, Bélanger R et al (1994) Synoviorthesis with colloidal 32P chromic phosphate for the treatment of hemophilic arthropathy. J Bone Joint Surg Am 76:482–488
4. Caviglia HA, Fernández-Palazzi F, Maffei E et al (1997) Chemical synoviorthesis for hemophilic synovitis. Clin Orthop 343:30–36
5. Wiedel JD (1996) Arthroscopic synovectomy of the knee in hemophilia: 10- to 15-year follow-up. Clin Orthop 328:46–53
6. Luck JV, Kasper CK (1989) Surgical management of advanced hemophilic arthropathy: an overview of 20 years´ experience. Clin Orthop 242:60–68
7. Smith MA, Urquhart DR, Savidge GF (1981) The surgical management of varus deformity in haemophilic arthropathy of the knee. J Bone Joint Surg Br 63:261–265
8. Ragni MV, Crossett LS, Herndon JH (1995) Postoperative infection following orthopaedic surgery in human immunodeficiency virus-infected hemophiliacs with CD4 counts < or = 200/mm3. J Arthroplasty 10:716–721
9. Rodríguez-Merchán EC, Lee CA (2002) Inhibitors in Patients with Haemophilia. Blackwell Science Ltd, Oxford
10. Rodríguez-Merchán EC, Wiedel JD, Wallny et al (2003) Elective orthopaedic surgery for inhibitors patients. Haemophilia 9:625–631
11. Rodríguez-Merchán EC. Rocino A, Ewenstein B et al (2004) Consensus perspectivas on surgery in haemophilia patients with inhibitors: summary statement. Haemophilia 10(Suppl 2): 50–52
12. Rodríguez-Merchán EC (2007) Total knee replacement in haemophilic arthropathy. J Bone Joint Surg Br 89(2):186–188
13. Rodríguez-Merchán EC, Quintana M, Jimenez-Yuste V, Hernandez-Navarro F (2007) Orthopaedic surgery for inhibitor patients: a series of 27 procedures (25 patients). Haemophilia 13:613–619
14. Rodríguez-Merchán EC (2007) Haemophilic synovitis: basic concepts. Haemophilia 13 (Suppl 3):1–3
15. Rodríguez-Merchán EC, Quintana M, De la Corte-Rodriguez H, Coya M (2007) Radioactive synoviorthesis for the treatment of haemophilic synovitis. Haemophilia 13 (Suppl 3):32–37
16. Rodríguez-Merchán EC, Valentino L, Quintana M (2007) Prophylaxis and treatment of chronic synovitis in haemophilia patients with inhibitors. Haemophilia 13(Suppl 3):45–48
17. Rodríguez-Merchán EC (2007) Total joint arthroplasty: the final solution for knee and hip when synovitis could not be controlled. Haemophilia 13(Suppl 3):49–58

Chapter 21
Treatment of Knee Flexion Contractures using Casts and Hinges

Paulo J. Llinás Hernández

Introduction

A knee flexion contracture is an articular complication frequently found in severe hemophilia patients. Fernández-Palazzi and Batistella reported having found a knee contracture in every patient they assessed in hemophilia centers [1]. Since such facilities offer specialized care to hemophilia patients, their finding suggests that even despite moderate access to expert medical care, factor concentrates, and rehabilitation, contractures are difficult to prevent.

This condition changes the gait pattern and sports ability of patients with severe hemophilia, adversely affecting their psychological wellbeing, social life, and work performance, and impairing their quality of life. The deformity produces an obvious shortening of the limb, requiring the patient to use external support devices, which induce both articular bleeding and impairment of the elbows and shoulders [2]. Thus, besides restricting ambulation, lower limb flexion contractures may contribute to upper limb skeletal impairment; consequently, correcting them is essential.

Pathophysiology of Knee Flexion Contractures

Contractures are defined as a loss of articular movement. Generally, they can be classified as acute (secondary to hemarthrosis) or chronic, resulting from a series of complex events involving the joint and surrounding structures. The development of flexion deformities of the knee has multiple causes, among which intra-articular/intramuscular bleeding is the main triggering factor. When experiencing hemarthrosis, keeping the knee in flexion relieves pain due to enhanced articular compliance. Without adequate replacement therapy to avoid repeated bleeding, the hamstring muscles, the iliotibial band, and the posterior capsule all undergo retraction, which prevents proper extension of the knee [3]. In addition, the articular distension leads to a reflex muscular inhibition caused by intracapsular mediators, which prevents the normal performance of the quadriceps [4].

H.A. Caviglia, L.P. Solimeno (eds.), *Orthopedic Surgery in Patients with Hemophilia.*

If the process continues, the contracture turns into a fixed flexion deformity, impairing the patient's support, and resulting in shortening of both ligaments and tendons. The final result is increased pressure by unit of area in the posterior condyles over the tibial plateau, subluxating the tibia towards the back, and impairing the cartilage irreversibly. This initiates an arthritic process with reduced articular spaces, osteophytes, and the deformities that are typical of hemophilic joint disease [5].

Treatment of Knee Flexion Contractures

There are several treatment options, which include physical therapy, corrective devices, and surgical procedures [6]. Some key parameters that should be considered when choosing the best therapeutic option include: the patient's age, contracture severity, the presence of surrounding contractures, duration of the condition, muscular development, gait pattern, the presence of an articular subluxation, radiological findings, willingness of the patient to cooperate, and availability of health care [7].

Treatment options may be included in three groups: (1) physical therapy; (2) orthotic therapy and corrective devices; and (3) surgical procedures. This chapter will focus on the second category, and will describe the management of knee flexion deformities by using corrective casts with hinges.

Corrective Casts with Hinges

Having been used (with certain variations) for many years in different parts of the world, this method has stood the test of time. Over recent decades, its use has declined in countries where access to primary prophylaxis is readily available, and where articular contractures have consequently become less frequent. However, it is still a useful tool in countries that rely on secondary prophylaxis or that lack regular availability of either factor concentrates or cryoprecipitate. We suggest its use for managing chronic knee flexion contractures greater than 30° resulting from intra-atricular or extra-articular bleeding. We also suggest using hinges in the post-operative treatment of acute flexion deformities in patients who have undergone either total knee replacement or osteotomies close to the knee.

For contractures measuring less than 30° and showing no improvement following physical therapy, we have used serial casts to correct the deformity by replacing the cast every third day until reaching the desired knee extension. In order to avoid replacing the cast so frequently, the system has been modified by opening wedges in the back area of the knee. The system is covered by a plaster layer, which delays the time of replacement for up to a week [1]. The use of dynamic splints is an effective therapeutic option that can be carried out on an outpatient basis and controlled by the patient himself.

Definition

Hinges are an adjustable corrective system used for managing knee flexion contractures (Fig. 21.1). They include two screws, one with a coarse thread and one with a fine thread, which allow the correction of both anteroposterior and flexion/extension deformities.

While the large screw with the coarse thread is being screwed, the tibia is pushed anteriorly, elongating the posterior structures of the knee, and improving the posterior subluxation of the tibia over the femur. Once the posterior subluxation of the tibia is corrected, the patient will proceed to work on the small screw with the fine thread. While being screwed, the screw with the fine thread extends the knee, correcting the flexion contracture (Fig. 21.2).

Hinges are incorporated in two cast segments (over the thigh and leg), while the knee is left uncovered.

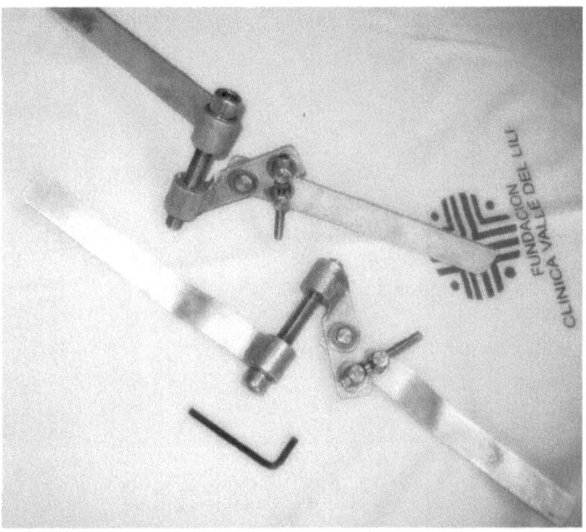

Fig. 21.1 Hinges

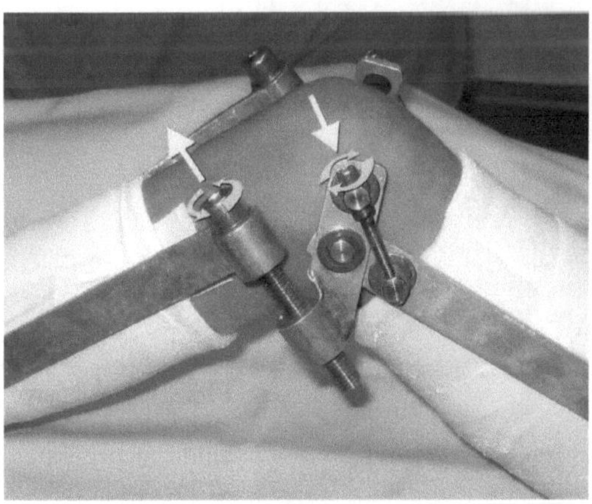
Fig. 21.2 Hinges with a large and small screw

Procedure

1. Benzoin dye is applied to the skin of the lateral and medial calf and thigh, to prevent irritation and enhance the adhesive properties of the skin. Adhesive tape is placed underneath the laminated cotton using sufficient length to travel about 10 cm distal to the knee and ankle joint line (Fig. 21.3). The distal segments of the adhesive tape at the knee and ankle will be everted and incorporated in either cast segment to prevent distal migration of the structure upon knee extension, which would injure both the suprapatellar area and the ankle (Fig. 21.4). Once the treatment has been concluded, the patient should remove the adhesive tape, using lukewarm water or alcohol to avoid skin detachment and resultant bleeding.

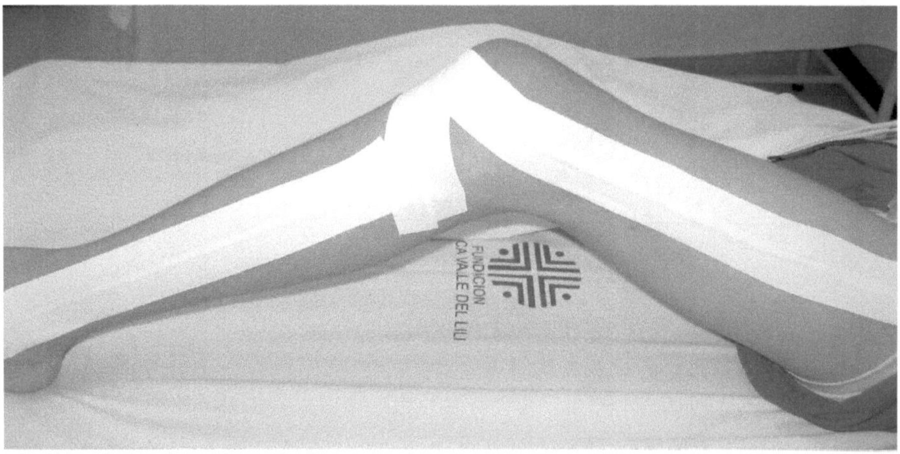

Fig. 21.3 Adhesive tape

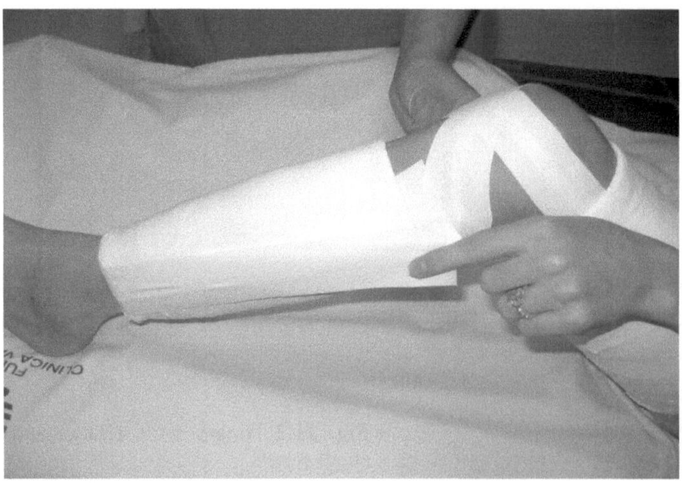

Fig. 21.4 Adhesive tape at the knee and ankle incorporated in the cast

2. Four layers of laminated cotton are positioned. Plush is used on the sites undergoing the highest pressure (anterior surface of the thigh and both anterior distal and posterior proximal surfaces of the leg), in order to make the patient more comfortable and to prevent blisters from appearing (Fig. 21.5).
3. A plaster layer is placed on the thigh and the leg, leaving the knee free (Fig. 21.6).
4. Hinge angles are adapted to the patient's contracture (Figs. 21.7 and 21.8). Hinges are placed at each side of the thigh and the leg while being incorporated in a new plaster layer in such a way that the articular line of the knee corresponds with the flexion/extension center of the hinges (Figs. 21.9 and 21.10).

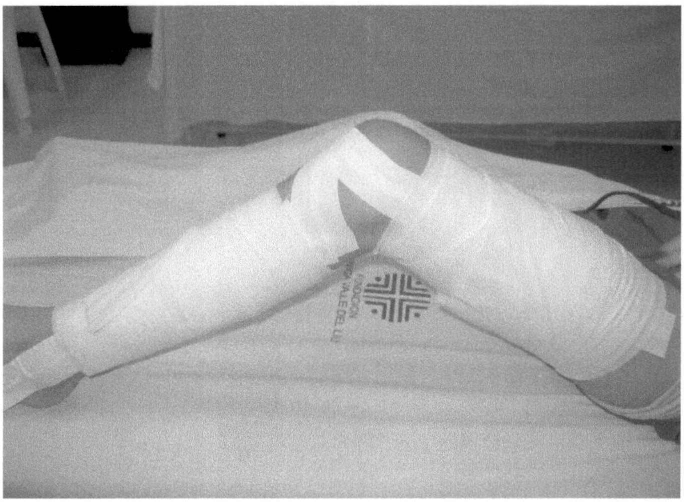

Fig. 21.5 Layers of laminated cotton

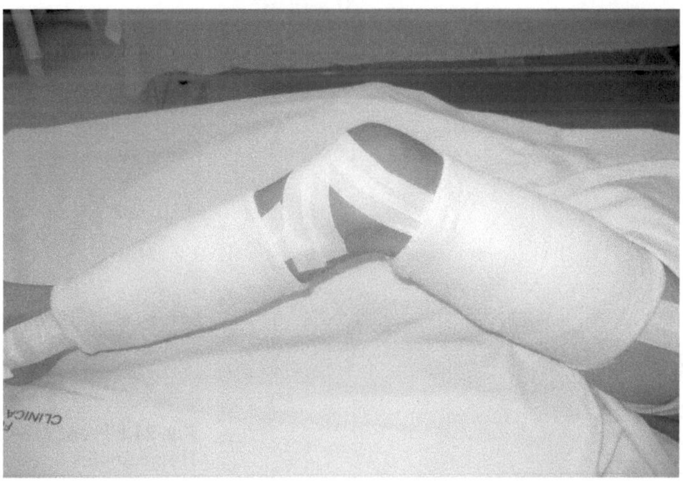

Fig. 21.6 A plaster

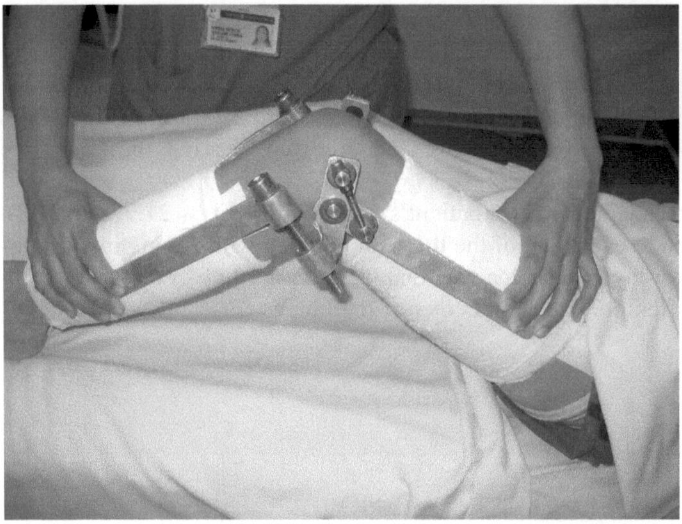

Fig. 21.7 Side view. Hinge angles

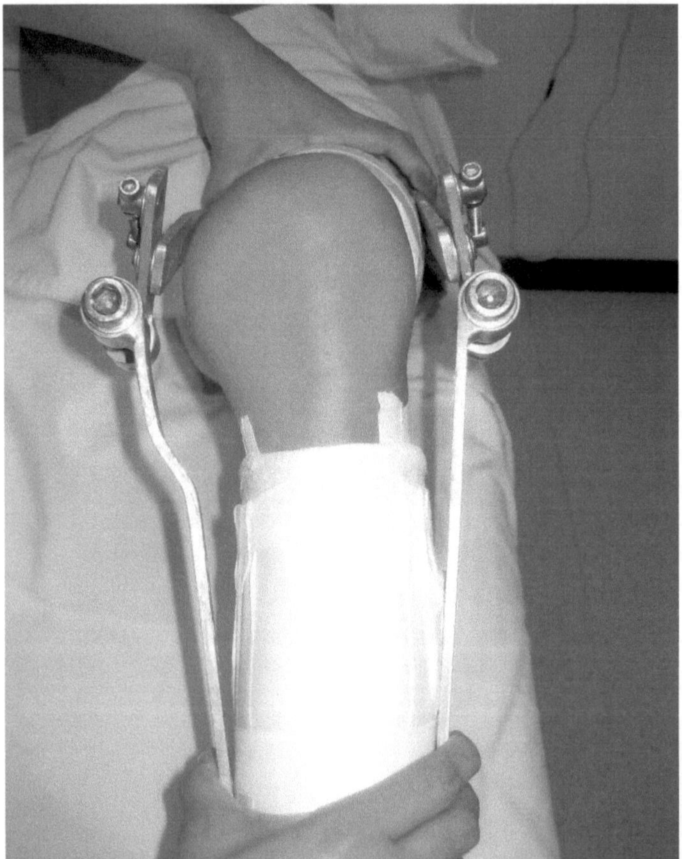

Fig. 21.8 Front view. Hinge angles

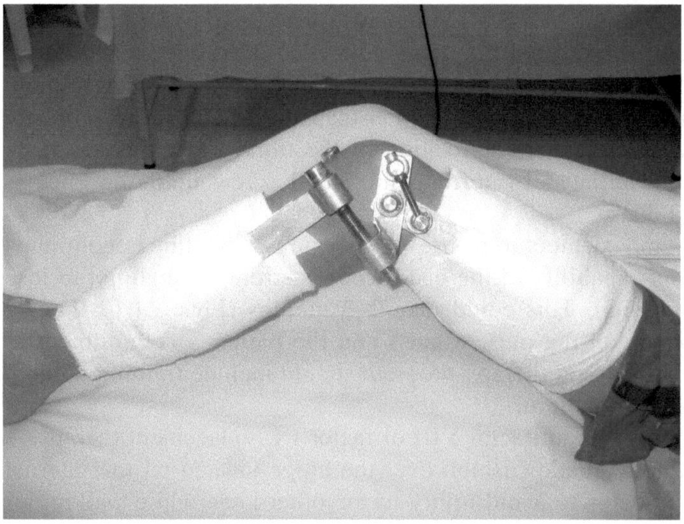

Fig. 21.9 Side view. Hinges incorporated in a new plaster layer

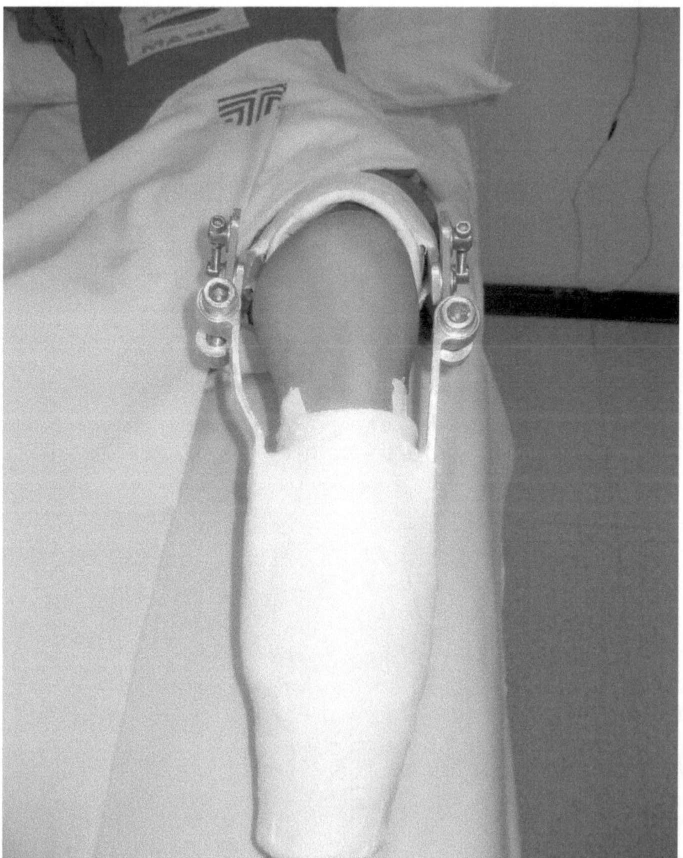

Fig. 21.10 Front view. Hinges incorporated in a new plaster layer

5. The patient is taught how to use a hexagonal Allen key in order to continue correcting the contracture according to his tolerance. The process is initiated by turning the large screw, which creates an anterior tibial drawer, both allowing elongation of posterior structures (capsule and posterior cruciate ligament), and correcting the subluxation of the tibia. Once this has been done, extension is initiated by turning the small screw until the knee is extended (Fig. 21.11).
6. Following cast removal, nocturnal use of an extension splint is continued until the extending capability of the quadriceps is strong enough not to lose the achieved correction. This could take 2–3 months (Figs. 21.12–21.14). However, it depends on the muscle mass and the patient's commitment to rehabilitation. The physical therapy program should include training on both propioception and gait pattern.
7. Procedures are done without factor VIII or factor IX replacement therapy.
8. Placing a small, home-made cushion over the hinge located on the internal aspect of the knee helps to avoid injury to the other knee while walking or lying on the side.

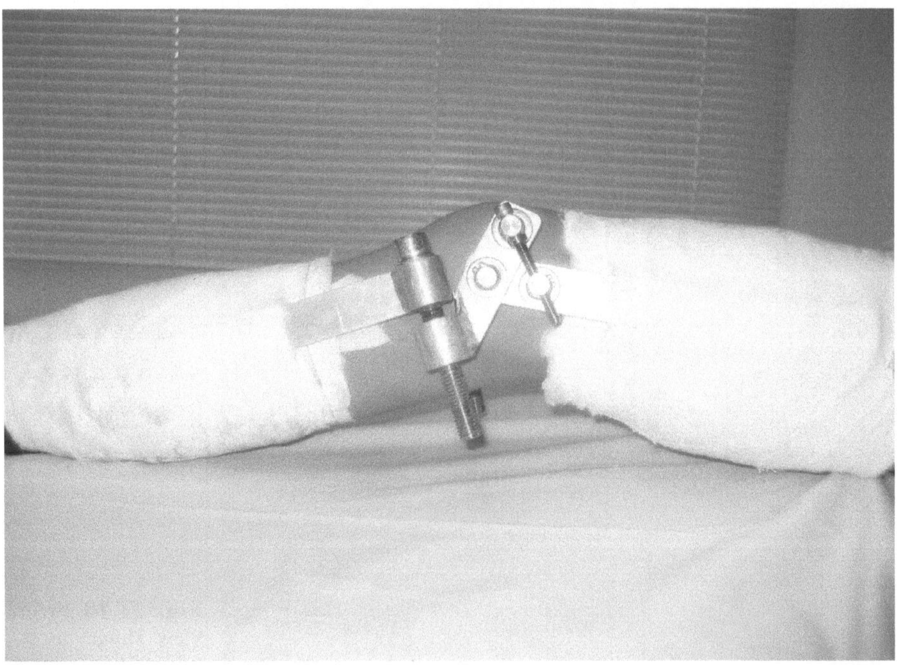

Fig. 21.11 Extended knee

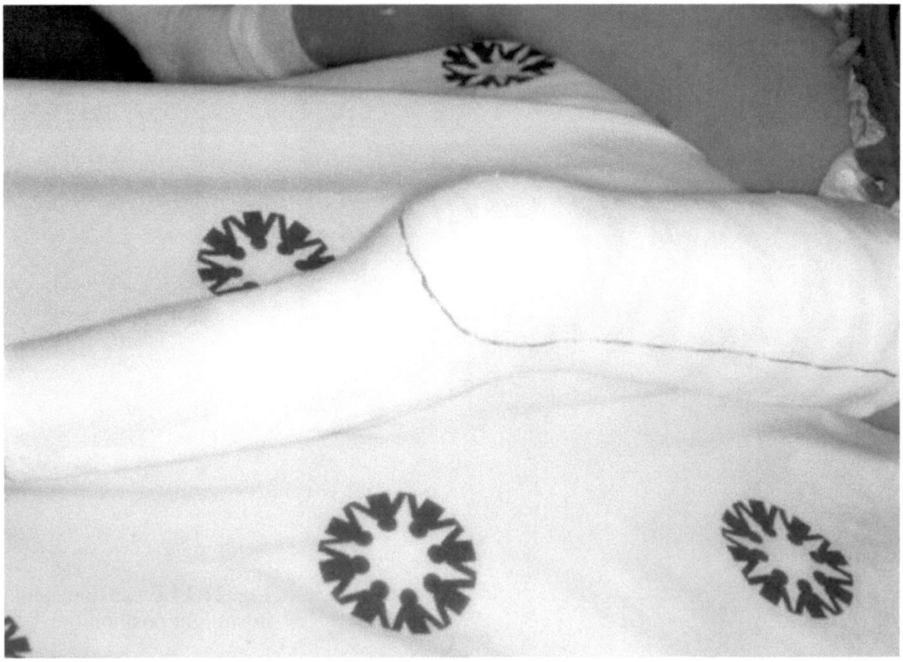

Fig. 21.12 Extension splint for nocturnal use

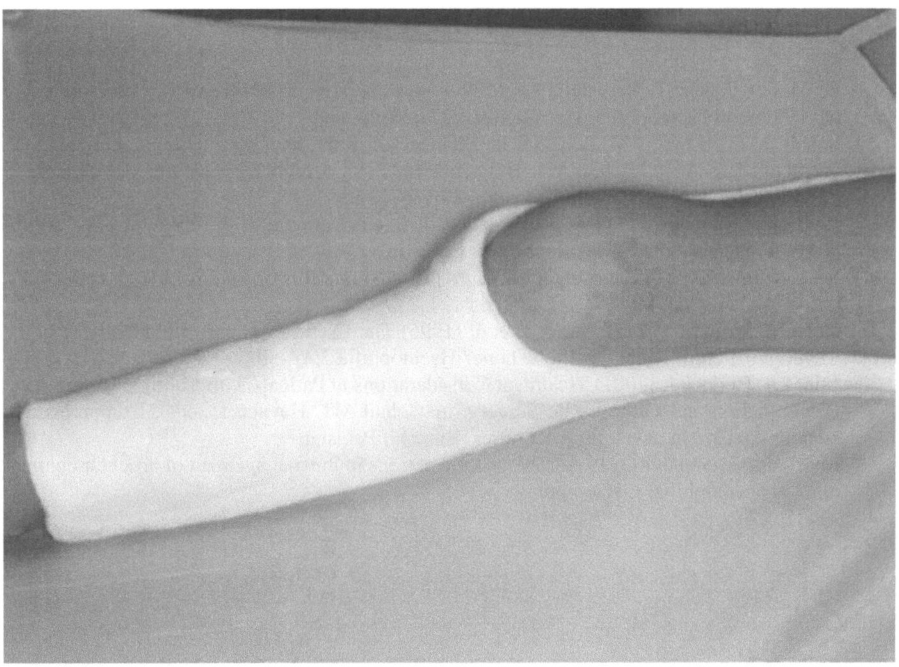

Fig. 21.13 Extension splint with femoral window

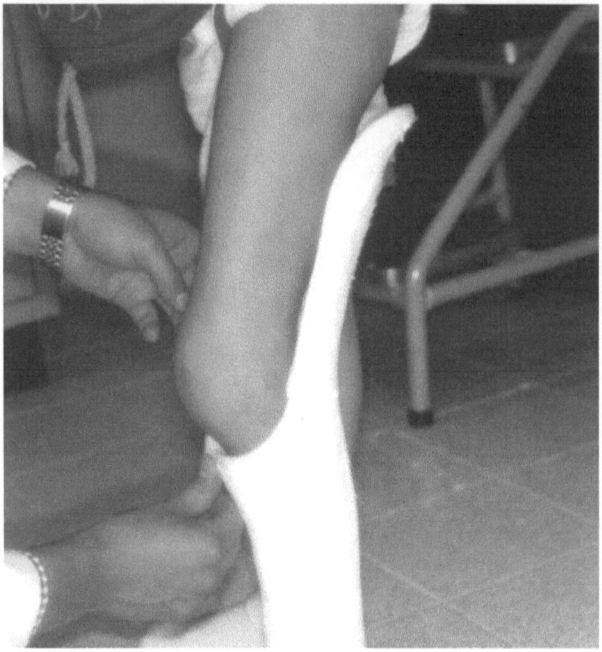

Fig. 21.14 Extension splint in straight position

References

1. Fernández-Palazzi F, Battistella LR (1999) Non-operative treatment of flexion contracture of the knee in haemophilia. Haemophilia 5(1):20–24
2. Sohail MT, Akhtar ZM (2001) Management of joint and soft tissue contractures in haemophilic patients. Sohail MT, Heijnen L (eds). In: Comprehensive hemophilia care in developing countries. Karachi, Pakistan, 20:166–177
3. Rodríguez-Merchán EC (1999) Correction of fixed contractures during total knee arthroplasty in haemophiliacs. Haemophilia 5(1):33–38
4. Spencer JD, Hayes KC, Alexander IJ (1984) Knee joint effusion and quadriceps reflex inhibition in man. Arch Phys Med Rehab 65:171–177
5. Heim M, Horoszowski H, Varon D et al (1996) The fixed flexed and subluxed knee in the haemophilic child: what should be done? Haemophilia 2:47–50
6. Llinás A, Heijnen L (2001) Treatment Considerations in Patients with Multiple Deformities: Rehabilitation and Orthopaedic Surgery. In: Sohail MT, Heynen L (eds). Comprehensive hemophilia care in developing countries. Karachi, Pakistan
7. Rodríguez-Merchán EC (1999) Therapeutic options in the management of articular contractures in haemophiliacs. Haemophilia 5(1):5–9

Chapter 22
Arthroscopic Evaluation of the Knee

Gaetano Torri, Luigi P. Solimeno and Emilia Lozej

Introduction

On the point of writing this short chapter of the book that so many friends would like to dedicate to the memory of Henri Horozowski, I asked myself how such an expert surgeon, as I remember him, would evaluate the use of arthroscopy as a routine surgical procedure for the treatment of hemophilic arthropathy of the knee.

Actually, Professor Horozowski lived in the "heroic times" of orthopedic surgery in hemophiliacs, in which a relatively "insufficient" and less-effective replacement therapy with factor VIII and IX concentrates made every open surgery a high-risk procedure. Horozowski was a pioneer of this kind of surgery: he tested every surgical option (such as multiple joint surgery in a single operation session) or new devices (such as laser scalpel, or fibrin seal), that could reduce surgery-related bleeding and the amount of factor replacement.

Today, many of those procedures have become "mini-invasive", so that even hemophilic pseudotumors can be dealt with by percutaneous treatment. At present, the indications for performing a knee arthroscopy in hemophiliac patients could be considered the same as those commonly indicated in patients not affected by bleeding disorders. Arthroscopic lavage, meniscal resection, removal of loose bodies, cartilage shaving, resection of plicae and adhesions, and synovectomy are common procedures, and are often performed in the same surgical session, since in hemophilic arthropathy of the knee all articular structures may be involved at the same time.

Kim and Wiedel [1, 2] reported their first experiences in the treatment of chronic synovitis of the knee by arthroscopic synovectomy in 1983, at the XVth WFH (World Federation of Hemophilia) Congress in Stockholm. From 1984 to 1997, many authors [1–6] stated the main advantages of arthroscopic synovectomy of the knee, which in comparison with open synovectomy, shows a minor reduction of the range of motion, though the final outcome is related to the stage of arthropathy [5, 6]. The procedure effectively reduces — and in most cases stops — recurrent bleeding episodes, offering, at the same time, lower incidence of the well-known post-operative stiffness of the joint; on the other hand, arthroscopic synovectomy did not prove to be effective in arresting the progression of

H.A. Caviglia, L.P. Solimeno (eds.), *Orthopedic Surgery in Patients with Hemophilia.*

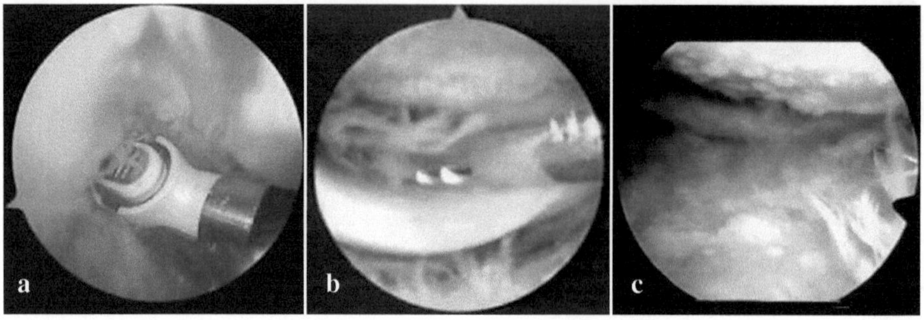

Fig. 22.1 a Bipolar radiofrequency device, **b, c** motor-powered instrument for cartilage shaving or débridement

arthropathy, though it can slow it in some cases [5, 6]. Arthroscopy allows multiple procedures, such as meniscal resection or (very often) the removal of the hypertrophic synovial tissue that can give an "impingement"-like lesion around the menisci, with features suggestive of meniscal lesion. All degrees of hyaline cartilage degeneration, with "flaps", ulcers with loose borders, mixed with scar tissue, can be observed at patellofemoral and femorotibial level, and can be treated by shaving devices (Fig. 22.1). The major surgical difficulties of an arthroscopic procedure to treat hemophilic arthropathy of the knee are the narrowed joint space filled with hypertrophic synovium, the presence of adhesions, and impaired distension of the cavity. For this reason, motor-powered instruments are needed, especially at the beginning of the arthroscopic approach: the surgeon should be prepared to perform a kind of limited or complete joint débridement, as this is the only way to allow progression of the arthroscope and enlarge the field of vision inside the joint.

Since 1995, 37 patients affected by hemophilic artrhopathy of the knee have undergone 40 arthroscopic procedures at the Orthopedic Clinic of Milan University. Thirty-five were hemophilia A patients, and two had hemophilia B. The average age was 34 years (range: 18–50 years). Standard knee X-rays and magnetic resonance imaging (MRI) scans were carried out in each patient before the arthroscopic procedure. Patients selected for arthroscopic synovectomy for chronic synovitis proved to be unresponsive to a long period of prophylaxis with the deficient clotting factor, physiotherapy, intra-articular corticosteroid therapy, and synoviorthesis with rifampicin.

Surgical Technique

On the day of operation, factor VIII or IX is given to produce a factor level of 100%. During the post-operative period, the factor concentration should be kept at 50% until the end of second week.

Anesthesia

General anesthesia remains the most frequently used method. In our department, anesthesiologists do not like spinal anesthesia in patients affected by bleeding disorders. Recently, they performed a block of sciatic and femoral nerve ("4 in 1" block with nerve stimulator) in six arthroscopic procedures for hemophilic arthropathy.

Patient's Position

The patient is placed supine on an ordinary table, with no support device. The use of a leg holder at the root of the thigh, with the possibility of folding down the end leaf of the table, are conditioned by the residual range of motion of the involved knee.

Irrigation

Saline is the fluid most commonly used, and in our experience irrigation can be carried out by simple gravity (also for synovectomies).

In every knee arthroscopy, a tourniquet is placed before starting the procedure. At the end of the procedure, three or four ampoules of an antifibrinolytic agent can be added to the washing fluid.

Arthroscopic Procedure

A wide-angle arthroscope 4.5 mm in diameter with 25° to 30° oblique angle is usually inserted at the anterolateral portal, and a probe at the anteromedial one. We use suprapatellar portals in very few cases. At the beginning of procedure, hypertrophic synovial villi, scar tissue, and adhesion should be treated by motorised instruments.

When vision is unobstructed, a standardized exploration of the knee should be done, bearing in mind the following characteristic features of hemophilic knee arthropathy:

- Hyperthrophic synovial tissue looks different when observed at a suprapatellar pouch, around the anterior cruciate ligament, and around the menisci (Fig. 22.2)
- All the degrees of hyaline cartilage degeneration can be observed in the same joint, and in different areas, with splitting of cartilaginous tissue, mixed with plentiful scar material and white areas of fibrocartilaginous tissue. A cartilage "shaving" or a limited resection, can be performed with motor-powered cutting instruments or with a bipolar radiofrequency device (Fig. 22.1)

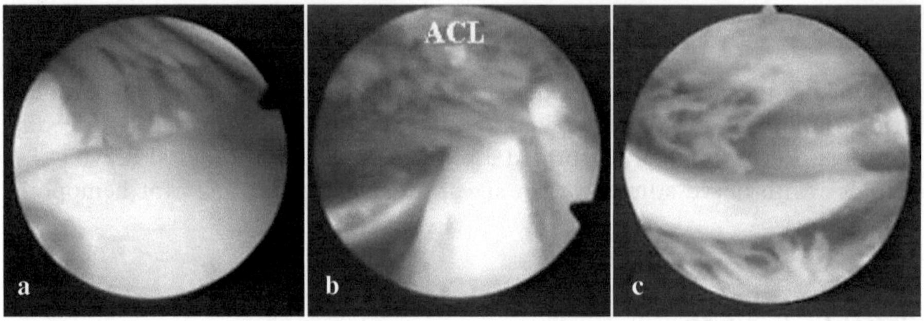

Fig. 22.2 Aspect of hypertrophic synovia around the menisci and anterior cruciate ligament

- Meniscal resection (when indicated) and removal of loose bodies can be performed using grasping and "basket" forceps. Limited synovectomy around menisci or complete débridement are carried out by motorized instruments (Fig. 22.2).
- After washing the joint, an intra-articular drain is placed for at least 24 h if needed and then a compression bandage is applied.

Rehabilitation Schedule

Continuous passive motion on a machine starts the first day after knee arthroscopy with sessions of 20 min (0–90°) three times a day.

References

1. Kim H, Klein K, Hirsch S et al (1984) Arthroscopic synovectomy in the treatment of hemophilic synovitis. Scand J Haematol 33:271–279
2. Wiedel JD (1984) Arthroscopic synovectomy in hemophilic arthropathy of the knee. Scand J Haematol 33(40):263–270
3. Wiedel JD (1985) Arthroscopic synovectomy for chronic hemophilic synovitis of the knee. Arthroscopy 1:205–209
4. Klein KS, Aland CM, Kim HC et al (1987) Long term follow-up of arthroscopic synovectomy for chronic hemophilic synovitis. Arthroscopy 3:231–236
5. Wiedel JD (1996) Arthroscopic synovectomy of the knee in hemophilia: 10 to 15-year follow-up. Clin Orthop 328:46–53
6. Eickhoff HH, Koch W, Raderschadt G, Brackmann HH (1997) Arthroscopy for chronic hemophilic synovitis of the knee. Clin Orthop 343:58–62

Chapter 23
Lengthening of Hamstring Tendons in Knee Flexion Contractures

Muhammad Tariq Sohail and Wazahat Hussain Warraich

Introduction

Contractures of joints are usual sequelae of hemophilic arthropathy. These contractures result from a combination of recurrent hemarthroses which cause fibroblastic proliferation of the capsule, progressive arthropathy, and extra-articular intramuscular bleeding episodes leading to fibrosis. Hypertrophied synovium promotes fibrillation and erosion of articular cartilage. Progressive fibrosis of synovium leads to pain, spasm, and shortening of muscles, resulting in joint contractures and restriction of joint motion [1].

The prevalence of joint contractures in patients with severe hemophilia has been reported to be between 50% and 95% [2].

Pathogenesis

Recurrent hemarthrosis may result in a fixed flexion deformity of the knee due to increased intra-articular pressure and distension of the joint capsule. Joint distension causes reflex inhibition of the quadriceps. With the knee held in flexion, the knee flexors overcome the weakened knee extensors, pulling the tibia into posterior subluxation on the femoral condyles. This progressive posterior traction causes a shortening and tightening of the posterior knee capsule [3].

When a fixed knee flexion deformity is established, the abnormal position of the joint seems to cause an increased number of intra-articular bleeding episodes. Hamstring release is a useful procedure, not only to extend the knee, but also to diminish the number and intensity of hemarthroses.

Indications for Hamstring Tendon Lengthening

- Flexion contracture >30°.
- Failed physiotherapy and rehabilitation program.

H.A. Caviglia, L.P. Solimeno (eds.), *Orthopedic Surgery in Patients with Hemophilia.*

- Hemophilic arthropathy of grade I and II.
- Increased bleeding tendency.
  Results are better results in young patients.

Contraindications for Hamstring Tendon Lengthening

- Gross degenerative and unstable joints.
- Presence of inhibitors.

Diagnostic Workup

Hemophilia Workup

- Factor level assessment (50–100%).
- Inhibitor status.

Imaging Studies

- *Plain X-rays*: anteroposterior and lateral views of involved joints show joint space narrowing, subchondral bone cysts, marginal sclerosis, erosions, and cartilage loss.
- *Ultrasonography*: this is useful for evaluation of fluid, and inflammation of the synovium, cartilage, ligaments, and capsules of the joints.
- *Magnetic resonance imaging (MRI)*: being multi-planar, this provides excellent soft tissue contrast and supporting qualitative volumetric assessment of synovial hyperplasia. MRI evaluates cartilage and bone abnormalities earlier and more rapidly than ultrasonography.

Differential Diagnosis

- Intrapopliteal soft tissue hemorrhage.
- Subperiosteal bleeds.
- Juvenile rheumatoid arthritis.
- Osteoarthritis.

Surgical Procedure: Hamstring Lengthening and Posterior Capsulotomy

1. Prior to surgery, deficient factors are corrected until the patient has a normal activated partial thromboplastin time.

2. All operations are performed under general anesthesia.
3. A tourniquet is applied in every case.
4. After antiseptic measures and proper draping, patients are placed in a prone position, and the knee opened with a straight incision made in the midline to the distal one-third of the thigh, ending at the popliteal crease.
5. The posterior capsule is débrided.
6. The semitendinosus tendon is z-lengthened.
7. The lateral aspect of the distal end of the semimembranosus is freed of fat and connective tissue to expose the whole of its aponeurosis, which is then incised in a V shape.
8. As the knee is extended, the ends of the aponeurosis pull apart and the muscle fibers also glide apart.
9. Aponeurosis on the lateral aspect of the biceps femoris is exposed and similarly incised as the knee is extended.
10. In severe contractures the gracilis tendon is also cut.
11. Once the posterior capsule of the knee has been released, the popliteus tendon and posterior cruciate ligament are also released, after protecting the neurovascular bundle in the region and the peroneal nerve in particular.
12. Intra-operatively, a tissue sealant such as fibrin glue is also used for better hemostasis.
13. A suction drain is placed, the wound is closed in layers, and a pressure bandage is applied.

Post-operative Care

1. A long leg plaster with ample soft padding over the posterior aspects of the knee is placed on the leg in order to bring the knee gradually into complete extension.
2. Active, gentle physiotherapy is initiated 48 h after the drain has been removed.
3. The posterior splint is removed for intervals after the eighth post-operative day.
4. Intensive physiotherapy is started in the hospital once the wound has healed, and continued after the patient's discharge.
5. A posterior splint is used during the night.
6. Physiotherapy, including stretching exercises, is advised three times a week during the first 2 months, and close observation for the first 6 months, post-operatively.
7. Approximately 50% of the level of the deficient factor is maintained throughout the follow-up.

Rehabilitation

Intense physiotherapy and a high level of patient cooperation are essential to keep the increase in knee extension and improve the total arc of motion. Continuous passive motion may be useful part-time during the day. Physiotherapy should be performed twice daily in the hospital, then 5 days a week for the first 2–3 months after leaving the hospital, and then 3 days a week, usually for a period of 6 months [4].

References

1. Silva M, Luck JV (2003) Flexion contractures of the knee in haemophilia. In Rodríguez-Merchán EC (eds) The haemophilic joints – New prospectives. Blackwell Publishing, Oxford, pp 99–105
2. Atkins RM, Handerson NJ, Duthie RB (1987) Joint contractures in the haemophilia. Clin Orthop 219:97–105
3. Heim M, Horoszowki H, Varon D et al (1996) The fixed flexed and subluxed knee in the haemophilic child; what should be done? Haemophilia 2:47–50
4. Heijnen L, de Kleijn P (1999) Physiotherapy for the treatment of articular contractures in haemophilia. Haemophilia 5(Suppl 1):16–19

Chapter 24
Knee Osteotomy

Luciano da Rocha Loures Pacheco, Maurício Alexandre de Meneses Pereira and Cyro Kanabushi

Introduction

Classic hemophilia is the most common of the inherited disorders of blood coagulation that are transmitted in a sex-linked, recessive manner. The incidence of hemophilia A is approximately 0.1 in 1000 male births and for hemophilia B it is 0.02 in 1000 male births.

Diagnosis is only possible after laboratory tests, because the two disorders are very similar in clinical presentation. Hemarthrosis is the most disabling manifestation of hemophilia, particularly in the knees, elbows, and ankles.

The early synovial reaction to intra-articular bleeding is similar to rheumatoid arthritis: synovial hypertrophy, hemosiderin deposition in phagocytic cells, perivascular infiltrates of inflammatory cells, and early fibrosis of the subsynovial layer. The hypervascularity and friability of the synovium probably cause an increased tendency to further bleeding, which may become cyclical. It is unlikely that the excess clot formed by chronic hemarthrosis will be completely removed by the fibrinolytic system, and organization of the remaining clot leads to the development of fibrous adhesions, capsular fibrosis, and joint contracture.

With knee involvement, there are several appropriate radiographs: standing anteroposterior and lateral views, tangential patellar view, panoramic views of the lower limb, and tunnel views.

The indications for osteotomy are: knees in fixed flexion, with articular contracture or valgus or varus deformities, and without intra-articular cartilage destruction.

Arnold and Hilgartner's classification system, which separates hemophilic arthropathy into five stages, is as follows:

- *Stage 0*: normal knee
- *Stage I*: soft-tissue swelling
- *Stage II*: soft-tissue swelling, osteopenia, epiphyseal overgrowth, no narrowing of the joint space
- *Stage III*: no significant narrowing of the joint space, subchondral cysts, osteopenia

H.A. Caviglia, L.P. Solimeno (eds.), *Orthopedic Surgery in Patients with Hemophilia.*

- *Stage IV*: destruction of cartilage and narrowing of the joint space
- *Stage V*: end stage, with destruction of the joint and gross bony changes.

Arthropathy is clinically reversible only in stages I to III, and stage III is the best time to plan osteotomies. After stage IV, osteotomies can be performed, but only with the objective of palliative treatment and to postpone a possible total knee arthroplasty.

The indications for proximal tibial osteotomy are: pain and disability resulting from osteoarthritis that significantly interfere with employment or recreation, evidence of degenerative arthritis that is confined to one compartment with a corresponding varus or valgus deformity (Figs. 24.1 and 24.2), the ability of the patient to use crutches after the operation, the possession of sufficient muscle strength and motivation to carry out a rehabilitation program, and good vascular status without serious arterial insufficiency or large varicosities.

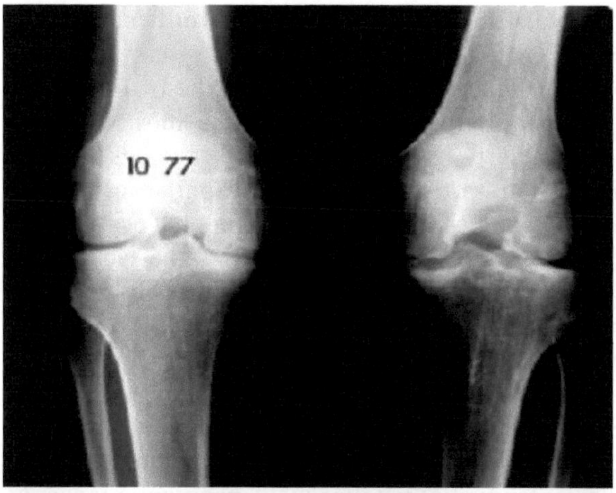

Fig. 24.1 Patient with hemophilic arthropathy of the knees prior to surgery. Note the marked genu varum on the right side and genu valgum on the left side (the left side of the figure represents the right knee)

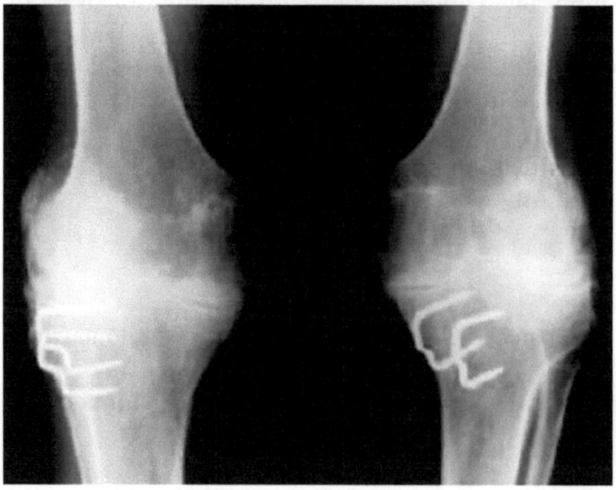

Fig. 24.2 Same patient as in Fig. 1, 22 and 23 years after high tibial osteotomy with valgization of the right, and varization of the left knee respectively. Internal fixation was performed using blunt staples. Despite the fact that radiographically visible joint space in some regions is less than 1 mm, the patient claimed to be free of pain in the left knee and complained of only slight pain in the right knee

Contraindications to a Coventry-type proximal tibial osteotomy are: narrowing of the lateral compartment cartilage space, lateral tibial subluxation of more than 1 cm, medial compartment tibial bone loss of more than 2 or 3 mm, flexion contracture of more than 15°, knee flexion of less than 90°, a need for more than 20° of correction, and rheumatoid arthritis.

The Coventry Technique for Proximal Tibial Osteotomy

1. Place the patient in the dorsal decubitus position with the knee at 90° of flexion.
2. Tourniquet.
3. Begin a curved lateral incision distally at the fibular head, carrying it proximally over the midlateral aspect of the knee joint, and ending it just proximal to the lateral femoral condyle.
4. Free the insertions of the fibular collateral ligaments and the biceps femoris tendon from the fibular head and reflect them proximally and anteriorly as a Y-shaped "conjoined tendon".
5. Divide the posterior 2.5 cm of the iliotibial band to expose the lateral tibial condyle and the knee joint. Incise the subcutaneous tissue, protect the peroneal nerve with a blunt retractor, and resect most of the fibular head.
6. Plan the tibial osteotomy, depending on the size of the wedge to be removed. Begin the proximal plane of the osteotomy at least 2 cm distal to the articular surface of the tibia. Begin the distal plane of the osteotomy at a level which, when the wedge of bone is removed, will permit correction of the deformity.
7. Carefully and neatly approximate the tibial fragment and check the alignment of the limb. Fix the osteotomy using one or two staples driven from laterally to medially just anterior to the fibula, or with a laterally applied contoured T-plate.
8. Release the tourniquet, cauterize all bleeding vessels, and insert a suction drain.
9. Suture the structures of the iliotibial band and close the wound.
10. Extend the knee and apply a large compression dressing and a knee brace.

Post-operative Treatment

The day after surgery the patient is allowed to walk on crutches with the foot touching the ground. The bulky compression dressing and knee brace are removed at 10–12 days, and a cylinder cast is applied with the knee straight. The cast is usually removed at 5–6 weeks if X-rays show early bony union. Protected weight-bearing and range-of-motion exercises are begun. Full weight-bearing on the extremity is allowed by 10–12 weeks.

Coventry recommends a distal femoral varus osteotomy rather than a proximal tibial varus osteotomy if the valgus deformity at the knee is more than 12–15°, or the plane of the knee joint deviates from the horizontal by more than 10°.

In Coventry's method, a medial approach is used. An anterior total knee incision can also be used by exposing the medial distal femur through a subvastus approach. This can avoid skin bridges if subsequent total knee arthroplasty is required.

The Coventry Technique for Distal Femoral Osteotomy

1. Place the patient in the dorsal decubitus position.
2. Tourniquet.
3. Use a medial incision to separate the rectus femoris and vastus medialis at their junction, expose the lower part of the femur, and displace the suprapatellar pouch distally without opening it until the base of the medial femoral condyle.
4. Insert the blade plate and cut the femur. Bring the plate into contact with the diaphysis after either removing a wedge or simply cutting across the bone and countersinking the distal end of the proximal fragment into the medullary cavity of the distal portion.
5. Correct any flexion deformity by appropriate placement of the nail plate.
6. Secure the plate to the proximal fragment with screws.
7. Insert a suction drain and close the wound.

Post-operative Treatment

The extremity is treated in the same manner as after proximal tibial osteotomy.

Examples of a knee joint before and after osteotomy are shown in Figures 24.3-24.6.

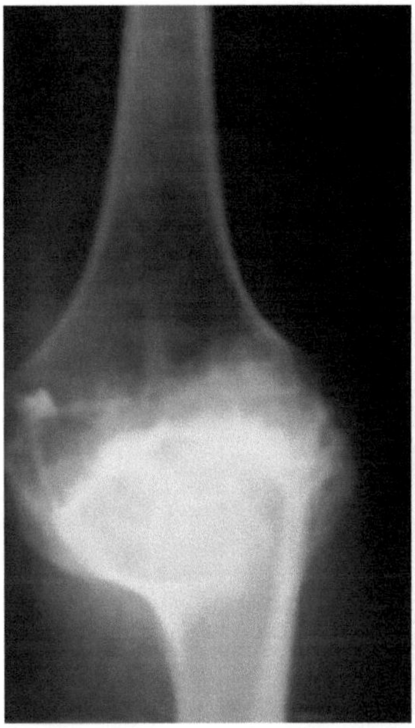

Fig. 24.3 Pre-operative anteroposterior view

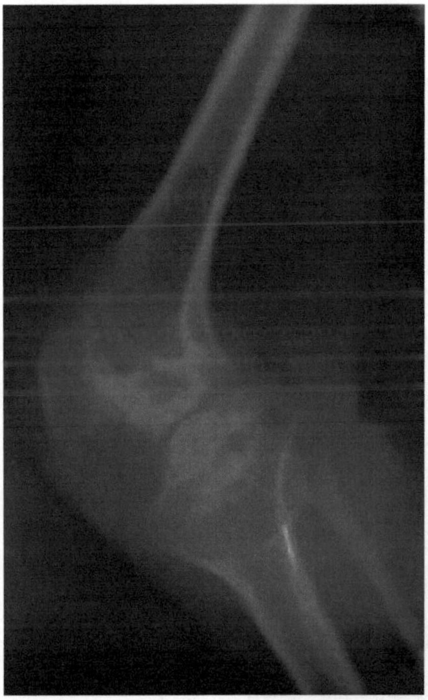

Fig. 24.4 Pre-operative lateral view: patello-femoral liberation

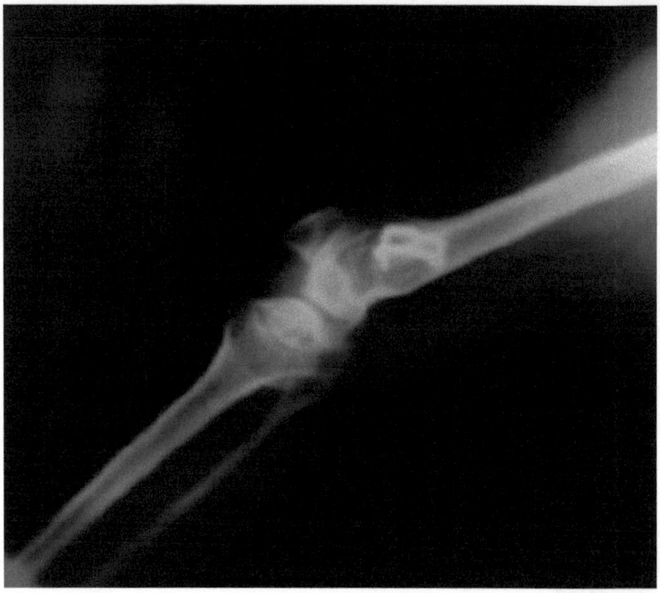

Fig. 24.5 Maximum extension 2 years post-surgery

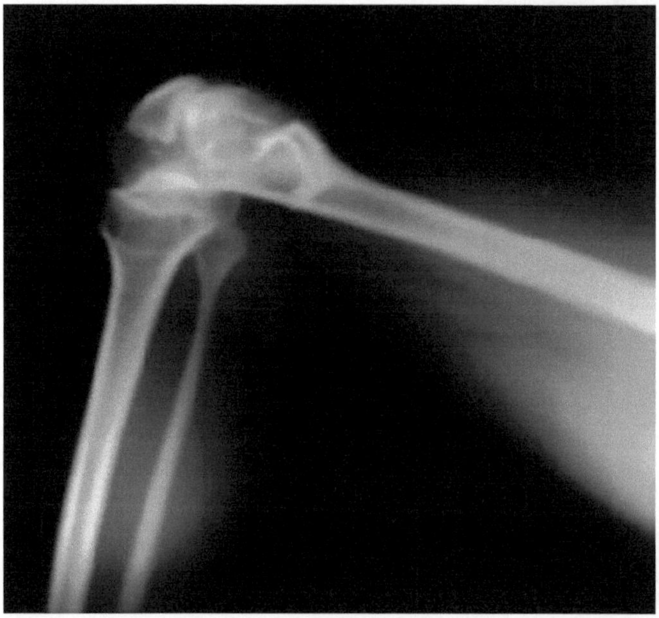

Fig. 24.6 Maximum flexion 2 years post-surgery

Suggested Readings

Canale ST, Campbell WC (2003) Campbell's operative orthopaedics 10th edition. Mosby, Philadelphia, 1:918–936

Caviglia HA, Perez-Bianco R, Galatro G et al (1999)Extensor supracondylar femoral osteotomy as treatment for flexed haemophilic knee. Haemophilia 5(Suppl 1):28–32

Caviglia HA, Rodríguez-Merchán EC (1994) An algorithm for the treatment of knee flexion contracture in haemophiliacs. In: Recent advances in rehabilitation in haemophilia. Medical education network sussex UK, 6:39–43

Insall JN, Scott WN (2001) Surgery of the knee. Churchill Livingstone, Philadelphia, 1134–1149

Rodríguez-Merchán EC (2002) Orthopaedic surgery of haemophilia in the 21st century: an overview. Haemophilia 8:360–368

Rodríguez-Merchán EC (1999) Therapeutic options in the management of articular contractures in haemophiliacs. Haemophilia 5:5–9

Rodríguez-Merchán EC (1999) Correction of fixed contractures during total knee arthroplasty in haemophiliacs. Haemophilia 5(Suppl 1):33–38

Schultz W (1999) Osteotomies near the knee joint – indications, operations, results. Arthroskopie 12:22–28

Wallny T, Saker A, Hofmann P (2003) Long-term follow-up after osteotomy for haemophilic arthropathy of the knee. Haemophilia 9:69–75

Chapter 25

Supracondylar Extension Osteotomy for the Treatment of Fixed Knee Flexion Contracture in Hemophiliac Patients

S.M. Javad Mortazavi

Introduction

Articular contractures in patients with hemophilia are the result of recurrent intra-articular and intramuscular hemorrhage [1, 2]. Since the knee is the joint that is most frequently affected in hemophiliac patients, flexion contracture of the knee is a frequent pathology in these individuals [2]. The muscular imbalance caused by repetitive hemarthrosis sometimes results in fixed flexion contracture in the hemophilic knee [3]. The extension deficiency not only leads to pressure peaks and progressive arthropathy, but it also increases the rate of hemarthrosis in the same joint and in the joints of other extremities [4]. On the other hand, this fixed flexion contracture of the knee results in secondary contractures in the same limb, including equinus deformity of the ankle, and flexion contracture of the hip and lumbar hyperlordosis. In addition, fixed flexion contracture of the knee intervenes with the patient's normal walking. In severe unilateral cases, the patient has to use an assistance device for walking, and in bilateral cases patients may become wheelchair bound. Therefore, flexion deformity of the knee should be corrected as soon as possible. This aim can be achieved conservatively by physiotherapy or mechanical corrective devices such as a wedging cast, and extension de-subluxation devices [2, 5, 6], or if these measures fail, operatively by different surgical methods [3, 4, 6–9].

Advanced or severe cases often require surgical correction in the form of soft tissue procedures, osteotomies, or mechanical distraction devices. Soft tissue procedures (hamstring release) are often insufficient to gain full correction [3, 4]. Also, mechanical distraction using external fixators is an effective way to correct deformity, with advantages such as as versatility and low risk of neurovascular complication [7]; it also has potential disadvantages including rebound phenomena after frame removal, decreased range of motion, and subluxation, and it is time consuming. Supracondylar extension osteotomy of the femur is a procedure that can be used to correct severe deformity [8]. This method may have several disadvantages. It creates a secondary deformity (shortening and angulation), and may lead to abnormal joint-loading forces in ambulatory patients [1]. It also makes the future total knee arthroplasty difficult, by

H.A. Caviglia, L.P. Solimeno (eds.), *Orthopedic Surgery in Patients with Hemophilia.*

distorting the anatomy of the distal end of the femur. In spite of these flaws, acute correction of the deformity, improvement in the patient's walking in both unilateral and bilateral cases, and an increase in total arc of motion of the joint in some patients are important advantages of this procedure. On the other hand, correction of deformity decreases the rate of hemorrhage in the same joint and the other joints.

We introduce a new technique of supracondylar extension osteotomy in which we use a trapezoidal wedge resection instead of a triangular one. This type of wedge resection not only decreases the rate of neurovascular injuries during the procedure, but also helps to release the extensor mechanism and increase the range of motion of the affected knee.

Indication

Supracondylar extension osteotomy is indicated for patients with severe fixed flexion contracture of the knee of more than 30°, which remains unchanged in spite of 3 months' conservative treatment.

Pre-operative Planning

Pre-operative planning is essential in this procedure. We recommend that the procedure should not be performed during the course of acute hemorrhage. The amount of deformity should be measured clinically using a goniometer (Fig. 25.1).

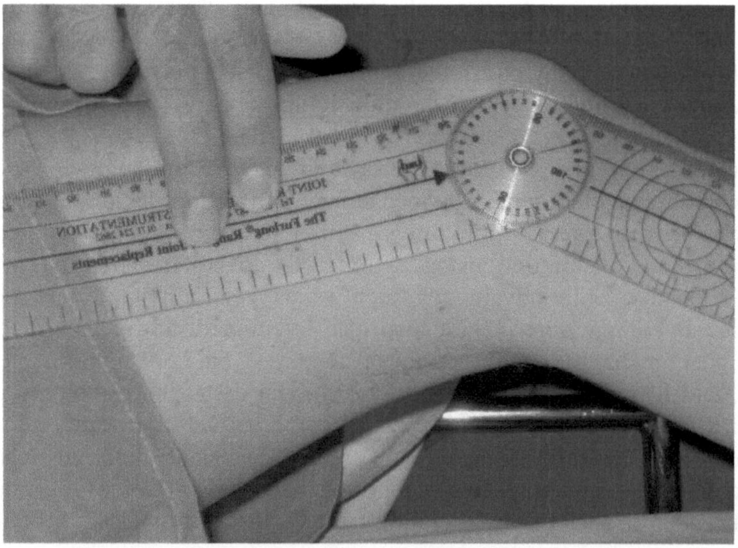

Fig. 25.1 Measurement of flexion contracture using a goniometer

It is best to measure the deformity while the patient allows his leg to fall at the side of the bed and tries to extend his knee as much as possible. By doing this, the femur is parallel to the bed and the measurement will be more accurate. Then good-quality true anteroposterior and lateral radiographs of the involved knee should be obtained. The true lateral radiograph of the knee should be performed in maximum possible correction of the flexion deformity. Then the optimum site for osteotomy should be determined. The osteotomy should be made as near the joint as possible. The more distal the osteotomy, the greater the chance of union, and the lower the risk of secondary deformity. On the other hand, in patients with open growth plate we prefer to put the osteotomy site and fixation device above the physis.

Planning starts after determining the site of the osteotomy. Firstly, the angle of deformity should be measured again. It can be easily assessed by drawing the axes of the femur and tibia in lateral radiographs. Then at the planned osteotomy site, a line should be drawn perpendicular to the longitudinal axis of the femur on a lateral radiograph. This line will be the bisector of the trapezoidal wedge. Then the trapezoidal wedge can be illustrated with a 0.5–1 cm base on the posterior cortex (the more severe the deformity, the larger the base), and two equal superior and inferior lines which make equal angles (half of the correction angle) with the bisector line (Fig. 25.2). Adequate factor replacement is, obviously, essential during and after surgery.

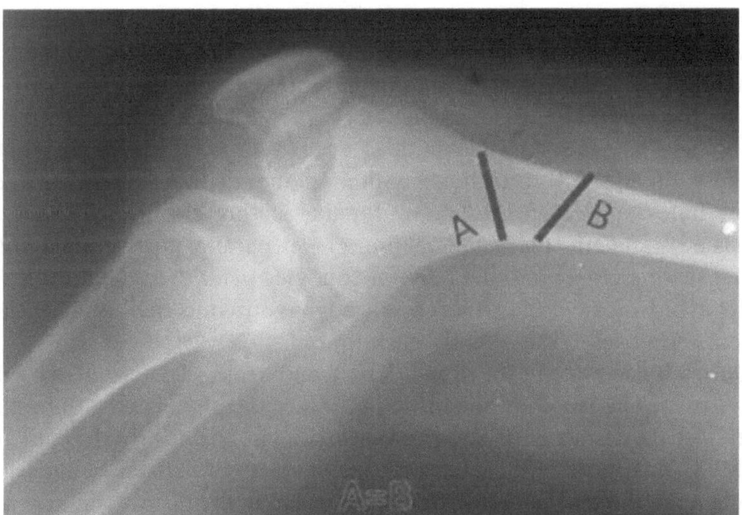

Fig. 25.2 Pre-operative planning to determine the site of the osteotomy and the size of the wedge

Surgical Technique

Place the patient supine on a radiolucent table and prepare and drape the entire injured extremity. Apply and inflate a tourniquet. Make a lateral longitudinal incision of 10 cm parallel to the shaft of the femur starting just proximal to the lateral femoral condyle. Divide the fascia lata and the vastus lateralis muscle and retract the latter anteriorly. Try to keep your dissection between the muscle and lateral intermuscular septum to save the muscles as much as possible. Then subperiosteally expose the supracondylar area of the femur laterally, and anteriorly and posteriorly.

According to the pre-operative planning, the site of the trapezoidal wedge should be marked on the lateral femoral cortex. The next step is placement of your fixation device which is usually an AO condylar blade plate. To obtain anatomical alignment, the seating chisel must be inserted accurately in the coronal, axial, and sagittal planes simultaneously. To accomplish this, insert a Kirschner wire transversely through the knee joint parallel to the surface of the tibial condyles to serve as a guide to the condylar articular surface. Pass a second Kirschner wire transversely posterior to the center of the patella, and a third Kirschner wire 1 cm above the articular surface of the lateral femoral condyle parallel to the first Kirschner wire. This wire should lie parallel to both the first and second wires, and serve as a guide for the blade of the condylar plate. Check the position using the AO condylar template if the AO condylar blade plate is being used.

Then the most important step of the procedure, placement of the chisel in the appropriate position, should be performed. The guide pin should clear the site of the chisel in both the coronal and axial planes, but the rotation of the chisel round the guide pin determines the corrected sagittal plane. As a rule of thumb, hold the knee in the maximum corrected position, then put the put the blade of the condylar blade plate on the third pin and rotate it until its side plate becomes parallel to the longitudinal axis of the leg (Fig. 25.3). This is the correct position for the blade. Place the AO triple guide sleeve parallel to the third Kirschner wire in this position and drill three holes with a 4.5 mm drill. Use a router to expand the three holes and create a window for the seating chisel. To ensure proper three-plane alignment, place the seating chisel parallel to the tibial shaft and insert the seating chisel into the femoral condyles parallel to the third Kirschner wire. To avoid incarcerating the chisel, advance it into the condyles in 1 cm increments and back it out slightly each time.

Choose a blade plate of the proper length and depth as determined by the preoperative plan. The length of the blade portion of the plate is critical because the distal end of the femur is narrower anteriorly than posteriorly. In patients with hemophilia, it is more critical because the shape of the distal femur is significantly changed in these patients. On the other hand, the distal femur seems larger on anteroposterior radiographs because the flexion contracture increases the distance of the distal femur from the cassette, and this results in magnification. On anteroposterior X-ray, the end of the blade should be approximately 8–10

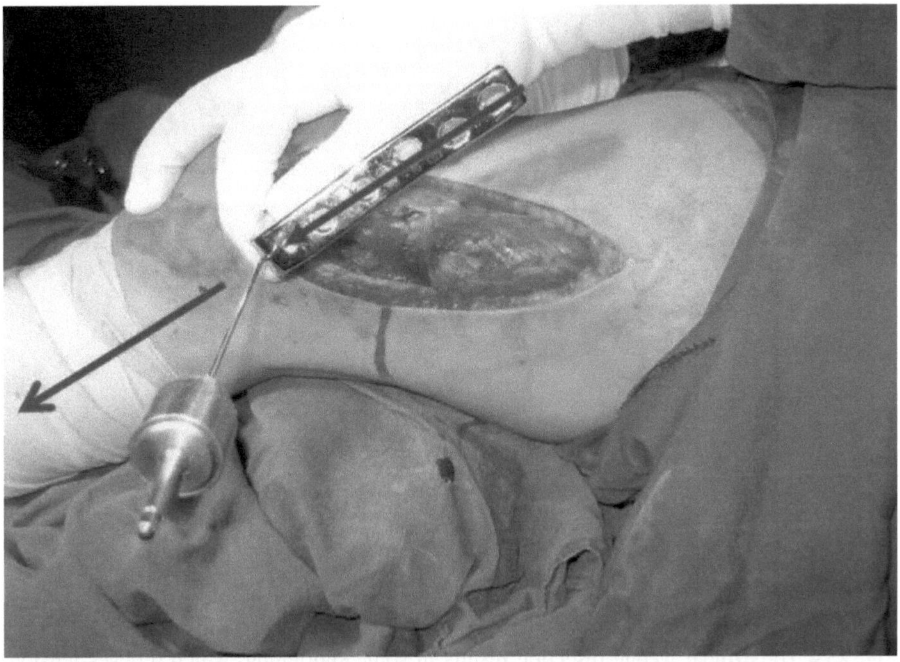

Fig. 25.3 As a rule of thumb, to determine the rotation of the angle blade while inserting, put the side plate along the long axis of the leg when the knee is placed in maximum possible extension

mm short of the medial cortex to prevent penetration and resultant irritation of the tibial collateral ligament. The proper length of the blade can be measured by drilling a hole adjacent to the blade and measuring with a depth gauge. Insert the 95° AO condylar blade plate into the path created by the chisel without fully seating it. With a reciprocating motor saw, cut the lateral, anterior, and posterior cortices of the proximal and distal borders of the trapezoidal wedge (Fig. 25.4). It seems to be safer to cut the medial cortices using osteotomes or rongeurs.

After removal of the wedge, correct the deformity, then fully seat the condylar blade plate and secure the side plate the femoral shaft with a bone clamp. At this point you should release the tourniquet and check the vascular status of the limb. If there is any problem, further shortening is essential to relieve the tension of the neurovascular structure. This shortening is best done by removing slices of bone parallel to the proximal cutting edge. If no vascular problem is observed, obtain meticulous hemostasis at this point using electrocautery. Then inflate the tourniquet again and secure the side plate to the femoral shaft with 4.5 mm cortical screws (Fig. 25.5a and b). After irrigation, close the wound in routine fashion over a suction drainage tube. Apply a large bulky dressing and then a long posterior plaster splint in 20° of knee flexion as an external support.

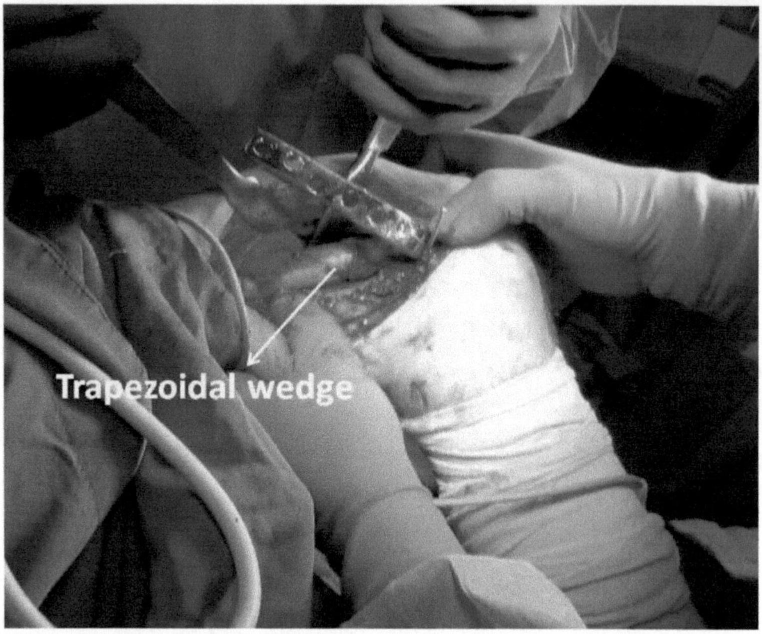

Fig. 25.4 Trapezoidal wedge resection results in some shortening, which relieves tension from the neurovascular bundle after correction

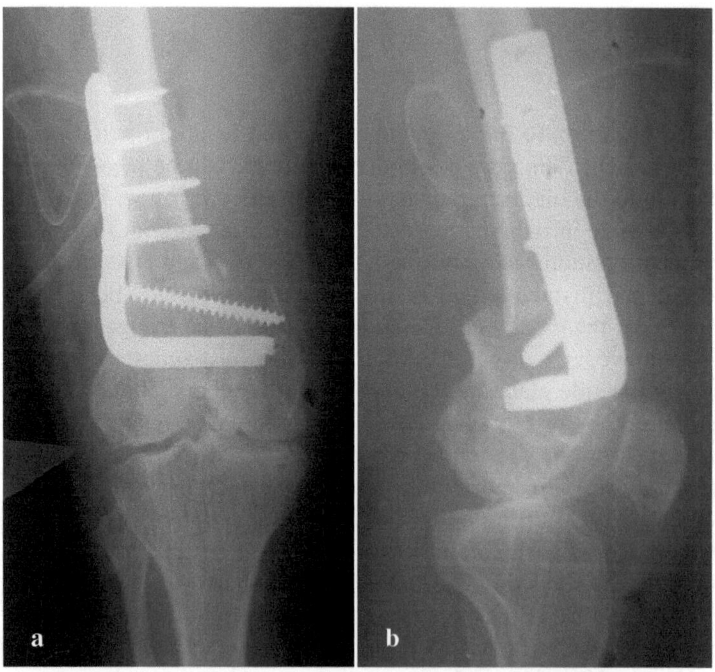

Fig. 25.5 Post-operative radiographs: **a** anteroposterior, **b** lateral

Rehabilitation

Active quadriceps and hamstring exercises are started 2 days after surgery. Range-of-motion exercises also can begin at this time if fixation is stable.

References

1. Rodríguez-Merchán EC (1999) Therapeutic options in the management of articular contractures in haemophiliacs. Haemophilia 5(1):5–9
2. Fernandez-Palazzi F, Battistella LR (1999) Non-operative treatment of flexion contracture of the knee in haemophilia. Haemophilia 5(19):20–24
3. Rodríguez-Merchán EC, Magallon M, Galindo E, Lopez-Cabarcos C (1997) Hamstring release for fixed knee flexion contracture in hemophilia. Clin Orthop 343:63–67
4. Wallny T, Eickhoff HH, Raderschadt G, Brackmann HH (1999) Hamstring release and posterior capsulotomy for fixed knee flexion contracture in haemophiliacs. Haemophilia 5(1):25–27
5. Kale JS, Ghosh K, Mohanty D et al (2000) Use of the dual force system to correct chronic knee deformities due to severe haemophilia. Haemophilia 6(3):177–180
6. Heijnen L, De Kleijn (1999) Physiotherapy for the treatment of articular contractures in haemophilia. Haemophilia 5(1):16–19
7. Kiely PD, McMahon C, Smith OP, Moore DP (2003) The treatment of flexion contracture of the knee using the Ilizarov technique in a child with haemophilia B. Haemophilia 9(3):336–339
8. Caviglia HA, Perez-Bianco R, Galatro G et al (1999) Extensor supracondylar femoral osteotomy as treatment for flexed haemophilic knee. Haemophilia 5(1):28–32
9. Rodríguez-Merchán EC (1999) Correction of fixed contractures during total knee arthroplasty in haemophiliacs. Haemophilia 5(1):33–38

Chapter 26
Primary Total Knee Replacement

Jerome Wiedel

Introduction

With the long-term success of total knee arthroplasties performed for osteoarthritis, and the availability of factor concentrates allowing safe major surgical procedures to be performed in hemophilia, total knee arthroplasty is considered the procedure of choice for the patient with chronic hemophilic arthropathy of the knee. The primary indication for total knee arthroplasty in a person with hemophilia is severe disabling pain. Deformity and poor functional range of motion are contributing indications, and may by themselves be the main indication when severe pain is not present.

The characteristics of chronic hemophilic arthropathy of the knee are restricted range of motion and fixed deformities causing severe functional impairment. Pain due to the advanced degenerative arthritic condition contributes to the loss of function.

The most common deformity associated with chronic hemophilic arthropathy of the knee is a fixed flexion contracture. This develops because the painful knee assumes a flexed position for comfort. With recurrent bleeding episodes, the patient with hemophilia will tend to keep the knee in a flexed position for comfort, and as the disease progresses with severe cartilage and subchondral bone damage the knee eventually assumes a fixed position of flexion.

Although flexion contracture may exist alone, it is probably more common to have associated deformities, particularly external rotation and posterior subluxation of the tibia on the femur. With these deformities a valgus deformity is common. Associated with each of these deformities is contracture of the soft tissue structures on the concave side of the deformity. With the severe destruction of articular cartilage and subchondral bone damage due to cysts and erosions, asymmetric bone loss may also be seen on the concave side of the deformity.

The evaluation of a person with hemophilia who is facing a total knee arthroplasty requires a thorough physical examination of the affected lower extremity. This begins by observing the patient's gait and his ability to change positions, particularly from seated to standing positions. Associated deformities at the hip, foot, and ankle, and of the opposite extremity should be documented. It is not

H.A. Caviglia, L.P. Solimeno (eds.), *Orthopedic Surgery in Patients with Hemophilia*.

uncommon to see multiple joint involvement, which will greatly influence surgical decision making.

Specific aspects of the knee examination should include defining the type of deformity and determining if it is passively correctable or whether it is a fixed deformity. Both passive and active range of motion should be measured and recorded. Particular attention must be paid to the extensor mechanism. This includes observing for the degree of quadriceps atrophy, the degree of tendon and capsular contracture, and the position and mobility of the patella.

Radiographic evaluation of the knee should include an anteroposterior and lateral standing view, and a notch and sunrise view. It is preferable that this should include both knees. If possible, the anteroposterior view should be taken on a long film, which would include the hip to the ankle. The important radiographic features to evaluate in preparation for the surgical procedure include the deformity and associated bone loss. The information that is gathered from this observation will help determine the need for soft tissue release and also the potential need for accommodating bone loss with either bone graft or prosthetic augmentation. Common findings in chronic hemophilic arthropathy are large subchondral bone cysts which may need bone graft augmentation. Segmental bone loss of femoral or tibial surfaces may require prosthetic augmentation or structural allograft.

It is very important to determine the status of the patellofemoral joint radiographically, as this will provide important information regarding the surgical approach as well as the functional outcome. The patellofemoral joint may present in two abnormal ways. One is a lateral subluxation of the patella and the other is a central location of the patella, but with erosion centrally into the patellar groove of the femur.

Prior to considering any major surgical intervention in a person with hemophilia, medical clearance must be obtained. A thorough medical evaluation by the hematologist should be performed. Basic studies include factor levels, testing for the presence of inhibitors, liver function studies, and viral studies, which should include HIV and hepatitis C (HCV). The presence of an inhibitor is considered a contraindication to elective surgery. A patient with known viral disease (HIV and HCV) must be medically stable. This surgery, when performed, should be done in a hemophilia center where a comprehensive team approach can be provided.

Surgical Technique

In preparation for the surgery, appropriate factor concentrate should be given immediately pre-operatively to achieve a 100% level during surgery. Peri-operative antibiotic prophylaxis should begin with the first dose administered 30 min prior to tourniquet inflation. Antibiotics should be continued for 48 h post-operatively. The procedure should be performed under tourniquet control and the entire involved lower extremity should be draped free to allow full visualization of the leg.

The skin incision is made vertically and midline, with the length depending on the need. The capsule is entered through a medial parapatellar incision extending from the tibial tubercle distally to the superior pole of the patella. At this point a surgeon's choice is either to extend the capsular incision along the quadriceps tendon proximally, or to extend the incision in line with the fibers of the vastus medialis obliquus. The decision on the direction of the proximal extension of the deep incision will be the surgeon's preference, but will also be determined by the condition of the quadriceps muscle and tendon unit. If severe intra-articular fibrosis and extensor mechanism contracture exists, a release of the extensor mechanism will be necessary in order to gain adequate exposure to the joint. The choices for releasing the quadriceps contracture are a proximal release or a distal tibial tubercle osteotomy. A proximal release would involve cutting the quadriceps tendon in a V–Y fashion, or performing a quadriceps snip. Releasing the extensor mechanism with a tibial tubercle osteotomy has the advantage that it does not disturb the quadriceps mechanism as a proximal muscle release would.

Once the extensor mechanism is mobilized by whatever method, it can be retracted laterally providing full exposure of the distal femur and the proximal tibia. At this time débridement of the joint should be performed, removing any residual chronic hemophilic synoviums, and prominent marginal osteophytes from the distal femur and proximal tibia.

The following steps are probably the most common ones used for performing the bony cuts at the knee; however, the surgeon should be prepared to change the routine based upon any difficulties encountered at any time in the procedure. Cutting the patella first helps relieve some of the tension encountered when the extensor mechanism and the patella are retracted laterally. Cutting of the distal femur is the next step, and if a significant flexion contracture exists, I usually remove an additional 2 mm of distal femur from the standard amount that is recommended for a normal resection. An intramedullary alignment system is used for the distal femur providing there are no deformities of the shaft, otherwise an extramedullary system would have to be used.

I next resect the proximal tibia using an extramedullary system. Having resected both the distal femur and the proximal tibia, additional mobility of the joint is possible which provides better exposure so that one can complete the preparation of the distal femur and proximal tibia.

At this time the flexion and extension spaces created by the surgical bone resections need to be measured. The soft tissue contractures that are identified when measuring the flexion and extension will have to be addressed. For the valgus and external rotation contractures, the lateral capsule including the posterior arcuate ligament complex, the iliotibial band, popliteus tendon, and lateral collateral ligaments need to be evaluated. Initially a complete capsular release is accomplished from the entire lateral margin of the tibia. If the popliteal tendon is contracted it is released from its femoral attachment. The posterior arcuate ligament complex must be released and this may require developing a subperiosteal flap that extends proximally into the lateral intermuscular septum of the distal femur. Flexion contracture requires a posterior capsulotomy by releasing the posterior capsule close to the posterior aspect of the femur. A posterior cruciate ligament resection will be necessary in most cases when a flexion contracture is present, and particularly if associated posterior subluxation of the tibia on the femur is recognized. During the release of the posterior structures, the knee should be flexed at 90° with distraction of the joint. Once the soft tissue release has been performed and the flexion and extension gaps are made equal, trial prosthetic components should be placed for determining the alignment, soft tissue balance, and range of motion. The extensor mechanism with the prosthetic patella must be centrally located and tracking without subluxation. Lateral release may be necessary.

Bone loss, which was assessed as the bony cuts were made, has to be managed based upon the type of loss. A contained lesion such as a subchondral cyst may be filled with impaction bone grafting. Small defects may be filled with the bone cement used for the stabilization of the implanted prosthesis. Large segmental areas of bone loss will require either a structural bone graft or the use of prosthetic augments.

Prior to implantation of the implants I recommend that the tourniquet be deflated, which will allow controlling of bleeding with full view of the joint. Once hemostasis has been obtained, the tourniquet can be reinflated if the implants are to be cemented. The surgeon may want to consider using antibiotic-impregnated cement.

After the final implantation and irrigation of the joint, I place a wound drain which should be kept in place and functioning for 24–48 h post-operatively. Closure of the soft tissues is performed in a stepwise fashion, first using non-absorbable sutures to repair the capsule and extensor mechanism. Once this is completed, a range of motion of the knee should be performed passively to test the repair and to be certain that the extensor mechanism tracks centrally. Skin closure is probably best done with metal staples. The post-operative dressing should include a large compressive dressing and the knee should be immobilized with a splint holding the leg in extension for the first 24 –48 h. After that time, with supervised therapy, flexion should be encouraged; however, careful attention should be given to maintaining extension as there is a tendency for the patient to keep the leg in a flexed position because this is the position of comfort. Although the use of the continuous passive motion (CPM) machine is helpful in gaining flexion, it is difficult to obtain extension in a CPM machine. The CPM machine should, therefore, be only used intermittently on a daily basis, and initial emphasis should be on gaining active knee extension. It is expected that a fairly prolonged rehabilitation period will be necessary for the patient to obtain complete recovery. Goals of the total knee replacement are to gain pain relief and to improve the functional range of motion. Gaining and maintaining the functional range of motion will be the most difficult thing the patient encounters in this procedure and he must understand this before undertaking it.

It is important for the patient, surgeon, and physiotherapists to understand that a gain in range of motion is not usually obtained. What is important to understand is that the range that is obtained should be a functional range of motion, meaning 0° extension to the best level of flexion that the patient can obtain. Usually the amount of flexion obtained is determined by the status of the extension mechanism. The goal is flexion past 90°.

Suggested Readings

Goddard NJ, Rodriguez-Merchan EC, Wiedel JD (2002) Total knee replacement in haemophilia. Haemophilia 8(3):382-386

Rodríguez-Merchán EC (2007) Total joint arthroplasty: the final solution for knee and hip when synovitis could not be controlled. Haemophilia 13(3):49-58

Silva M, Luck JV Jr.(2005) Long-term results of primary total knee replacement in patients with hemophilia. JBJS 87(1):85-91

Chapter 27
Pitfalls in Primary Total Knee Replacement

Adolfo Llinás

Introduction

Total knee replacement is a demanding surgical procedure, with high morbidity and cost. Often patients and their families as well as healthcare personnel experience a false perception of low risk, extrapolating from the rather uneventful operative and post-operative courses of primary total knee replacement in the non-hemophiliac patient. When performed in hemophilia treatment centers in the hands of experts, a total knee arthroplasty may yield moderate results, with infection rates of about 13% in HIV-negative patients and survival rates of about 77% at 10 years [1–3]. However, reproducing these results requires a sophisticated medical environment and an experienced hemophilia treatment group. An inexperienced surgeon may engage in this procedure, wrongly assuming that as long as the patient's coagulopathy has been corrected, everything else will be the same as in a non-hemophiliac patient. This is not the case. Total knee arthroplasty in the hemophiliac requires additional planning, deviation from the standard surgical routine, and familiarity with a combination of technical difficulties seldom found in other conditions. My purpose in this chapter is to outline the technical difficulties that co-exist in total knee arthroplasty in hemophilia, so the reader may prepare for the surgical procedure.

Idiosyncratic Elements of Total Knee Arthroplasty in the Hemophiliac Patient

Approach

A three-dimensional deformity of the knee is often the first difficulty the surgeon will encounter, with ankylosis or considerable loss of range of motion, a flexion contracture, and some angulation and/or translation of the tibia. An ample exposure will be needed to address any of the aforementioned conditions. A semicircular osteotome will aid in the development of a joint line in case of fusion or ankylosis.

H.A. Caviglia, L.P. Solimeno (eds.), *Orthopedic Surgery in Patients with Hemophilia*.

When the ankylosis or severe loss of range of motion is associated with scarring of the quadriceps, the surgeon should foresee difficulty in achieving flexion during surgery, and later during rehabilitation. If a quadriceplasty will be considered at a later point, performing it at the beginning of the procedure will allow the surgeon to bring the quadricipital tendon and the patella down, making the exposure of the femur and tibia easier (Fig. 27.1). Dislocating the patella and bringing the knee into deep flexion is also troublesome, placing the insertion of the patellar tendon on the tibia at risk. Alternatively, the surgeon may consider elevating the tibial tubercle to aid exposure and prevent avulsion.

Definition of the Location of the Joint Line

A common finding in severe arthropathy of patients, who bleed into the joint early in childhood, is a patella baja or infera. Therefore, before starting the bone cuts the surgeon must decide whether the joint line of the arthroplasty will be placed where it belongs or if it must be lowered artificially, to prevent the lower pole of the patella or the patellar component from impinging on the tibial insert. Typically, there is little room to maneuver, since the fibular head is often prominent,

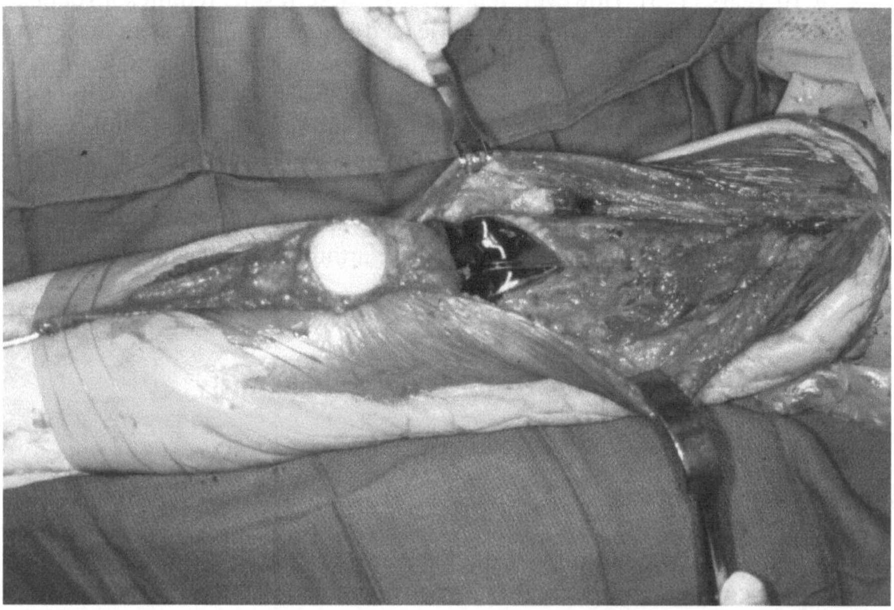

Fig. 27.1 When the ankylosis or severe loss of range of motion is associated with scarring of the quadriceps, the surgeon should foresee difficulty in achieving flexion during surgery, and later, during rehabilitation. If a quadriceplasty will be considered at a later point, performing it at the beginning of the procedure will allow the quadricipital tendon and the patella to be brought down, making the exposure of the femur and tibia easier

resulting from bone loss of the tibial plateau; consequently, in order to lower the joint line at the expense of tibial bone, a partial resection of the fibular head should be performed. One should avoid contact of the fibular head with the tibial tray to prevent pain during ambulation, since there is motion at the tibiofibular proximal joint with gait. Alternatively, the patellar button may be placed eccentrically, displacing it proximally to move it away from the tibial polyethylene.

Bone Cuts

The surgical feel of the bone cuts in the hemophilic knee is reminiscent of that felt during revision surgery. Some of the anatomic landmarks for orientation of the guides will be absent, and when attempting to cut through some of the guide slots, the saw blade will only find air on the opposite side. The surgeon must be prepared to use augmentation blocks or structural bone graft even in primary knee replacement.

The Femur

One of the most challenging idiosyncratic elements of the hemophilic knee is the disproportion between the mediolateral dimension and the anteroposterior dimension of the femur. The former is usually large and the latter small, forcing the surgeon to compromise while sizing the implant (Fig. 27.2). Under these conditions, sizing the knee requires additional care, since the anteroposterior dimension may seem artificially small because of the wear of the posterior condyles or the presence of a deep patellofemoral groove (Fig. 27.3). If striking a balance

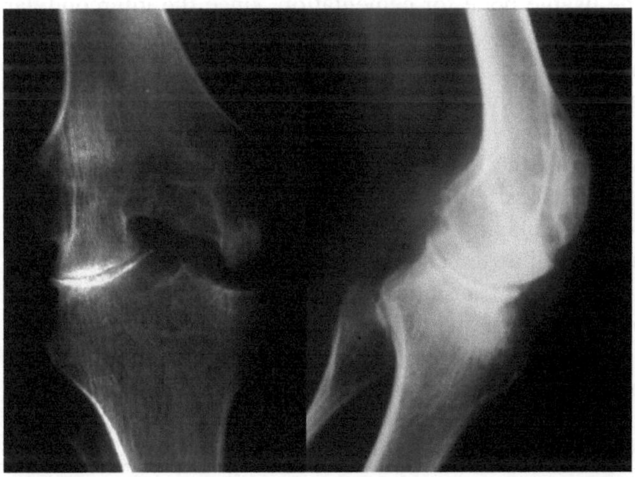

Fig. 27.2 One of the most challenging idiosyncratic elements of the hemophilic knee is the disproportion between the mediolateral dimension and the anteroposterior dimension of the femur. The former is usually large and the latter small, forcing the surgeon to compromise while sizing the implant

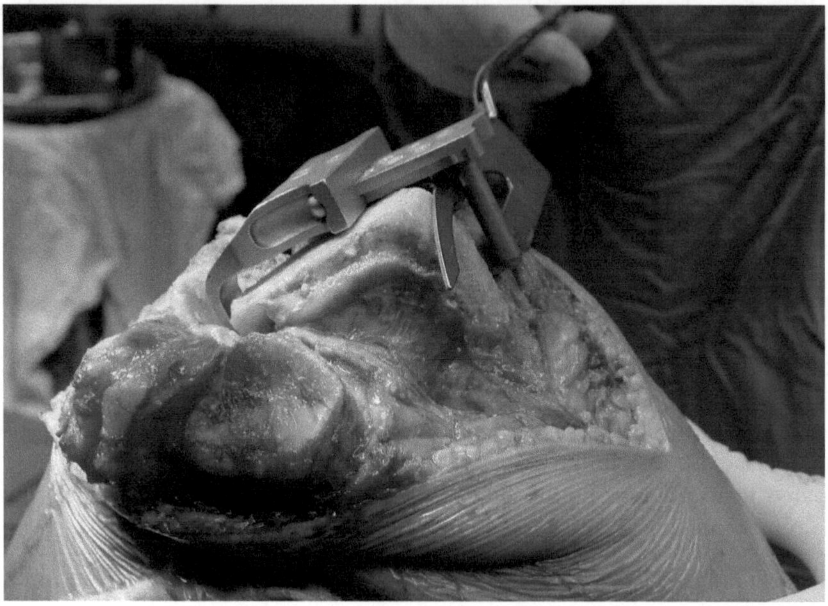

Fig. 27.3 Sizing guides usually take into account only the anteroposterior dimension, thus undersizing the femoral component. Note the angel-wing probe being placed under the guide to prevent it falling into a deep — pathological — femoral groove, again running the risk of biasing the measurement towards undersizing

between the two dimensions is not possible, posterior augmentation or grafting of the femoral condyles will be required.

Oversizing the femoral component will result in a tight flexion gap due to the shortness of the collateral ligaments in flexion and in difficulty in achieving extension because of the lack of posterior space to accommodate them and the resulting posterior capsule tightness. Undersizing the femoral component will result in a decrease in the usable bone for cementation, since the intercondylar notch is usually large and the mediolateral dimension of the implant small. The possibility of a tibiofemoral mismatch has to be addressed before making a final selection of the femoral component, for undersizing the tibial tray is not an option, if long-term survival of the implant is a concern.

The small anteroposterior of the femur may be the result of small posterior condyles and a deep patellofemoral groove. This combination is especially difficult to handle, because while placing the guide required to make the anterior and posterior femoral cut as well as the chamfer cuts, the surgeon may inadvertently slide it posterior. A posterior translation of the cutting guide will produce a posterior translation of all the cuts, and during the final anterior cut there will be a high probability of producing notching of the anterior distal femoral cortex. If the guide is placed correctly in this circumstance, the saw will only find bone to cut when in the chamfer slots. Anterior augmentation with bone graft or cement may be required in addition to posterior augmentation.

The increased width and depth of the intercondylar notch, as well as the low density of bone in this area, requires attention to prevent fractures extending to the supracondylar region during femoral component impaction. This is more apparent when using components with large intercondylar boxes such as semi-constrained implants.

Decades of wear of the distal femoral condyles results in a unique condition seldom seen elsewhere in arthroplastic surgery, where the distance from the insertion of the femoral collateral ligaments to the joint line is short, such that the regular distal femoral cut may injure the collateral ligament insertion. This may require partial elevation of the insertion of the collateral ligaments to avoid injury by the oscillating saw during distal femoral condyle resection (Fig. 27.4).

The Tibia

A three-dimensional tibial proximal metaphyseal deformity is the norm in patients who bled in early childhood. Centering the tibial cutting guide on the leg may seem awkward, because the shaft of the guide will not align harmonically with the diaphysis of the leg. It is critical to focus on a perpendicular cut

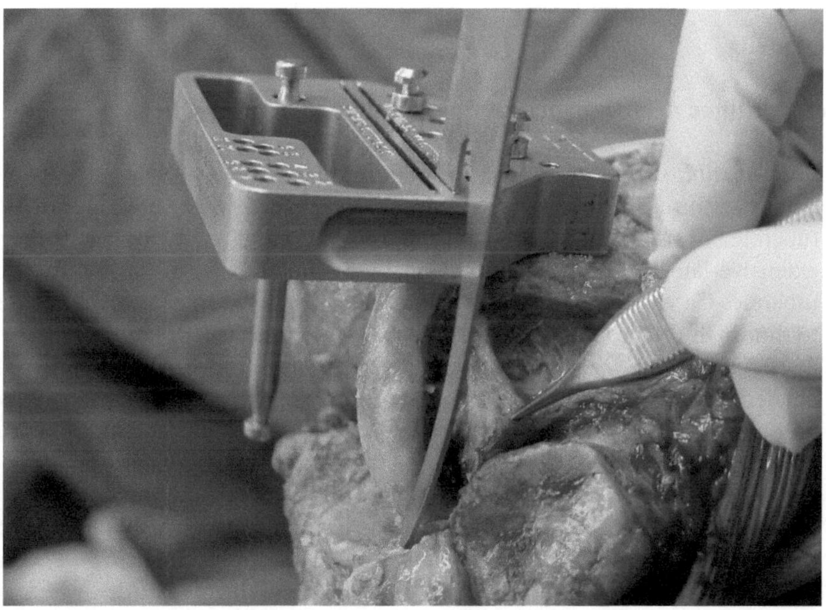

Fig. 27.4 Decades of wear of the distal femoral condyles results in a unique condition seldom seen elsewhere in arthroplastic surgery, where the distance from the insertion of the femoral collateral ligaments to the joint line is short, such that the regular distal femoral cut may injure the collateral ligament insertion. This may require partial elevation of the insertion of the collateral ligaments to avoid injury by the oscillating saw during distal femoral condyle resection.

of the tibial plateaus in reference to a central placement to the shaft of the guide on the distal tibia, about the level of the ankle. Further confusion may arise from the lack of the normal posterior slope of the tibia, or from the presence of a reverse anterior slope of the tibia. These deformities arise from physeal abnormalities due to bleeding in infancy, or from the permanent knee extension efforts from casts and wedges, manipulation, or apparatus used to treat flexion contractures. The reverse tibial slope should be ignored and the tibia cut in the usual fashion, which in this case will produce a thick anterior wedge of bone.

The preparation of the proximal tibia for the keel of the tibial tray must be approached with care, and the same is true for placement of the trial component, for the medial tibial cortex may not allow full entry of the tibial tray's keel. In this situation, a fracture of the medial tibial metaphysis may result or, alternatively, only partial seating of the tibial tray when cementing the permanent components.

Wear of the tibial plateaus during years of hemophilic arthrosis, but not of the proximal fibula, may make the proximal fibular head artificially prominent. Therefore, it may be necessary to trim the fibular head down to allow clearance between the proximal aspect of the tibial head and the tibial tray. The surgeon must resist the temptation to cement the tibial tray to the fibular head, since motion between the tibia and the fibula under load, and friction from the tibial tray may produce pain.

The Patella

There are three distinct patterns of patellofemoral abnormalities:

1. *Lateral subluxation or chronic dislocation*: these are usually associated with valgus deformities of the knee and a lateral placement of the anterior tibial tubercle. Consequently, achieving appropriate patellar tracking will require extensive lateral release, and occasionally medial transfer of the anterior tibial tubercle. Care should be taken to spare the supero-external geniculate artery, to diminish the probability of patellar necrosis and later fracture.
2. *Deepening of the femoral groove*: a deep femoral groove will not pose a big challenge when it comes to alignment of the extensor mechanism; however, it will make the placement of the first and second femoral guides difficult because of the lack of bone, and also will contribute to underestimating the anteroposterior dimension of the femur while sizing. Additionally, when the components are in place, and the patella is brought anteriorly by the new prosthetic femoral groove and patellar button, the extensor mechanism will become effectively shorter, and the patient will lose several degrees of flexion.
3. *Patella baja*: the combination of patella baja and worn tibial plateaus will leave little room for the required play to move away the tibial polyethylene insert from the lower pole of the patella. Lowering the joint line and proximal placement of the patellar button will be required to solve this problem. Lengthening of the patellar tendon should be avoided.

Often these patellofemoral abnormalities will be worsened by a small and/or thin patella that will require intra-operative customization of the patellar button, such as, drilling shallower bone anchor holes and shortening of the patellar pegs to prevent anterior cortical patellar penetration.

Ligament Balance

Operating on patients with flexion contractures and recutting the distal femur when the extension gap is inadequate is a frequent situation in knee arthroplasty. What is unique in hemophilia is the combination of wear of the distal femur and proximal tibia and the shortening of the collateral ligaments. Therefore, after all available distal femur and proximal tibia is resected, the leg will probably be in full extension, but without an extension gap. In this circumstance, there will be no room to fit the components, and after doing so, the flexion deformity will re-appear. This situation may be addressed with extensive, simultaneous distal-medial and proximal-lateral collateral ligament release, as well as with a proximal-posterior capsular release. This extensive dissection will be followed by considerable post-operative edema, pain, and the possibility of a large post-operative bleed within the first 10 days after surgery. When it is impossible to develop the extension gap, the collateral ligaments may be sectioned, the posterior capsule released, and a semi-constrained implant with femoral and tibial stems used (Fig. 27.5).

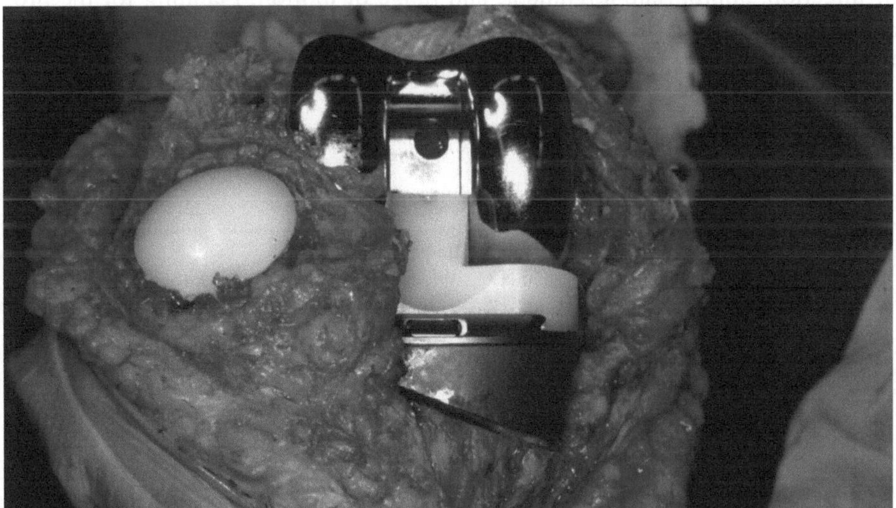

Fig. 27.5 A semi-constrained prosthesis was implanted because an adequate extension gap was not achieved. The collateral ligaments were sectioned and the posterior capsule released. Due to medial bone loss of the tibia, a full-width wedge was used, as well as a tibial stem

Procedure Checklist

The following are some elements to consider before embarking on a total knee replacement in a person with hemophilia:

- Template for the implant in the anteroposterior and lateral view. Emphasize the lateral view and beware of the need for small sizes.
- Verify the presence of femoral and tibial stems with built-in offset.
- Verify the presence of wedges and augmentation blocks for the femur and tibia.
- Use only antibiotic-loaded cement. If white, consider adding one drop of methylene blue per batch, because it makes removal of cement in case of revision easier.
- Plan having access to a semi-constrained prosthesis (one which substitutes the collateral ligaments) in case of collateral ligament rupture or inability to gain appropriate extension gap.
- Order structural bone graft if defects are not manageable with spacers or wedges.

Summary

Total knee arthroplasty in the person with hemophilia is a difficult procedure for the patient and surgeon. Predictably, the patient will get pain relief; however there is a large variation in the quality of other outcomes, for example, the lack of infection, appropriate alignment, and range of motion. Planning for the procedure and knowing the pitfalls associated with this condition should decrease the frequency of preventable adverse effects.

References

1. Cohen I, Heim M, Martinowitz U, Chechink A (2002) Orthopaedic outcome of total knee replacement in haemophilia A. Haemophilia 6(2):104–109
2. Goddard NJ, Rodríguez-Merchán EC, Wiedel JD (2002) Total knee replacement in haemophilia. Haemophilia 8(3):382–386
3. Silva M., Luck JV (2005) Long-term results of primary total knee replacement in patients with hemophilia. J Bone Joint Surg Am 87(1):85–91

Chapter 28

Arthroscopic Treatment of Hemophilic Arthropathy of the Ankle

Luigi P. Solimeno, Olivia Samantha Perfetto and Gianluigi Pasta

Introduction

In severe hemophiliacs, frequent bleeding and spontaneous hemarthroses occur. The ankle is a target joint in hemophiliac patients [1].

Repeated articular bleeding leads to hypertrophic and hypervascularized synovia. Almost simultaneously, the intra-articular bleeding produces proteolytic enzymes, cytokines, and oxygen metabolites which lead to direct damage of articular cartilage. Synovial and articular degenerative processes influence each other, contributing to end-stage hemophilic arthropathy. The clinical picture of hemarthrosis is characterized by pain, swelling, and restricted range of movement. Recurrent hemarthroses lead to significant hypertrophic synovitis with progressive restricted joint mobility, especially dorsiflexion, associated with soft tissue contracture, principally the Achilles' tendon. In the final stage of arthropathy there is significant functional impairment leading to subankylosis, which is often associated with reduced pain and bleeding.

Diagnosis

Standard X-ray generally leads to correct evaluation of articular involvement and allows us to use a staging system. We generally use the Pettersson score. If an anterior impingement is suspected, lateral dorsiflexion and plantar flexion views can help to confirm the diagnosis. Computerized tomography (CT) and magnetic resonance imaging (MRI) are useful for correct detection of subchondral cysts and soft tissue involvement.

Treatment

Conservative treatment has to be considered initially, and prophylactic treatment and a rehabilitation program are also recommended to reduce the frequency of hemarthrosis and preserve articular function

H.A. Caviglia, L.P. Solimeno (eds.), *Orthopedic Surgery in Patients with Hemophilia.*

Arthroscopic treatment is limited to initial arthropathy stages (Pettersson <5° to 6° [2]). In end-stage arthropathy, a prosthetic procedure or arthrodesis is necessary.

Open synovectomy is useful to reduce bleeding episodes, but has a high risk of subankylosis in the post-operative period.

Today we are able to speak of arthroscopic treatment in hemophiliac patients, because we not only perform synovectomy but also try to work on cartilage with condrectomy, coblation, and osteophyte removal, often with viscosupplementation.

It is important to perform a surgical procedure early in order to stop pathogenetic progression (synovial and cartilaginous) in the least-invasive way.

Surgical Technique

The factor levels are maintained at 80% for the operative procedure, and at approximately 50–80% for post-operative days 1 to 5.

The patient is placed supine in an arthroscopic leg holder, and a well-padded tourniquet is placed about the thigh.

The arthroscopic procedure is performed with manual distraction by anteromedial and anterolateral portals. Posterior portals are rarely necessary.

A 4 mm, 30° arthroscope is used. The procedure starts with the anterolateral portal where the arthroscope is introduced. In patients with extensive synovitis (Fig. 28.1), thorough observation of the joint requires the use of a full-radius resector (Fig. 28.2) through the anteromedial portal to perform partial synovectomy. In all patients a whisker-type blade should be used, but only after a better view has been obtained. We perform coblation in patients with early stages of arthropathy, and condrectomy and removal of osteophytes in patients with advanced stages of arthropathy.

When extensive synovectomy is performed, an intra-articular drain should be used and removed 24 h later.

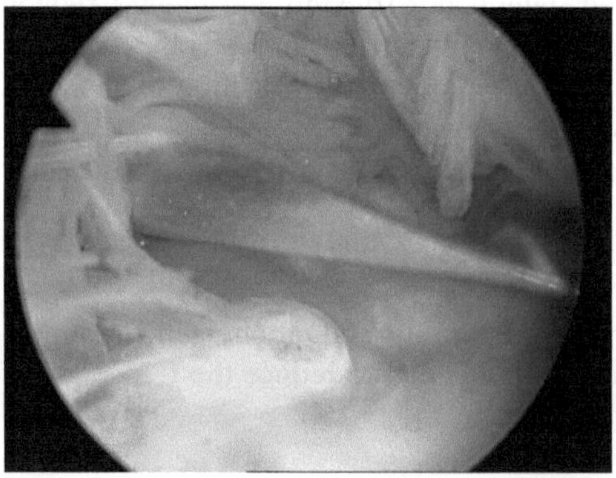

Fig. 28.1 Synovitis of the ankle

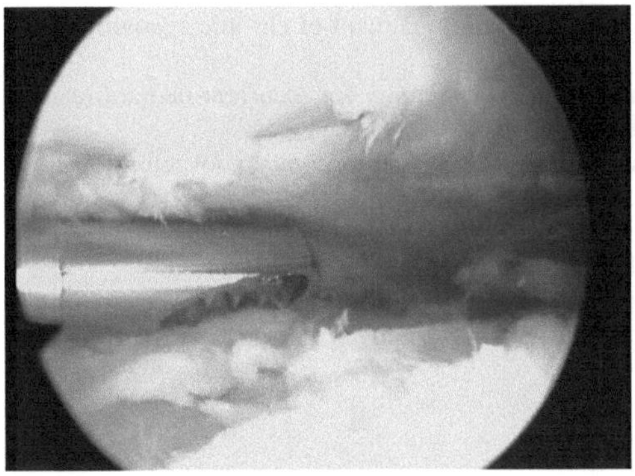

Fig. 28.2 The use of a full-radius resector to perform synovectomy

Post-operative Care

Post-operative care includes application of a compressive dressing and weight-bearing to tolerance with crutches for the first week. Then a progressive program of strengthening, range of motion, and functional agility exercises begins.

Results

Pain and the frequency of hemarthroses lessens considerably; the Pettersson score remains unchanged post-operatively. Any complications are recorded.

Conclusion

In our experience arthroscopic treatment of hemophilic arthropathy of the ankle provides a reduction of hemarthroses, with an unchanged or slightly augmented articular function.

Our findings coincide with those of the current international literature on radiographic evidence of halting articular degeneration [3–6].

Tamurian and coworkers [7] have demonstrated the economic benefits of reducing the frequency of bleeds, which diminishes the need for factor concentrate.

References

1. Gamble JG, Bellah J, Rinsky LA, Glader B (1991) Arthropathy of the ankle in hemophilia. J Bone Joint Surg Am 73:1008–1015
2. Pettersson H, Ahlberg A, Nilsson IM (1980) A radiological classification of hemophilic arthropathy. Clin Orthop 149:153–159

3. Martin DF, Curl WW, Baker CL (1989) Arthroscopic treatment of chronic synovitis of the ankle. Arthroscopy 5:110–114
4. Patti JE, Barry Mayo WE (1996) Arthroscopic synovectomy for recurrent hemarthrosis of the ankle in hemophilia. Arthroscopy 12(6):652–656
5. Journeycake JM, Miller KL, Anderson AM et al (2003) Arthroscopic synovectomy in children and adolescents with hemophilia. J Pediatr Hematol Oncol 25:726–731
6. Dunn AL, Busch MT, Wyly BJ et al (2004) Arthroscopic synovectomy for hemophilic joint disease in a pediatric population. J Pediatr Orthop 24:414–426
7. Tamurian RM, Spencer EE, Wojtys EM (2002) The role of arthroscopic synovectomy in the management of hemartrhosis in hemophilia patients: financial perspectives. Arthroscopy 18(7):789–794

Chapter 29

Surgical Resection of Osteophyte in the Ankle Joint

Horacio A. Caviglia, Pablo Nuova and Gustavo Galatro

Anterior osteophyte of the ankle can be located in the anterior part of the tibia bone or the superior part of the talus, and is secondary to arthropathy of the ankle joint.

Clinically, the patient shows limited dorsal flexion, which may also be seen in the equine position.

Diagnosis is by simple X-ray of the ankle joint from both frontal and lateral views. The anterior osteophyte is seen clearly, as shown in Figure 29.1.

Another X-ray view, taken in maximum dorsal flexion, allows us to see the impingement of the ankle joint (Fig. 29.2).

Surgery is needed when the patient experiences pain in the anterior part of the ankle while walking, which does not respond to physical therapy or oral analgesic. When the ankle X-ray does not show clear joint space, the patient is a candidate for arthrodesis. Pre-operative planning begins by determining the need for surgical excision of the tibia or talus osteophyte, or both.

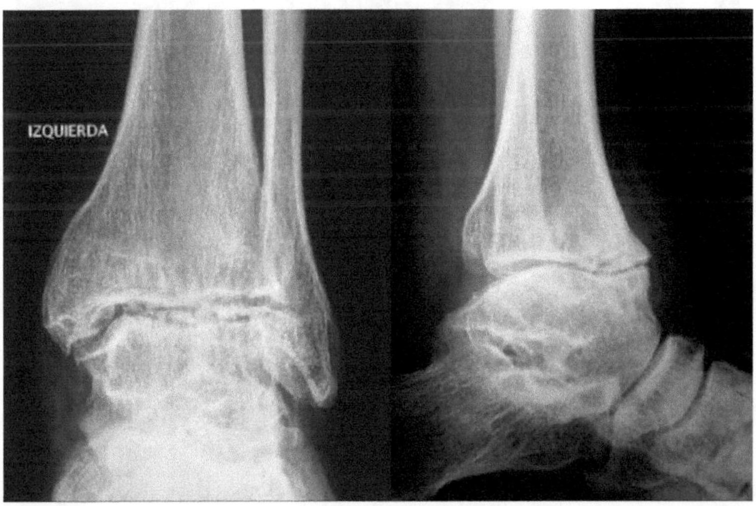

Fig. 29.1 Anterior osteophyte shown in X-ray of the ankle joint

H.A. Caviglia, L.P. Solimeno (eds.), *Orthopedic Surgery in Patients with Hemophilia.*

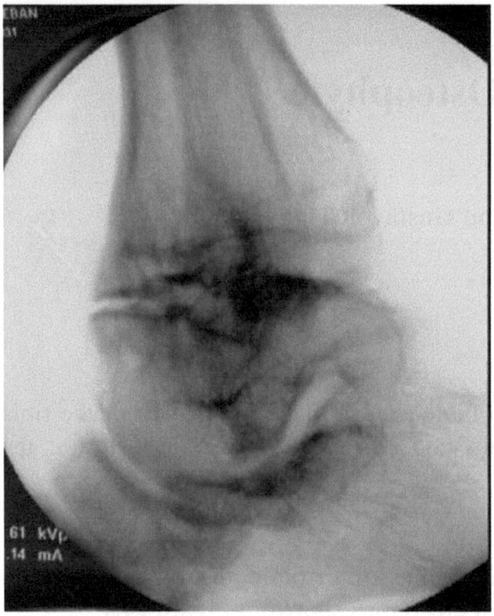

Fig. 29.2 Impingement of the ankle joint in maximum dorsal flexion

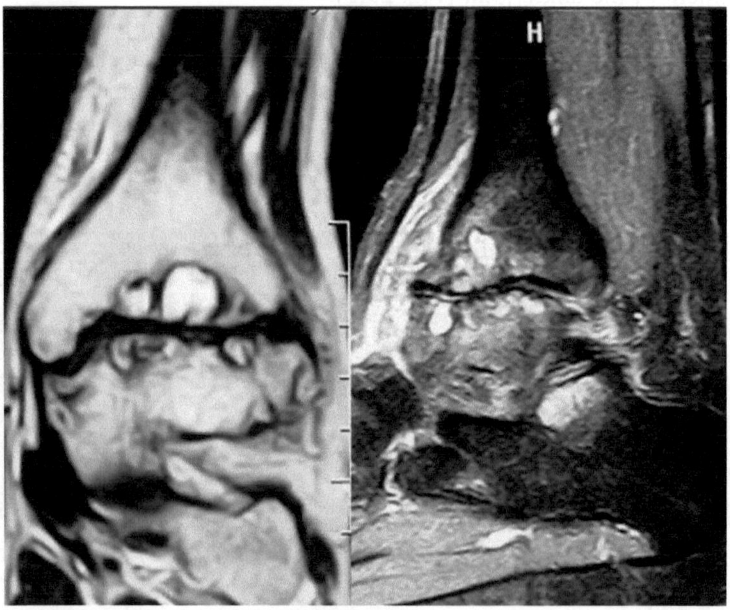

Fig. 29.3 Magnetic resonance imaging of the ankle

When the patient presents with associated cysts, it is necessary make the diagnosis by magnetic resonance imaging (MRI) to ascertain the number, location and size of the cysts (Fig. 29.3).

The patient is placed in a supine position with a pad beneath the buttocks to maintain the foot in a neutral position (Fig. 29.4).

A transparent surgical table must be used for fluoroscopy. A pneumatic tourniquet is not necessary.

The surgical approach is anterior, through a 4–5 cm anterior incision (Fig. 29.5).

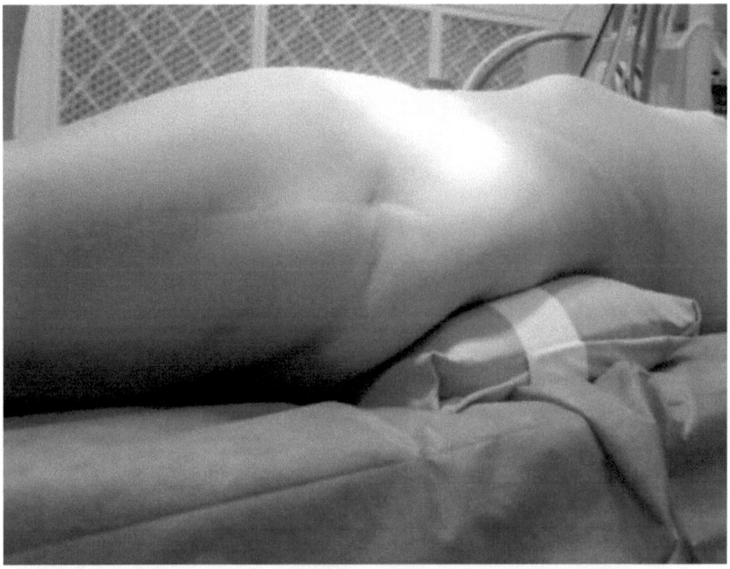

Fig. 29.4 Patient in a supine position with a pad beneath the buttocks

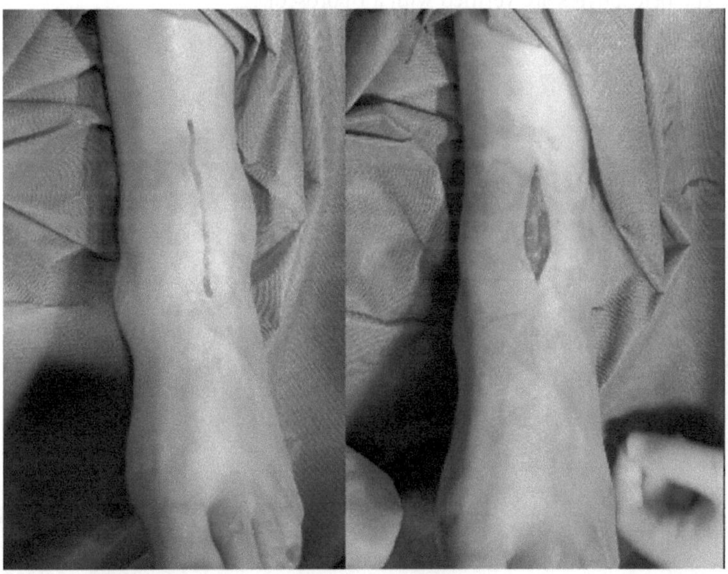

Fig. 29.5 The incision in the anterior surgical approach

The anterior tibial muscle is identified and the incision is parallel to its the external border. The articulation is incised and the osteophytes are identified (tibial, talus), verified with a fluoroscope (Fig. 29.6), and removed. The resection is completed with osteotomy, and the borders softened with a drill (Fig. 29.7). The resection can also be completed with bone-cutting forceps. It is verified with a fluoroscope, with the foot in a complete dorsal flexion position, to ensure the total absence of impingement (Fig. 29.8).

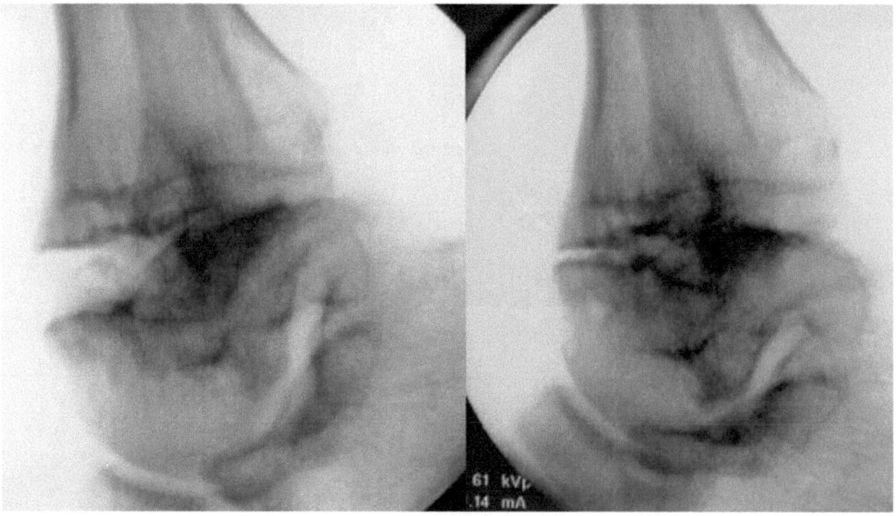

Fig. 29.6 The osteophytes are verified with a fluoroscope

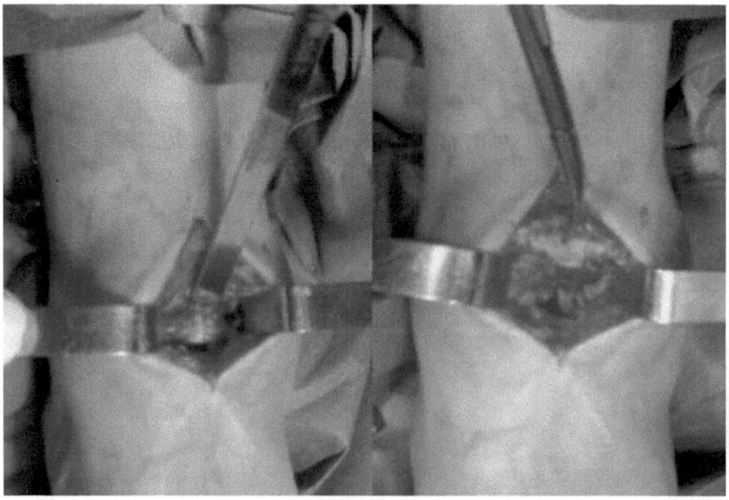

Fig. 29.7 Resection of the osteophyte by osteotomy

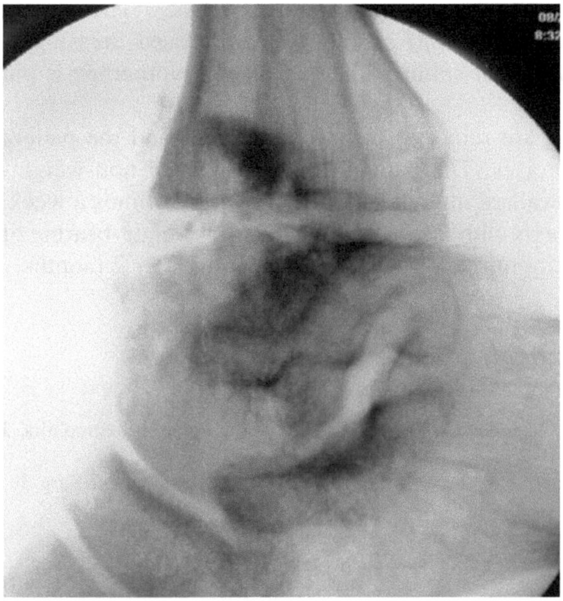

Fig. 29.8 Fluoroscope with the foot in a dorsal flexion position

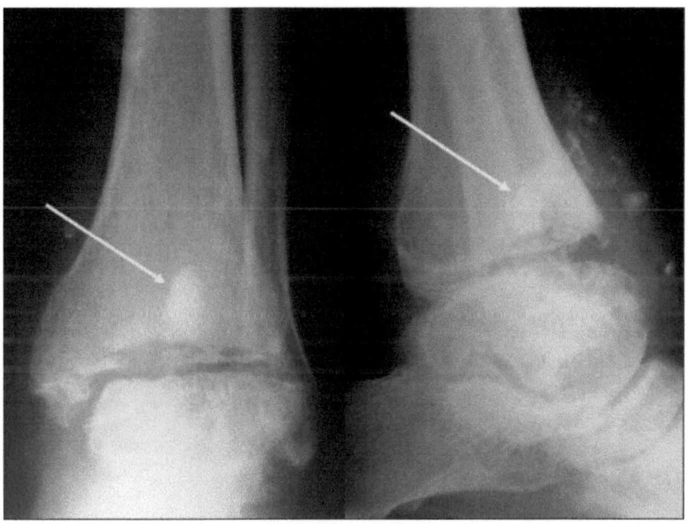

Fig. 29.9 The cyst in the subchondral area filled with bone substitute

The presence of a cyst in the subchondral area which affects more than 15% of the articular surface necessitates filling with bone substitute (Fig. 29.9).

The site of resection is covered with bone wax in order to achieve hemostasis and avoid the formation of heterotrophic bone.

The soft tissue closure is completed by its anatomic planes. The skin is closed with interrupted vertical nylon 3/0 sutures. A compressed dressing is applied to the wound, and a posterior splint with the desired cryotherapy is put in place.

The splint and the dressing are removed on the fourth day, and the patient begins active and passive exercises. The patient begins protected non-weight-bearing perambulation with a walker, attends physiotherapy three times a week, and receives secondary prophylaxis with factor substitute. Partial weight-bearing of the lower limbs begins after a month, and total weight-bearing after 2 months.

Suggested Readings

Gamble JG, Bellah J, Rinsky LA, Glader B (1991) Arthropathy of the ankle in hemophilia. J Bone Joint Surg Am 73:1008-1015

O'Donoghue DH (1957) Impingement exostoses of the tibia and talus. J Bone Joint Surg 39-A:835-842

Ribbans WJ, Phillips MA (1996) Haemophilic ankle arthropathy. Clin Orthop 328:39-45

Rodríguez-Merchán EC (2006) The haemophilic ankle. Haemophilia 12: 337-344

Chapter 30
Ankle Arthrodesis

Nicholas Goddard and M. Zaki Choudhury

Indications

Ankle arthrodesis should be considered for treatment for painful end-stage arthropathy of the talocrural joint. This is generally the result of progressive collapse of the dome of the talus with secondary degenerative change in the joint. The condition is usually associated with extensive osteophytes, both anteriorly and posteriorly, which in combination with the talar collapse, result in painful restriction of ankle movement [1, 2]. The sub-talar joint may be involved to a variable extent but mild-to-moderate sub-talar degenerative disease does not preclude ankle arthrodesis (Fig. 30.1).

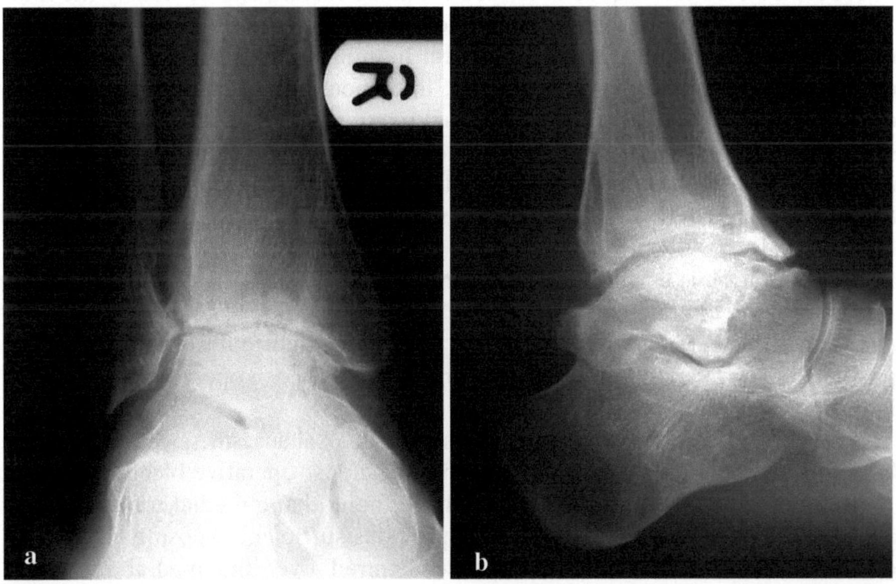

Fig. 30.1 Anteroposterior (**a**) and lateral (**b**) radiographs of an affected ankle showing flattening of the talus, cyst formation, and osteophytes

H.A. Caviglia, L.P. Solimeno (eds.), *Orthopedic Surgery in Patients with Hemophilia.*

Background

Fortunately in the majority of cases the ankle tends to adopt a relatively neutral position as the disease progresses, and as such it is necessary only to carry out an isolated, in-situ fusion of the talocrural joint. Occasionally it may be necessary to correct the position, especially if there is associated tightness in the Achilles' tendon with secondary equinus.

Alternatives

Prior to undertaking ankle fusion, it is important that all other complementary treatment methods have been considered. The natural history of ankle arthropathy is relentlessly progressive, but we have found that by providing simple orthotics, supporting the medial arch of the foot, and restoring a degree of supination of the forefoot, the rate of degeneration can be slowed [3]. In early cases the joint may remain reasonably mobile and congruent, and it may be possible to buy some time by performing a limited clearance of the anterior osteophytes by either an open or arthroscopic technique (O'Donoghue procedure, [4]).

Technique

There are over 20 techniques described for ankle fusion, and obviously the final decision of the technique employed is down to surgeon preference. However in making a decision the surgeon should bear in mind some of the basic principles of operating on patients with hemophilia. In particular there should be a minimal operative exposure, and the use of external fixation devices or percutaneous pins should be avoided. Thus in practice, the choices of technique become somewhat restricted, and we have found that staple fusion employing a medial approach and medial malleolar osteotomy is straightforward and successful in obtaining fusion [5–7].

The operation is performed under general anaesthetic with sterile conditions. It is possible to operate on the patient in a supine position. The limb is prepared and draped in the standard fashion and an upper thigh tourniquet is placed in position and inflated to a suitable pressure. It is possible to operate on the patient in a supine position.

I have found it helpful to infiltrate the skin with local anaesthetic and adrenaline, both for post-operative pain relief and to reduce post-operative bleeding.

In order to minimise the exposure I have found that a medial transmalleolar approach as described by Pridie (1969) provides sufficient exposure [5]. A longitudinal medial incision is then made, centred over the medial malleolus (Fig. 30.2). This can be curved anteriorly along the line of the tibialis posterior tendon which is identified (Fig. 30.3). A medial malleolar osteotomy is then performed using either a power saw or an osteotome. It is important to identify the

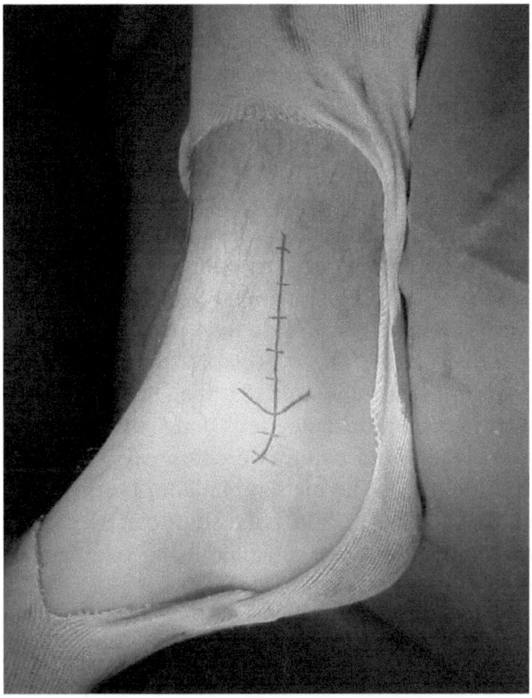

Fig. 30.2 Slightly curved medial incision centred over the medial malleolus

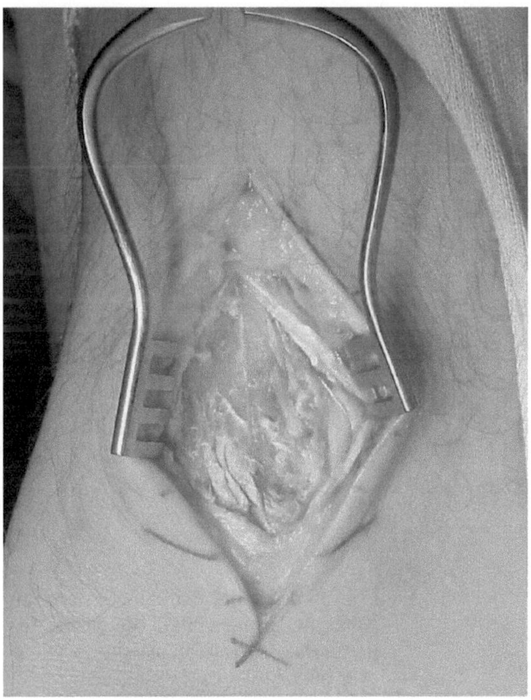

Fig. 30.3 Incision deepened and sub-periosteal exposure of the medial malleolus identifying the tibialis posterior tendon

distal limit of the osteotomy which corresponds to the superomedial aspect of the ankle joint at the junction between the dome of the talus and the lateral aspect of the medial malleolus (Fig. 30.4). The osteotomised fragment is then turned distally, hinging over the medial collateral (deltoid) ligament which is left in situ and attached to the medial aspect of the talus (Fig. 30.5). The talocrural joint can then be identified and a synovectomy performed if necessary.

I now use a modified dowel technique to perform an ankle arthrodesis as described by Baciu [7]. One or two dowels are taken using a Cloward drill (Fig. 30.6). This device is used by neurosurgeons for performing anterior cervical fusion, but there are proprietary devices available (precision bone grafting set). The dowels are taken across the talocrural joint, attempting to take an equal amount of articular surface from the respective bones. The dowels are then extracted, rotated axially through 90°, and re-inserted into the hole that they have just been lifted from, such that there is contact between the cancellous bone surfaces anteriorly and posteriorly. The position is then held using two compression staples and confirmed on intra-operative radiographs. The medial malleolus is then hollowed out to some degree and the harvested cancellous bone chips can be packed into the fusion site. The medial malleolus is then re-attached using two cancellous lag screws as for a large medial malleolar fracture (Fig. 30.7).

The tourniquet is then released, diathermy haemostasis secured and the wound is closed, ideally using a subcuticular suture, and a dressing applied. The limb is immobilised in a plaster backslab, and elevated in the post-operative period. I do not routinely use suction drains.

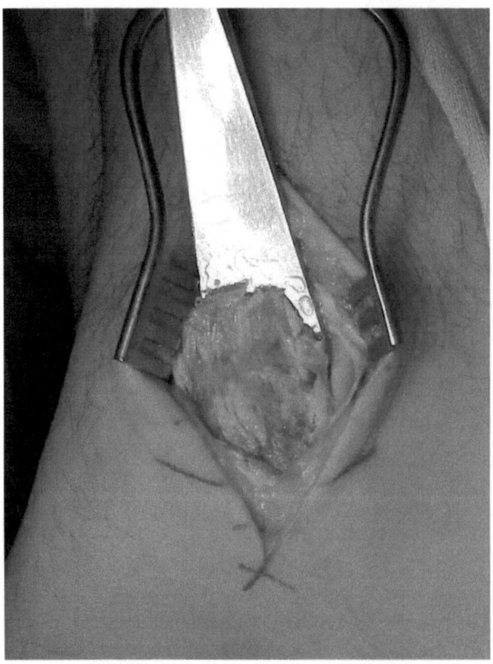

Fig. 30.4 Medial malleolar osteotomy performed using a broad osteotome. My preference is to use an osteotome whenever possible

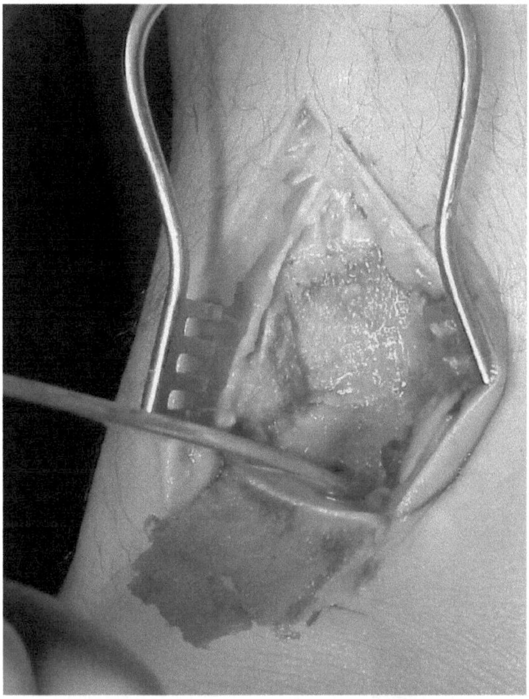

Fig. 30.5 The medial malleolar fragment is then reflected distally hinged on the medial ligament so exposing the talocrural joint

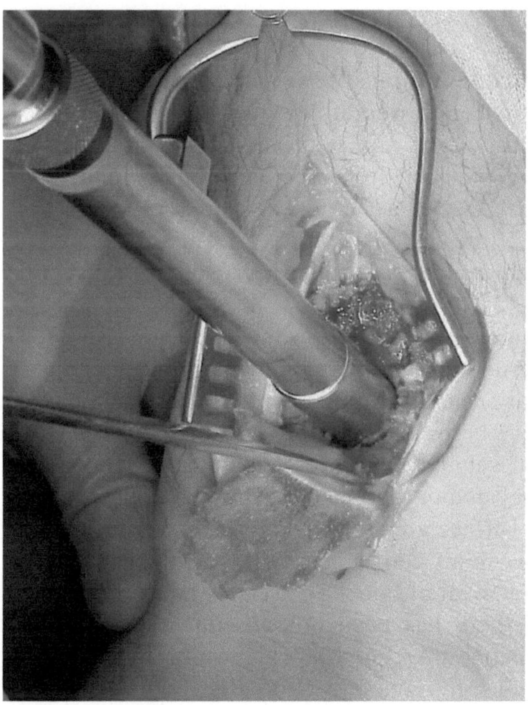

Fig. 30.6 Position of Cloward drill to take dowel

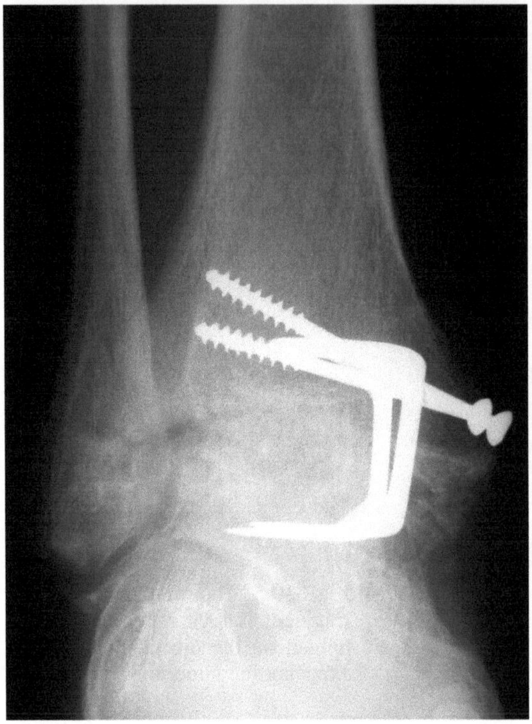

Fig. 30.7 Radiograph showing solid fusion. The position has been held with two compression staples and the medial malleolus re-attached using 3.5 mm cancellous screws

Care is taken to observe for complications, especially compartment syndrome. The patient is then mobilised, non-weight-bearing in the first instance, and discharged home once haemostatic control is ensured. The skin clips are removed at approximately 10 days, and a below-knee walking cast is applied, which remains in situ for 8 weeks.

Following removal of the cast, the patient continues to mobilise, weight-bearing as pain allows, with the ankle supported in either a soft elastic support or aircast support as pain dictates.

We believe that the medial malleolar approach to the ankle for arthrodesis affords many advantages over alternative techniques, including less potential for damage to posterior neurovascular structures, no compromise of the important lateral peroneal perforating vessels, better visualisation of the articular surface, especially if there is any degree of valgus, and preservation of the blood supply through the deltoid ligament which is not disrupted during this approach. The oblique osteotomy allows a large surface area for metaphyseal contact and subsequent healing. A thorough synovectomy can be performed and the dowel taken is re-inserted without additional removal of bone. The staples are placed underneath the medial malleolus and there has been no subsequent loosening or migration of these. No further incisions are required for screw placement or fibular shortening, with minimal overall soft tissue dissection. Cancellous bone graft can also be harvested from the medial malleolus and used as autograft to complement the fusion.

We have used this technique in ten patients, with satisfactory union achieved in all between 8 and 12 weeks. We feel that this method of ankle fusion is safe, minimally invasive, simple, and quick to perform, with good outcomes and a low complication rate. This method has proven useful in the haemophilic population with results at least comparable, and often superior, to other techniques [1, 8, 9].

References

1. Gamble JG, Bellah J, Rinsky LA et al (1991) Arthropathy of the Ankle in Hemophilia. J Bone Joint Surg Am 73:1008
2. Pettersson H, Ahlberg A, Nilsson IM (1980) A radiologic classification of hemophilic arthropathy. Clin Orthop 149:153–159
3. Ribbans WJ, Phillips AM (1996) Hemophilic ankle arthropathy. Clin Orthop 328:39–45
4. O'Donoghue DH (1957) Impingement exostoses of the talus and tibia. J Bone Joint Surg Am 39(4):835–852
5. Pridie KH (1953) Arthrodesis of the Ankle. J Bone Joint Surg Br 35:152
6. Thomas FB (1969) Arthrodesis of the ankle. J Bone Joint Surg Br 51(4):53–59
7. Baciu CC (1986) A simple technique for arthrodesis of the ankle. J Bone Joint Surg Br 68:266–267
8. Luck JV Jr, Kasper CK (1989) Surgical management of advanced hemophilic arthropathy: an overview of 20 years' experience. Clin Orthop 242:60
9. Schuberth JM, Cheung C, Rush SM et al (2005) The medial malleolar approach for arthrodesis of the ankle: a report of 13 cases. J Foot Ankle Surg 44(2):125–32

Section VI

Bone Defects

Chapter 31

Percutaneous Treatment of Hemophilic Cysts using "Fibrin Glue"

Federico Fernández-Palazzi, Freddy Chakal and Rafael Viso

Introduction

Pseudotumors in hemophilia are a clinical entity rather than a specific pathological injury, described for the first time by Starker in 1918 [1]. De Valderrama and Mathew have defined a pseudotumor as a subperiostic hemorrhage, Steiner and Mejía state that repeated bleeding causes lysis and expansion of the cortex and medulla [2–4], and Martínez and Vinageras believe pseudotumors are caused by various subperiostic hemorrhages over a period of several months [5]; others think that the bleeding is intra-osseous, subperiosteal, and intramuscular, and that it is a result of a traumatic episode. However, there is not always a cause–effect relationship, since in some cases the period of time between the trauma and the injury is very long, or there simply isn't any history of trauma. Either way, pressure seems to cause the injury, as Larsen demonstrated by injecting salt solution under the periosteum with a continuous pressure of 180 ml H_2O for 12 h [3, 6–8].

Hemophilic cysts can be described as encapsulated blood reservoirs with a tendency to grow. The increase in size can be slow or fast and, depending on their location, they may invade the surrounding tissue, imitating a neoplasm or tumor. This formation it is called a cyst if it is small or with little tuberculation, and a pseudotumor if it is large, lobulated, and invasive [5]. The incidence of hemophilic cysts and pseudotumors is 1.56%, and both appear frequently in the second or third decade of life in patients with severe factor VIII or IX deficiency [5, 9, 10]. Cystic hemophilic pseudotumors are caused by hemorrhages in adjacent bone, which produce areas of localized necrosis and progress to the pseudotumor. The most appropriate classification is the one proposed by Arnold: (a) pseudotumors originating only in soft tissue without including the bone; (b) pseudotumors clearly originating in the subperiosteum; and (c) pseudotumors evolving in the interior of osseous tissue [11]. Pseudotumors have been described in the long bones of the lower limbs, the pelvis, feet, and hand bones. Femoral location is the most frequent, followed by the pelvis, and, less frequently, the tibia [12]. Other less common locations are the mandible, radius, olecranon, and clavicle. Pseudotumors grow fast when they occur in the hands and feet of young patients with rapid epiphyseal growth. Conversely, in the pelvis and

H.A. Caviglia, L.P. Solimeno (eds.), *Orthopedic Surgery in Patients with Hemophilia.*

femur their growth and evolution are slow.

The pathogenesis is not well understood, but pseudotumors are preceded by trauma in most cases. Raised intercavity pressure causes the tumor to grow, provoking compressive injuries in surrounding structures and large areas of subperiosteal osteolysis [2, 13–16].

Diagnosis

X-rays are usually enough, although complementary studies may be needed to evaluate the soft tissue. In such cases we recommend magnetic resonance imaging (MRI), although if definition of the cyst and its cavities is the main objective, then a computerized tomography (CT) scan with three-dimensional reconstruction is preferable.

Percutaneous Treatment

Treatment should initially be conservative with administration of the deficient factor, in order to maintain its concentration at 25–30% for 8–10 weeks. It is important to immobilize the affected bone to avoid pathological fractures.

Tumors with uncontrollable growth require surgical treatment; this is discussed in the next chapter (Chapter 33).

Percutaneous treatment is a non-aggressive method, indicated when the cyst continues to increase in size despite preventive treatment, when the rupture of the hematoma is imminent, for the prevention of skin necrosis, and when there is evidence of neurovascular injury [11, 17–20].

In the 1960s Inmuno, Austria, developed a cryoprecipitation method to obtain highly concentrated fibrinogen solution with a high factor VIII content. This solution may be used to create a sealing system that works by forming a fibrin clot. This material was first used as a "fibrin glue" by Matras and Kuderna in 1973 in the Traumatology Center in Lorenz Bohler Hospital of Vienna, in order to suture medium-sized nerves. Fibrin glue consists of two different components: (1) fibrinogen: a high concentration of factor XII, plus other plasma proteins (albumin and globulin); and (2) a thrombin solution with calcium chloride, which precipitates the former components. The blend of these two components initiates the coagulation process. The resulting clot is stabilized by the union of the fibrin, causing the sealer to solidify. Fibrin glue may thus be used as an antihemorrhagic and adhesive material.

In 1986, we developed a procedure consisting of percutaneously filling the cyst with fibrin glue, using 1 ml of fibrin glue for each 4 ml of material removed. Prior to filling the cavity, the orthopedic surgeon should evaluate the stage of the pseudotumor, the existence of one or multiple cavities, and the need for curettage of the cavities. He should also determine whether clots need to be evacuated and, if so, a blood vacuum or small incision should be used.

Differential Diagnosis

It is important to correctly identify a hemophilic cyst; if it is very aggressive it can be mistakenly diagnosed as a malignant tumor — osteosarcoma. Other differential diagnoses that have been reported include hemangioma, osteomyelitis, giant cell tumor, aneurismic osseous cyst, chondroma, osteogenic fibroma, and chondromyxoid fibroma.

Case 1

We report a 14-year-old white male patient from white, from Carabobo State, Venezuela with a history of moderate hemophilia A (<3.3% factor VIII activity), diagnosed when he was 6 years old. He does not undergo regular checks or control. He was seen for a fusiform tumor of 8 months' duration, located in the first phalanx of the II finger of the left hand, with progressive growth accompanied by pain and changes in skin color (Fig. 31.1).

Clinical Examination

Tumor with deformity at the II finger left hand, with changes in skin color, pain while palpating, reduced phalangic and interphalangic metacarpal mobility, with greatly reduced flexion.

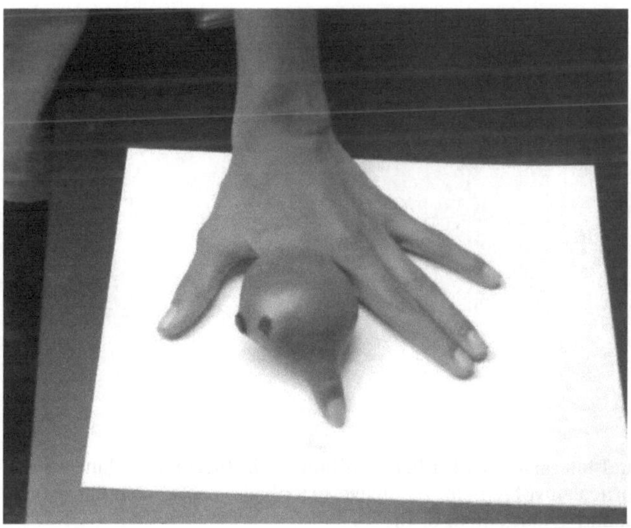

Fig. 31.1 Clinical presentation of fusiform tumor of the first phalanx of the middle finger

Radiology Findings

Areas with opacity at the edges, not well defined and mixing with surrounding tissue. Thin osseous cortical and medullary regions with extensive osteolysis, septal alveolar aspect with small areas of calcification. From one epiphysis to the other a reabsorption of phalanx I of finger II is seen (Fig. 31.2).

Surgical Intervention

Surgery is performed under local anesthesia, making a small incision to evacuate the the clot, perform curettage of the cavities, and fill them with fibrin glue to produce hemostasis (Fig. 31.3).

Procedure

1. Treatment with factor VIII.
2. Infiltration of the affected area with a local anesthetic without epinephrine.
3. Tourniquet in the forearm with a rubber band.
4. Small incision in the major area affected.
5. Clot evacuation and cavity curettage.
6. Filling of the cavities with home-made fibrin glue: 1 ml blood cryoprecipitate + 1 ml tranexanic acid + 1 ml thrombin + 1 ml calcium gluconate.
7. Application of a compression bandage.
8. Immobilization.

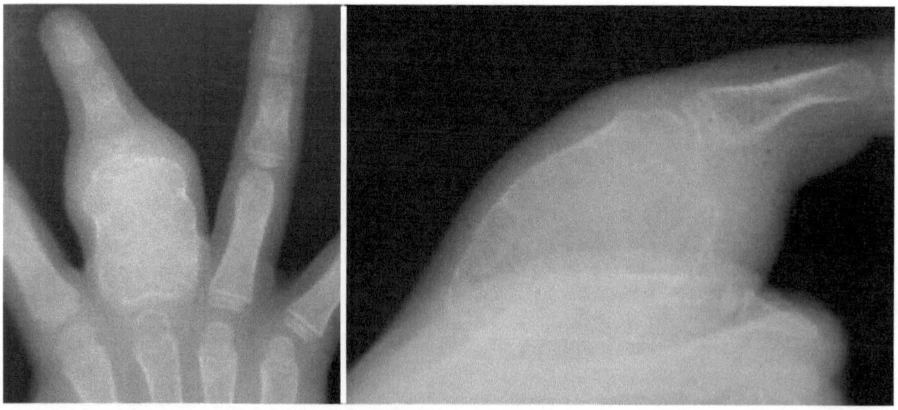

Fig. 31.2 Anteroposterior and lateral view of a hemophilic cyst in the first phalanx of the middle finger. Note the cortical involvement, extensive osteolysis, septal alveolar aspect from epiphysis to epiphysis, and enlargement of the bone

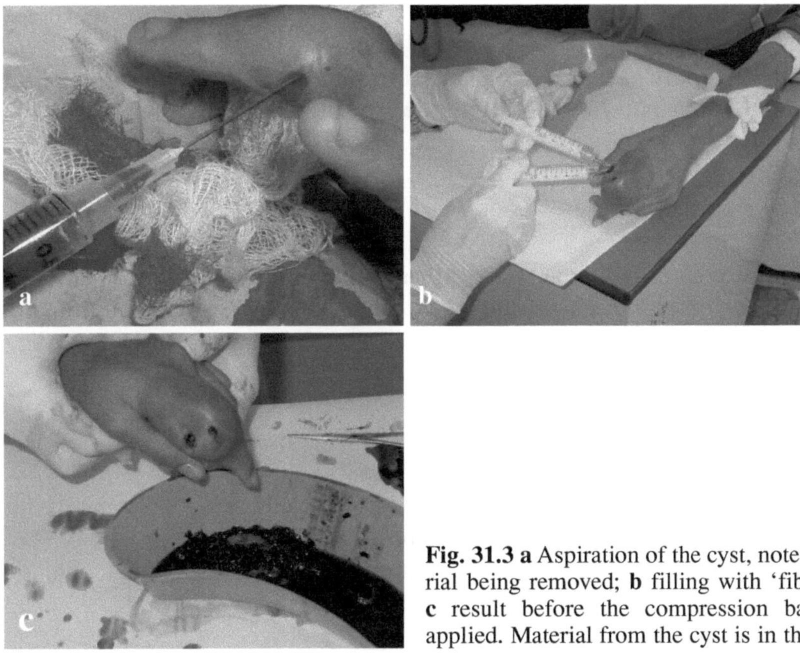

Fig. 31.3 **a** Aspiration of the cyst, note the material being removed; **b** filling with 'fibrin glue'; **c** result before the compression bandage is applied. Material from the cyst is in the tray

Case 2

The second case is a 12-year-old white male patient, from Maracay, Aragua State, Venezuela, with a history of moderate hemophilia A (<3.3% factor VIII activity), diagnosed when he was 3 years old. He undergoes regular control. He was seen for a tumor at the second phalanx of the ring finger of the left hand, of 5 months' duration, with progressive local growth accompanied by pain and functional limitation to flexion (Fig. 31.4).

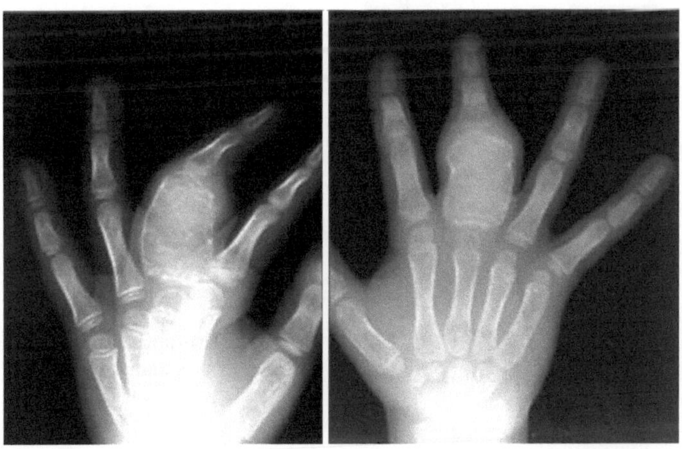

Fig. 31.4 Radiological images; note the bulging of the cortex and rarefaction of the bone

Clinical Examination

Tumor with deformity at the medial phalanx of the ring finger left hand, painful at palpation, interphalanagic mobility limited towards flexion.

Radiology Findings

Destruction of the cortical area, with extensive medullary osteolyis, and septal alveolar aspect of epiphysis to epiphysis of the medial phalanx of the ring finger.

Surgical Intervention

Surgery is performed, making a cavity vacuum with aspiration, filling the cavity with home-made fibrin glue to produce hemostasis.

To date, we have performed five procedures on fingers using this technique (Fig. 31.5).

Discussion

A hemophilic cyst is a severe bleeding complication in the bone or muscle and should be treated early before it grows to become a tumor of giant size (pseudotumor) that compromises the limb or threatens the patient's life. If a hematoma

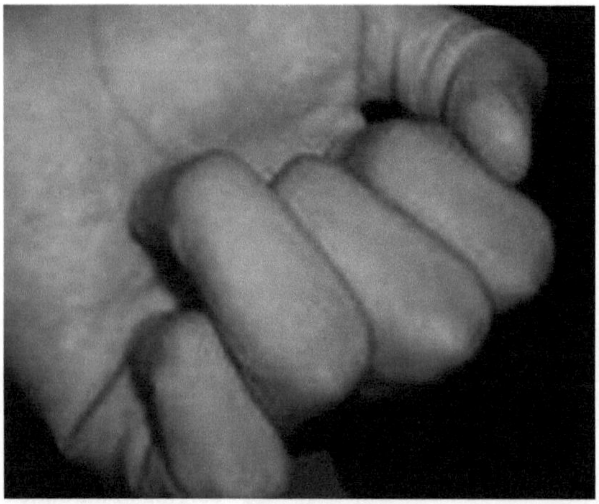

Fig. 31.5 Evolution in the sixth week after percutaneous surgery

does not respond to appropriate treatment or there is an osseous bleed that does not stop, the possibility of a cyst or a pseudotumor must be seriously considered. In our series, two cases with moderate hemophilia A are reported. The first patient did not attend for check-up, he lived a long way from the clinic so did not receive adequate treatment, and the cysts became a giant pseudotumor in the hand resulting in deformity, destruction of bone, and a high risk of amputation. With well-planned treatment with factor VIII by the staff of the National Hemophilia Center, and the consent of the patients and their parents, a percutaneous surgical procedure was performed for each patient, with evacuation of the clots, curettage of the cavities, and filling of the cavities with home-made fibrin glue, with satisfactory results. The home-made fibrin glue is made in the Orthopedic Unit National Hemophilia Center Municipal Blood Bank due to a lack of resourses to import the registered product. Treatment efforts should be focused on prevention of a pseudotumor, ensuring the patients and their parents and relatives are adequately educated, training health personnel, and eliminating the social barriers preventing access to adequate treatment for bleeding episodes. This is vital to avoid progression to a giant pseudotumor that necessitates radical surgery.

Conclusion

- Hemophilic cysts are is a rare complication observed in hemophiliac patients.
- Generally they are observed in patients who live far away from the treatment centers or who have no follow-up of their treatment, so they present late for adequate treatment.
- A significant proportion of the medical profession has insufficient knowledge of the pathology of hemophilic cysts, due to their low frequency.
- There is little application of preventive treatment in non-specialist centers, due to lack of knowledge and resources.
- In developed countries this pathology is not frequent because of better follow-up of hemophiliac patients and better resources for their treatment.
- In small tumors, early surgery should be performed (percutaneous draining and filling with fibrin glue) to avoid progression to a giant pseudotumor that necessitates radical surgery (Fig. 31.6).
- The adequate early treatment of a pseudotumor allows simpler surgery with rapid recuperation and return to the social and family environment.
- In the case of a giant psuedotumor, a resection or radical surgery is preferred.
- These patients should be treated by a multidisciplinary team, including hematologists, an orthopedic surgeon, physiotherapist, and a social worker for an adequate evaluation and to avoid complications.

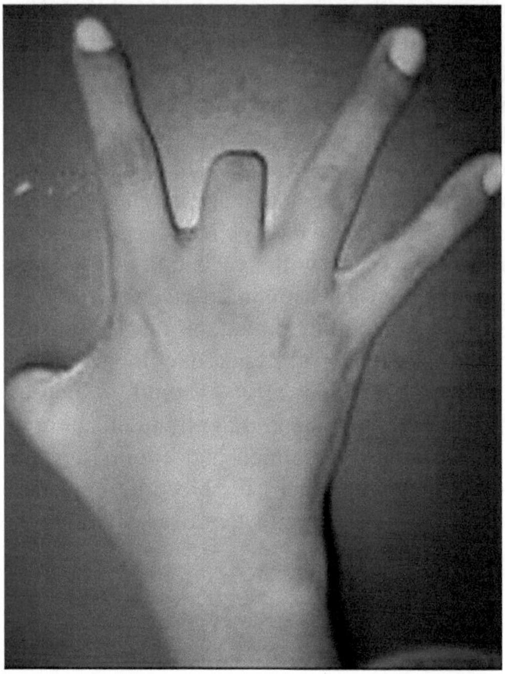

Fig. 31.6 Radical solution of amputation of the finger that should *never* be done and can be avoided with the percutaneous treatment

References

1. Astrup T, Sjolin J (1958) Thromboplastic activity of human synovial membrane and fibrous capsular tissue. Proc Soc Exp Biol Med 97:852
2. Starker L (1918) Knochenusur durch ein hämophiles subperiostales Hämatom. Mitt Grenzgeb Med Chir 31:381
3. Fernandez de Valderrama J, Mattews J (1965) The haemophilic pseudotumor or haemophilic subperiosteal haematoma. J Bone Joint Surg Br 47:2562–2565
4. Steiner GC, Mejía AR (1973) Hemophilic pseudotumor of intra-osseus origin in a child. Bull Hosp Jt Dis 34:139
5. Caviglia HA, Fernández-Palazzi F, Galatro G et al (2000) Percutaneous treatment of haemophilic pseudotumours. In: Rodríguez-Merchán EC, Goddard NJ, Lee CA (eds) Musculoskeletal Aspects of Hemophilia. Blackwell, Oxford, pp 971–1004
6. Martinson A (1976) Hemophilic pseudotumor. In: Boone DC (ed) Comprehensive Management of Hemophilia. Philadelphia, FA Davis, pp 94–99
7. Ahlberg A (1975) On the natural history of hemophilic pseudotumor. J Bone Joint Surg Am 57(8):1133-1136
8. Larsen RM (1938) Intra-medullary pressure with particular reference to massive diaphyseal bone necrosis. Ann Surg 108:127
9. Fernández-Palazzi F, Rivas S, Rupcich M (1985) Experience with fibrin seal in the management of haemophilic cysts and pseudotumor. Proceedings, mangement of musculoskeletal problems in haemophilia. Denver, pp 222–223
10. Fernández-Palazzi F, Rivas S, de Bosch NB et al (1991) Percutaneous treatment of haemophilic cysts and pseudo-tumors. In: Lusher JM, Kessler CM (eds) Hemophilia and von Willebrand's Disease in the 1990. Excerpta Medica, Amsterdam, 1576–1574
11. Arnold W, Hilgartner M (1977) Hemophilic arthropathy. Current concepts of pathogenesis and management. J Bone Joint Surg Am 59:2873–2905

12. Arnold WD (1976) Pseudotumor of hemophilia. In: Hilgartner MW (ed) Hemophilia in children, vol. 1. Progress in Pediatric Hematology & Oncology. MA: Publishing Sciences Group Littleton, 991–1008
13. Gilbert M (1990) The hemophilic pseudotumor. Prog Clin Biol Res 324:257–262
14. Gunning AJ (1966) The surgery of haemophilic cysts. In Biggs R, MacFarlane RG (eds): Treatment of Haemophilic and Other Coagulation Disorden Oxford: Blackwell, p 22
15. Horton D, Pollay M, Wilson A et al (1993) Cranial hemophilic pseudotumor. J Neurosurg. 79:936–938
16. Liu S, White W, Johnson P, Gauntt Ch (1988) Hemophilic pseudotumor of the spinal canal. J Neurosurg 69:624–627
17. Brant E, Jordan H (1972) Radiologic aspects of hemophilic pseudotumor in bone. AJR 115:5255–5239
18. Bryan G, Leibold D, Triplett R (1990) Hemophilic pseudotumor of the mandible report of a case. Oral Surg Oral Med Pathol 69:5505–5553
19. Ghormley R, Clegg R (1948) Bone and joint changes in hemophilia with report of cases of so-called hemophilic pseudotumor. J Bone Joint Surg 30:5896–6000
20. Jensen P, Putman C (1975) Hemophilic pseudotumor. Diagnosis, treatment, and complications. Am J Dis Child 129:717

Chapter 32
Intraosseous and Subchondral Cysts

Horacio A. Caviglia, Gustavo Galatro and Pablo Nuova

Introduction

Intraosseous and subchondral cysts have different pathophysiology.

Subchondral cysts are related to arthropathy. The first sign of arthropathy on X-ray is narrowing of the joint space and small abnormalities in the subchondral bone. The subchondral cysts appear later, and are multiple, irregularly distributed, and larger than others that appear in children or adolescents. These cysts are connected and exposed in the joint, and accompanied by disintegration of the subchondral bone [1–4]. Sometimes the cyst progression results in an osteolytic lesion that may lead to a pathological fracture (Fig. 32.1).

Intraosseous cysts are caused by intraosseous bleeding; this is generally located in the bone metaphysis and is not related to arthropathy (Fig. 32.2).

In both types of cyst, front and lateral views of the affected region are used for diagnosis.

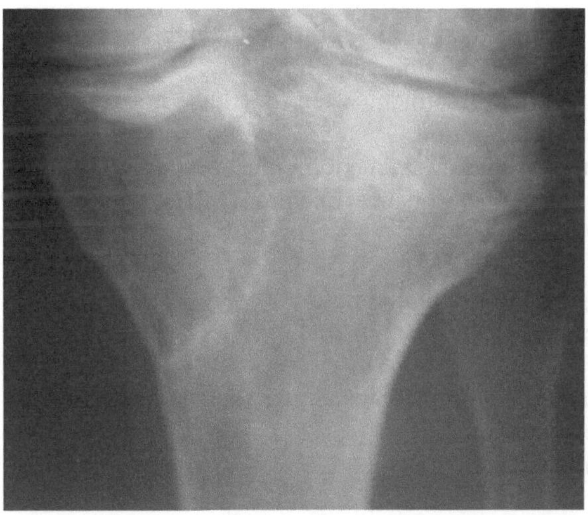

Fig. 32.1 Subchondral cyst of the proximal tibia

H.A. Caviglia, L.P. Solimeno (eds.), *Orthopedic Surgery in Patients with Hemophilia.*

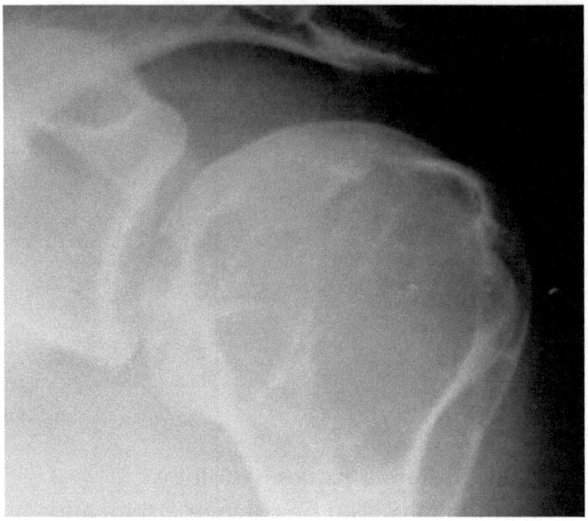

Fig. 32.2 Intraosseous cyst of the proximal humerus

Treatment

Surgery is indicated for subchondrals cysts when:

- The size of the cysts is greater than 15% of the area of the joint, particularly if they include the load articulations. In the knee and elbow, each medial and lateral compartment is considered to be separate and should therefore be evaluated separately.
- A control X-ray shows that the cyst size has progressed, even if its subchondral extension is less than 15%.

The purpose of treatment is to avoid crumbling of the joint and to reconstruct bone stock when necessary to carry out definitive arthroplasty.

Intraosseous cysts require surgical treatment when they have not responded to replacement therapy of 6 weeks' duration.

In both subchondral and intraosseous cysts, the joint must be studied by computed tomography (CT) and magnetic resonance imaging (MRI), which allow appropriate pre-operative planning.

The CT scan (Fig. 32.3) gives information about:

- The three-dimensional location of the cyst.
- The number of cavities it possesses.
- The thickness of its walls and the presence of fractures that are not visible on X-rays when the walls are very thin.
- Communication between the cavities.

The MRI (Fig. 32.4) shows:

- The contents of the cyst.

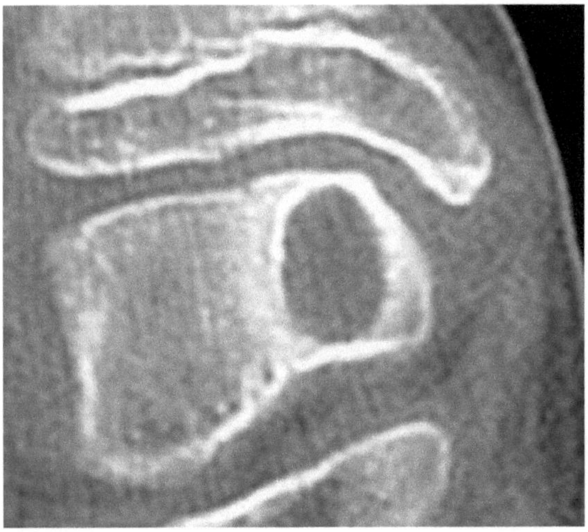

Fig. 32.3 Subchondral cyst of the talus. The CT scan shows only one big cyst that occupies over 15% of the articular joint

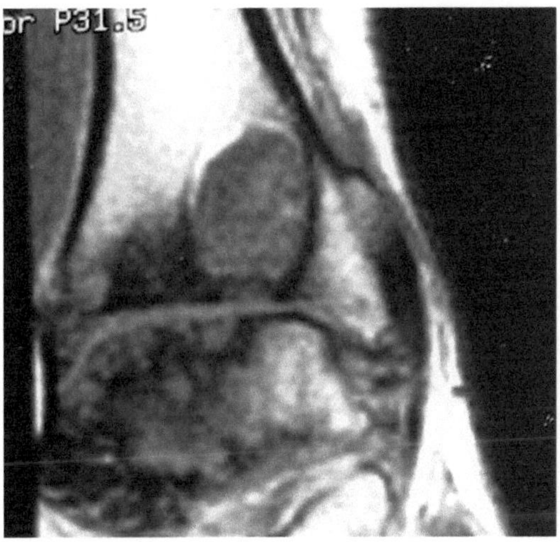

Fig. 32.4 Subchondral cyst of the distal tibia. The MRI image shows only one cyst which communicates with the joint

- Its size.
- The number of cavities.
- Communication with the articulation of the subchondral cysts.

Hemophilic intraosseous and subchondral cysts have a different origin but their treatment is similar [5–7].

Surgical Technique

1. Pre-operative planning, X-ray, CT scan: in an example case, X-ray shows subchondral cysts of the distal tibia in the ankle joint (Fig. 32.5), and CT scan shows the location of the cysts (Fig. 32.6).

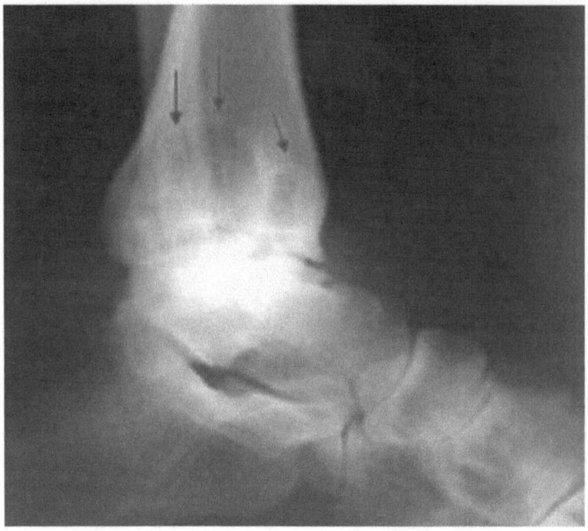

Fig. 32.5 X-ray shows multiple cysts of the tibia

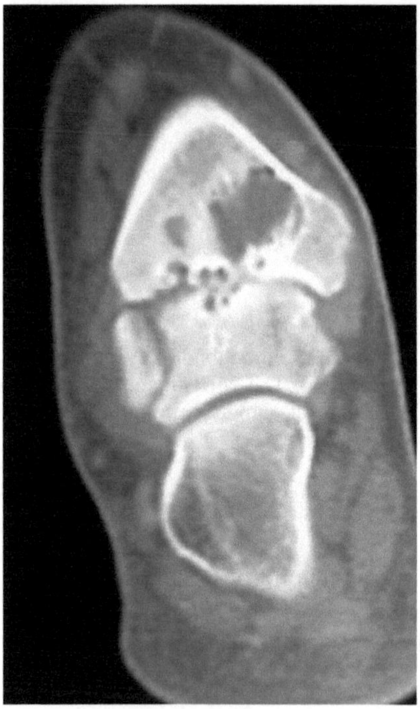

Fig. 32.6 CT scan shows the location of the cysts

2. The patient should be placed on a translucent operating table.
3. A hemostatic tourniquet is not necessary.
4. The area of the cyst should be identified clearly by means of an image intensifier (Fig. 32.7).

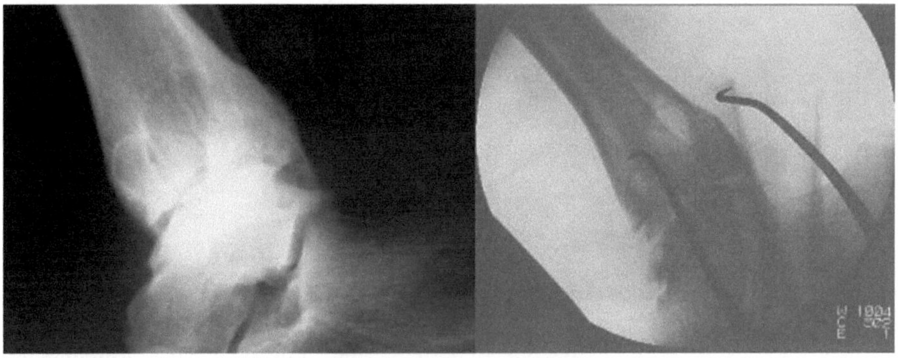

Fig. 32.7 Localization of the cyst with an image intensifier

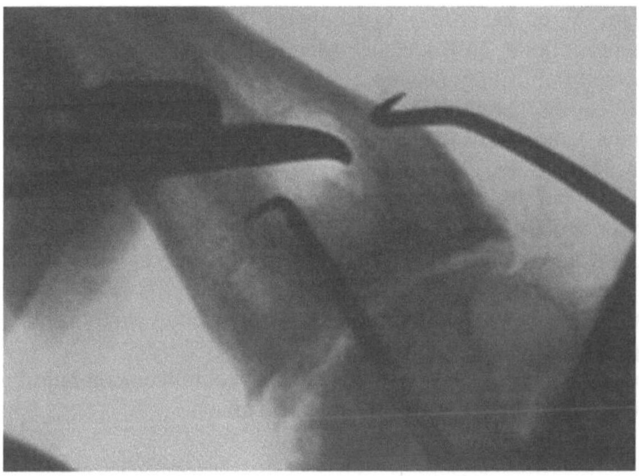

Fig. 32.8 Percutaneous approach and localization of the cyst

5. The incision is carried out percutaneously (Fig. 32.8), allowing the surgeon to approach the cyst in a region that will not generate any damage to the tendons, nerves, or blood vessels.
6. The contents of the cyst are aspirated, and it is filled with coralline hydroxyapatite (Fig. 32.9).
7. The incision is closed with separate sutures.
8. No suction drainage is necessary.
9. The rehabilitation program starts 48 h post-operatively.

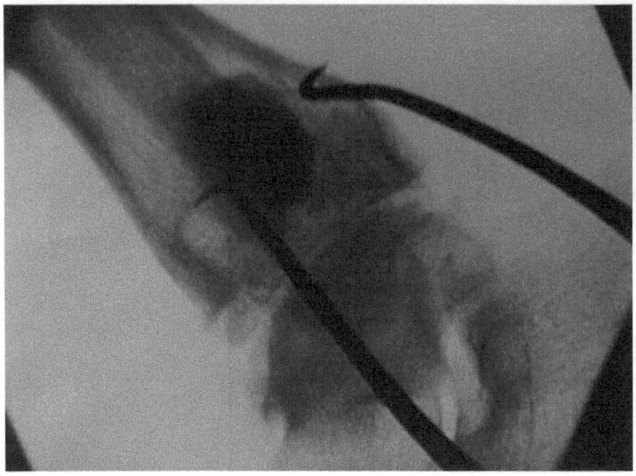

Fig. 32.9 After aspiration of the contents, the cavity is filled with coralline hydroxyapatite

References

1. Caviglia HA, Galatro G,Vatani N et al (2003) Osteophytes, subchondral cyst and intraosseous cyst of the haemophilic joint. In Rodríguez-Merchán (ed). The haemophilic joints. New perspectives: Blackwell Publishing, Oxford, pp 181–186
2. Swanton Mc (1959) Haemophillic arthropathy in dogs. Lab Invest 8:1269–1273
3. De Palma AF (1967) Haemophilic arthropathy. Clin Orthop 52:145–152
4. Jaffe HL (1972) Hemophilia. In: Jaffe HL (ed) Metabolic, degenerative, and inflamatory diseases of bone and joints. Lea & Fabiger, Philadelphia, pp 728–732
5. Galatro G, Perez Bianco R, Pascual Garrido C et al (2001) Cysts and Pseudotumors bone restaurations by means of coral [Abstract]. 7th Musculoskeletal Congress of World Federation of Haemophilia, Pakistan
6. Gustavo G (2002) Lesiones quísticas y pseudotumorales en pacientes hemofilicos. Asociación Argentina de Ortopedia y Traumatología. Buenos Aires
7. Caviglia HA (2005) Tratamiento de los quistes Hemofílicos mediante el relleno con hidroxiapatita coralina. XX World Congress – SICOT/ SIROT Istanbul, Turkey

Chapter 33

Surgical Treatment of Hemophilic Pseudotumors

Federico Fernández-Palazzi and Salvador Rivas

Introduction

In order to understand what a hemophilic pseudotumor is we refer the reader to the introduction of our previous chapter (Chapter 32), where a definition, the difference between a cyst and a pseudotumor, the pathology, evolution, diagnosis, and proposed treatments are explained. In this chapter we will deal only with those pseudotumors that, because of their size, cannot be treated percutaneously and require open, usually extensive, surgery

Indications for Surgery

Treatment should be initially be conservative with administration of the deficient factor in order to maintain its concentration at 25–30% for 8–10 weeks. It is important to immobilize the affected bone to avoid pathological fractures.

Tumors with uncontrollable growth require surgical treatment; they must be extirpated if the integrity of the affected bone or the patient's life is at risk, and when pathological fractures occur.

Preparation for Surgery

Before deciding on surgery a complete *imaging study* must be performed:

- Simple X-rays.
- Axial computerized tomography to examine the tumor's margins and lobulation and determine whether it has infiltrated soft tissues.
- Magnetic resonance to differentiate the layers of the mass which is to be extirpated (Fig. 33.1).

A complete set of *laboratory tests* and all coagulation controls should be performed, and extra replacement materials should be on hand as there is often excessive bleeding with this type of surgery.

H.A. Caviglia, L.P. Solimeno (eds.), *Orthopedic Surgery in Patients with Hemophilia.*

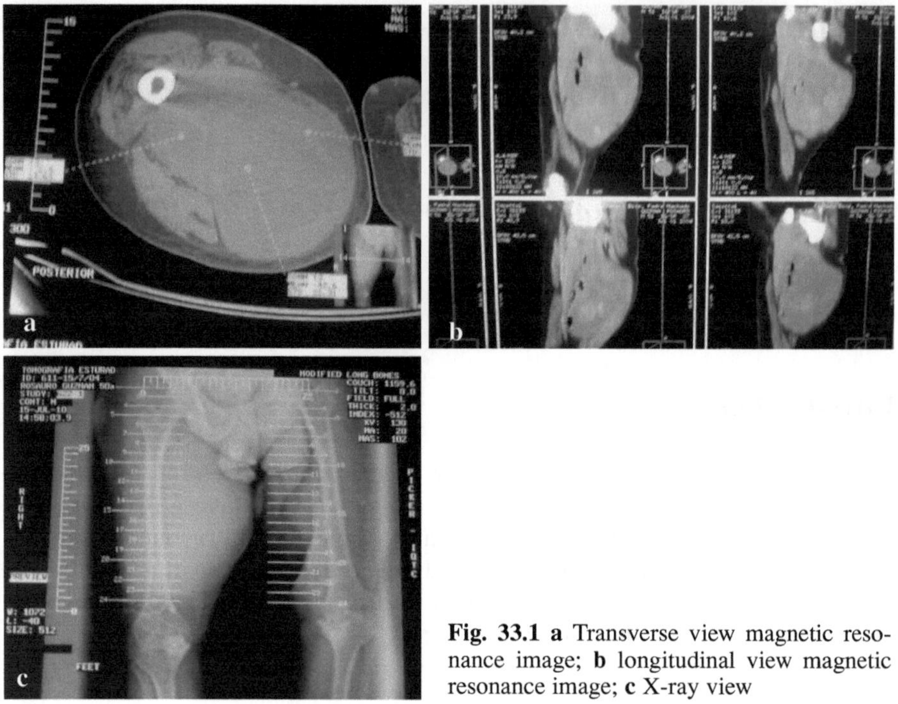

Fig. 33.1 **a** Transverse view magnetic resonance image; **b** longitudinal view magnetic resonance image; **c** X-ray view

A general or vascular surgeon should assist the orthopedic surgeon in some cases, particularly in pseudotumor surgery of the lower limbs.

Surgery

Pseudotumor surgery consists of voiding the mass and resection of the thick capsule, filling the resulting space with hemostatic and fibrous material such as "fibrin glue" (see Chapter 32), Spongostan® or another type of hemostatic tissue.

Surgical Technique

The patient must be positioned on the operating table with the part of the limb where the pseudotumor is located positioned above the table level (Fig. 33.2).

1. The surgical incision must be made in the apex of the deformity, and be long enough to allow complete resection of the mass.
2. Careful dissection must be done in the periphery of the tumor, in order to separate the infiltrated thick capsule from normal tissue (generally muscle), while trying not to open the mass. This is quite difficult, and if the mass is big it is usually necessary to open it, void it, and hold the borders of the open tumor with strong forceps in order to pull it from adjacent tissues and continue the dissection (Figs. 33.3–33.6).

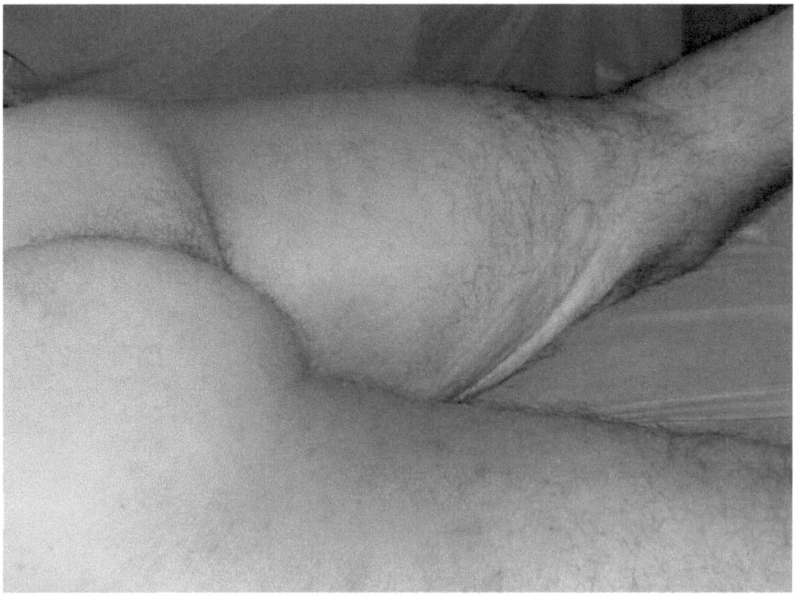

Fig. 33.2 Position of the patient for surgery

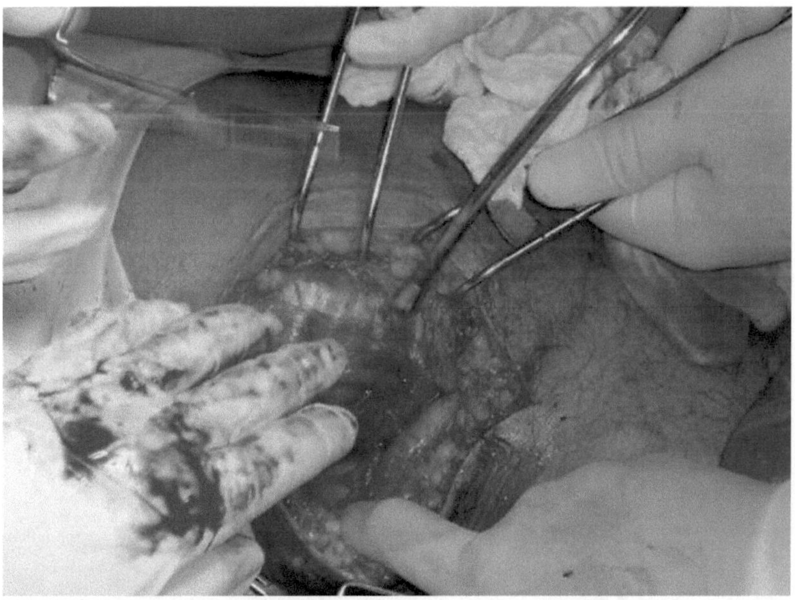

Fig. 33.3 Incision and dissection of the mass

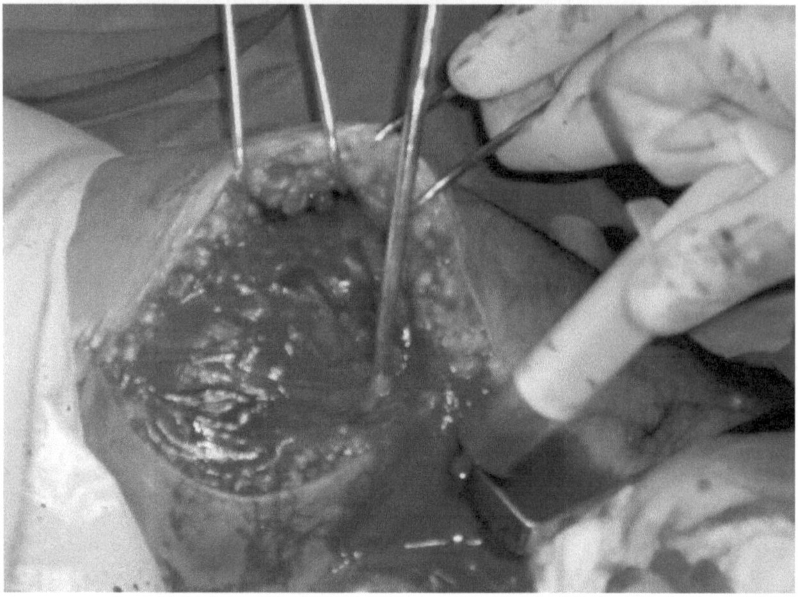

Fig. 33.4 Opening of the mass, notice the material coming out

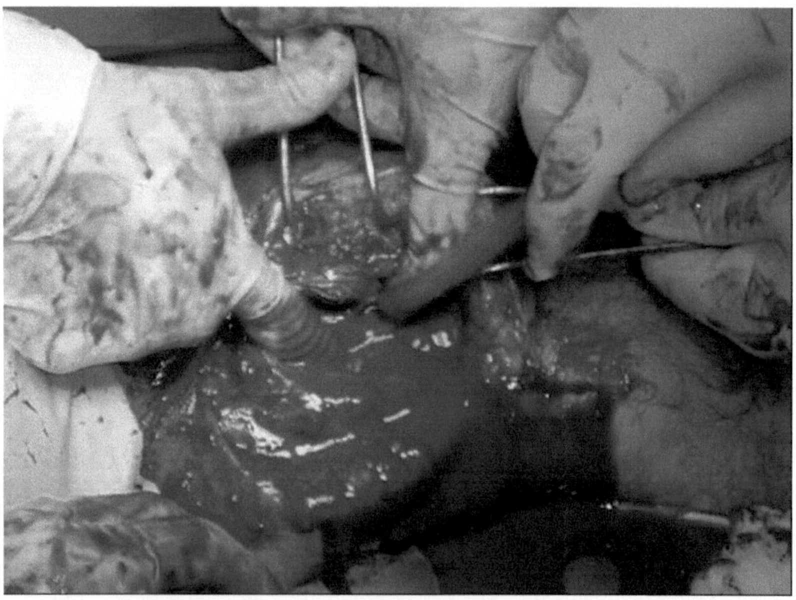

Fig. 33.5 Aspiration and voiding of content

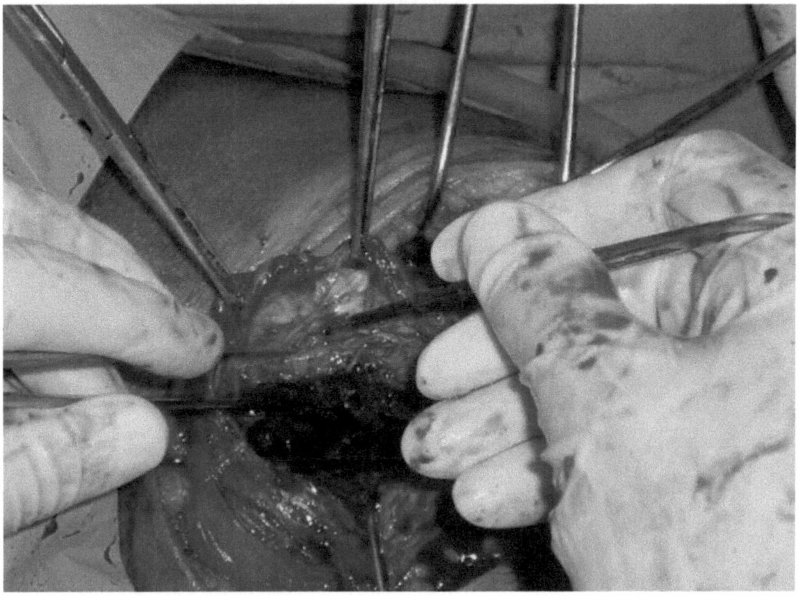

Fig. 33.6 Dissection of the capsule

3. The material that comes from inside is an undifferentiated mass of clots, necrotic tissue, and old, concentrated blood, that can sometimes weigh, as in one of our cases, up to 7 kg (Fig. 33.4).
4. The inside of the cavity should be carefully curetted, and as many bleeding vessels as possible should be electrically coagulated (Fig. 33.7). The crust from this coagulation generally falls off before the 21st post-operative day, when the patient is usually covered with anti-hemophilic factor well above 50% of anticoagulation level, and thus no further bleeding will occur.
5. Next, a layer-by-layer suture is performed from inside out, filling the gaps with enough fibrin seal to permit hemostasis and healing (Fig. 33.8).
6. Depending on the size of the space left, one or two thick, closed, drainage vacuums should be left in place for careful post-operative bleeding control.
7. The skin must be closed with thick non-absorbable sutures in double-stitch back-and-forth technique (Fig. 33.9). Figure 33.10 shows a resected pseudotumor.
8. A heavy compression bandage (Robert Jones type) should be applied and left in place for 1 week, at which time the wound can be examined and a new compression bandage applied.
9. The *most important item* of surgery is a correct calculation of the required anti-hemophilic factor. This is usually 100% on the day of the operation, above 80% for 2 weeks, and can then be lowered to 50% for 2 or 3 more weeks depending on the patient's progress. Ample intravenous coverage with different antibiotics should also be given for 3 weeks.
10. The patient must start isometric exercises as soon as possible in the case of a lower limb, and proceed with partial weight-bearing with crutches when able to stand up. Upper limbs should be used when pain permits.

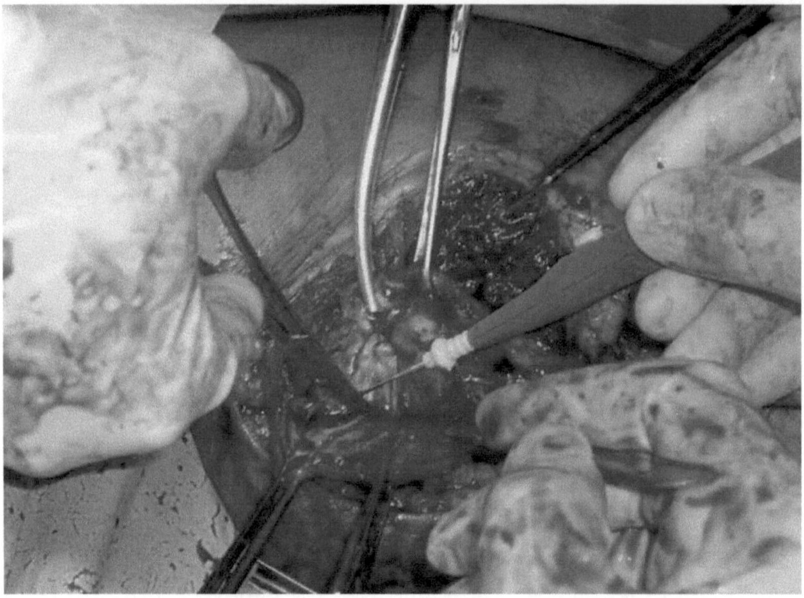

Fig. 33.7 Electrocoagulation

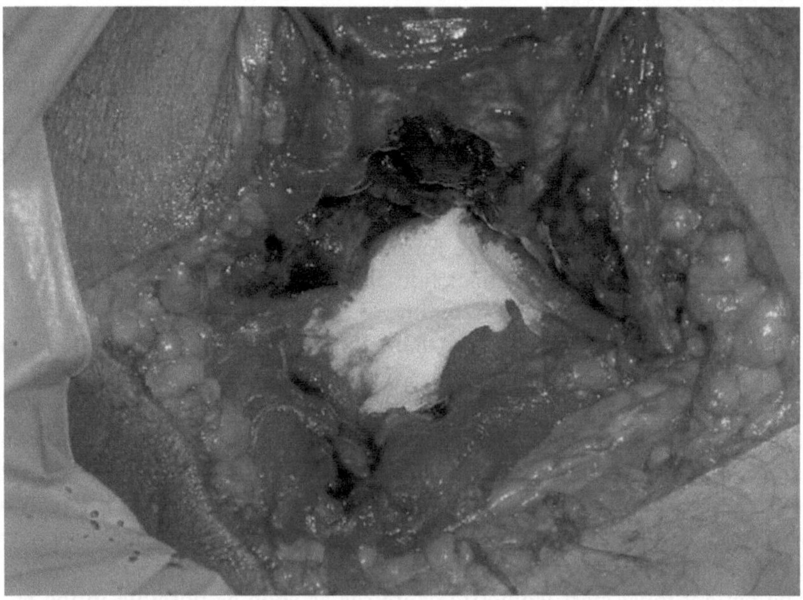

Fig. 33.8 Hemostasis

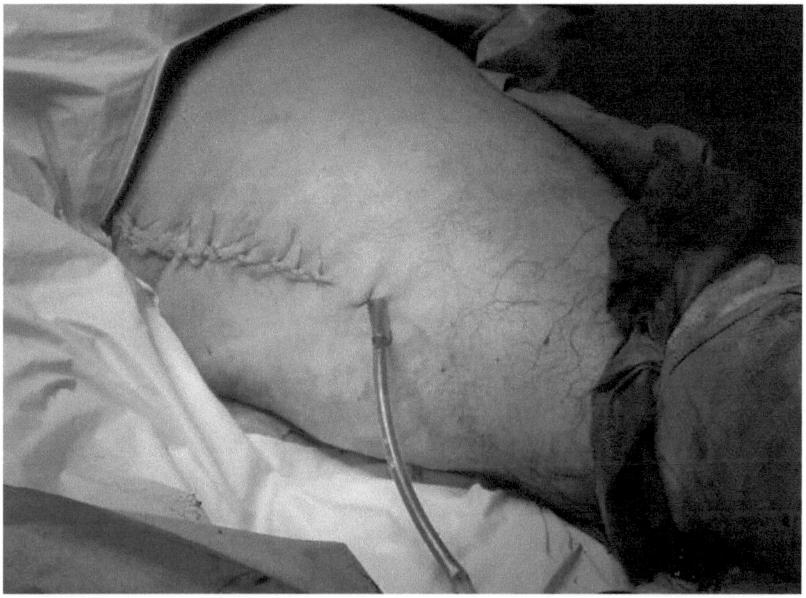

Fig. 33.9 Wound closure and closed drainage

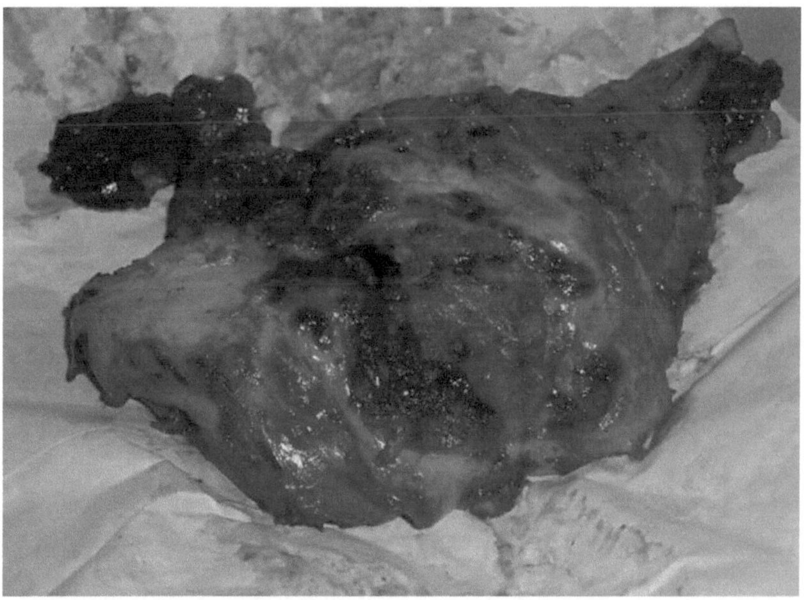

Fig. 33.10 Resected pseudotumor

Suggested Readings

Gilbert MS (2000) Surgical management of the adult haemophilic blood cyst (pseudotumour). In: Rodriguez-Merchan EC, Goddard NJ, Lee CA (eds) Musculoskeletal. Aspects of Haemophilia Oxford: Blackwell Science Ltd, 92–96

Rodríguez-Merchán EC (2002) Haemophilic cysts (pseudotumours). Haemophilia 8(3):393-401

Sagarra M, Lucas M, de la Torre E et al (2000) Successful surgical treatment of haemophilic pseudotumour, filling the defect with hydroxyapatite. Haemophilia 6:55– 56

Chapter 34

Percutaneous Treatment of Hemophilic Pseudotumors

Horacio A. Caviglia, Gustavo Galatro and Nosrallat Vatani

The specialist who treats this pathology must understand the importance of a multidisciplinary treatment approach in achieving a successful result.

Pre-operative Evaluation

1. *Clinical presentations*: type of pseudotumor, age of the patients, region (limbs or pelvis), location (proximal or distal), length of time of evolution, and damage to soft tissue.
2. *Radiology*: radiographs enable us to find out whether the tumors involve bone or not. When the bone is affected, X-rays will help reveal the location of the pseudotumor (epiphysis, metaphysis, diaphysis), its size, the degree of cortical destruction (thinning, erosion, or pathological fracture), and the presence of local osteoporosis. Radiography will also give information about compromise of the proximal and distal joint (Fig. 34.1).

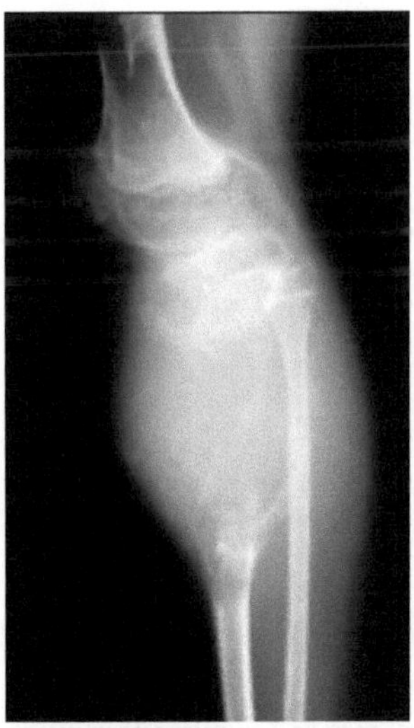

Fig. 34.1 Pseudotumors

H.A. Caviglia, L.P. Solimeno (eds.), *Orthopedic Surgery in Patients with Hemophilia.*

3. *Ultrasound*: ultrasound is a suitable method for diagnosing tumors of soft tissue. It provides information about the size in the three spatial planes, location, and associated vascular compression.
4. *Computed tomography (CT) scan*: the CT scan can be extremely useful in true pseudotumors, since it provides exact information on their location, number of cavities and their possible interconnections. It also shows the degree of cortical involvement and the spread of the pseudotumors towards soft tissue.
5. *Magnetic resonance imaging (MRI)*: this provides information about the location, size, and number of cavities of the pseudotumors, as well as the characteristics of the cavity contents (liquid or solid), and the involvement of soft tissue. An adequate reconstruction will permit evaluation of the interconnections between cavities (Fig. 34.2).
6. *Hematologist evaluation*: the hematologist should perform pre-operative corrective tests with factors VIII or IX to define the most adequate doses and detect whether any inhibitors are present. In the presence of high-responder inhibitor patients, an alternative strategy for the replacement therapy, for example recombinant factor FVIIa, is necessary.
7. *Evaluation of infection*: every patient's immune status (presence of HIV or hepatitis C should be evaluated. When the patient presents with a CD4 count of <400 cells/mm, the possibility of conservative treatment should be evaluated and prophylaxis with the deficient factor considered. Liver function tests give information about the type of anesthetic drugs that can be used, and in cases of severely impaired liver function, give a definite contraindication for surgical treatment.

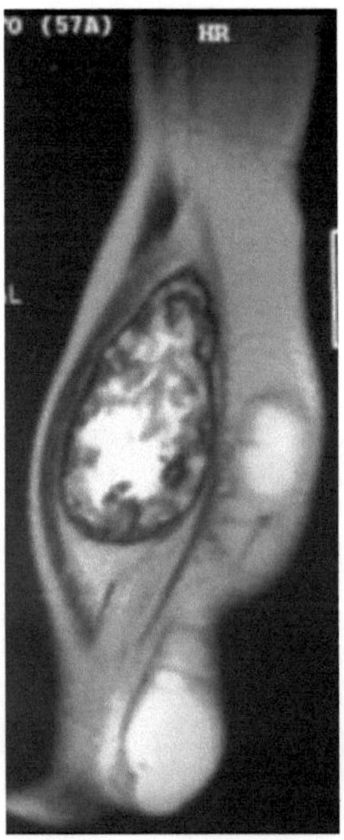

Fig. 34.2 MRI showing the location, size and number of cavities in a pseudotumor of the thigh

8. *Nursing evaluations*: the nurse should evaluate the degree of cooperation of the patient, and the presence of access routes for the administration of replacement therapy.
9. *Physiotherapist evaluation*: the role of the physiotherapist is to evaluate the degree of musculoskeletal compromise, and gain the cooperation of the patient in designing a suitable rehabilitation program.
10. *Psychological evaluation*: the psychologist will determine the psychological profile of the patient and the need for pre-operative and post-operative help.
11. *Social worker evaluation*: the social worker should ensure that the patient and their family have access to treatment with no discrimination in relation to their social circumstances or place of residence.

Treatment

Pre-operative Replacement Therapy

The purpose of this treatment is to reduce the size of the lesions before surgery and to determine the degree of the aggressiveness of the pseudotumor. Every patient requires pre-operative replacement therapy with a daily dose of 50–100 IU/kg of factor VIII or IX.

In adults the treatment is for 6 weeks, and in children for 12 weeks; after that a repeat MRI is carried out. If the pseudotumor has reduced to less than 50% of its original size, surgery is indicated. On the other hand, reduction in pseudotumor size of less than 50% is grounds for continuing the procedure (factor replacement), which must be repeated for another 6 weeks, followed by a repeat MRI.

More specifically, a reduction of at least 25% of the original size indicates that replacement therapy should be continued for 6 weeks, and a new MRI scan for control carried out. At this point, if the pseudotumor has disappeared, it can be considered cured (Fig. 34.3). However, if it is still present, and has reduced to less than 25% of its original size, it should be treated surgically.

The hematologist will decide on the length of time for continuous infusion according to the pseudotumor type and the need for catheter implants.

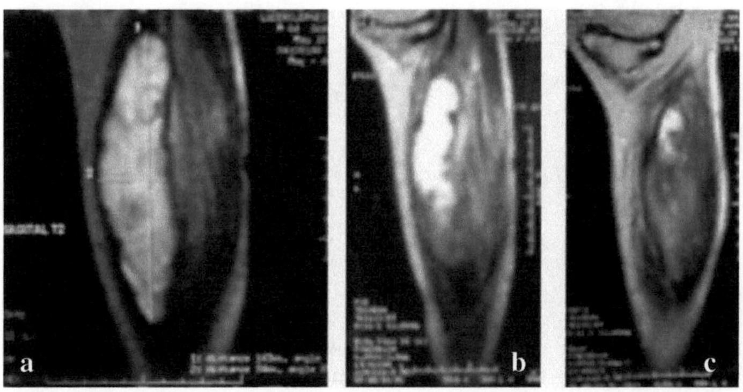

Fig. 34.3 Soft tissue pseudotumors of the leg treated with replacement therapy

Surgical Treatment

The treatment consists of four steps: opening the cavity, washing, aspiration, and filling with different products according to the location and size of the pseudotumor.

- *Antibiotic prophylaxis*: each patient should receive 1 g of cephalosporin preoperatively, and an equal dose 6 h later.
- *Tourniquet*: no tourniquet is used to control intracavity bleeding.

Soft Tissue Pseudotumor

- *Technical devices*: ultrasound is necessary to check the location and evacuation of the pseudotumor.
- In the presence of a *tumor in soft tissue*, the existence of a single cavity or multiples ones and their contents should be determined. In single cavities less than 3 cm in size, it is important to know the characteristics of the contents. Liquid contents can be aspirated with the guidance of ultrasound and thereafter the cavity filled with fibrin seal, whereas the treatment procedure for dense contents will necessitate a small incision, opening, washing, removal of solid contents by means of a curette, and posterior filling with fibrin seal.
- In the case of *single cavities >3 cm*, a small incison is made to introduce a laparoscopic cannula and the cavity is washed and filled with spongostane under video control (Fig. 34.4).
- *Multiple cavities* without clear routes of communication should be evacuated separately using ultrasound control.

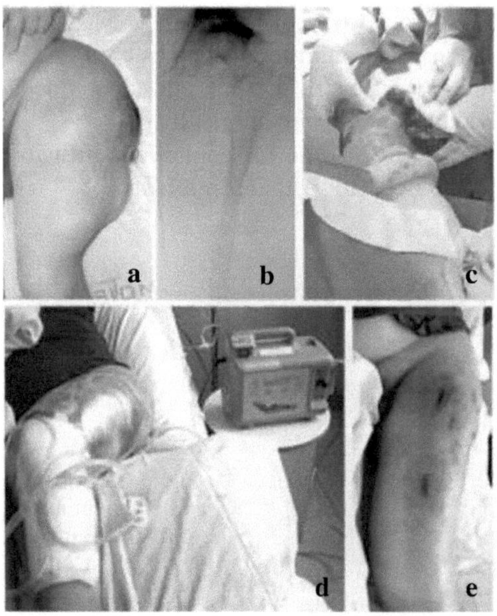

Fig. 34.4 Pre- and post-operative results in a giant pseudotumor

Bone Pseudotumor

- *Technical devices*: image intensifier.
- The location, size, and degree of cortical compromise of a pseudotumor in bone should be evaluated to confirm the true loss of bone stock. When the pseudotumor is diaphyseal or diaphymetaphyseal, it usually consists of a single cavity. In contrast, with a pseudotumour that is epiphyseal or epimetaphyseal (cancellous bone), there are multiple cavities.
- *Approach routes*: the numbers of approaches is equal to the numbers of cavities, except when a CT or MRI scan shows extended communication between them.
- The incision is located in the top of the cavity. A small incision (3–5 cm) can be made. If the cortical bone is broken, then the laparoscopy cannula can be introduced inside the lesion, whereas if the cortical bone it is not broken, a hole is drilled to enable the introduction of the cannula.
- *Aspiration and washing*: if the cavity content is liquid it is easy to aspirate, but solid contents (hemosiderin deposits) cannot be evacuated by aspiration and will need to be washed out and removed with curettes.
- *Filling the cavities*: cavities <3 cm may be filled with fibrin seal, whereas larger cavities should be filled with lyophilized bone graft or bone substitute such as coralline hydroxyapatite. The filling procedure is performed by manually pressing the graft into the cavity (bone packing), and the surgeon must achieve total filling of the cavity to the cortical bone (Fig. 34.5).

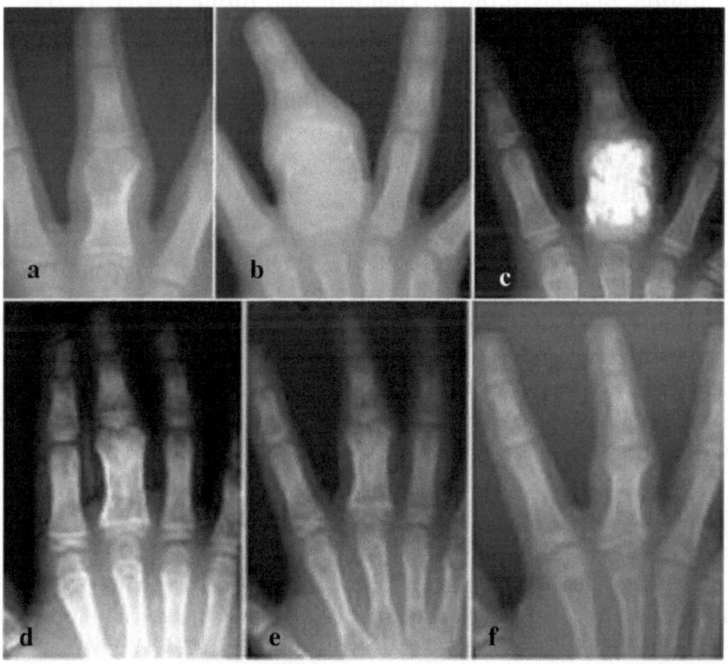

Fig. 34.5 Pseudotumors filled with hydroxyapatite (**a-f**)

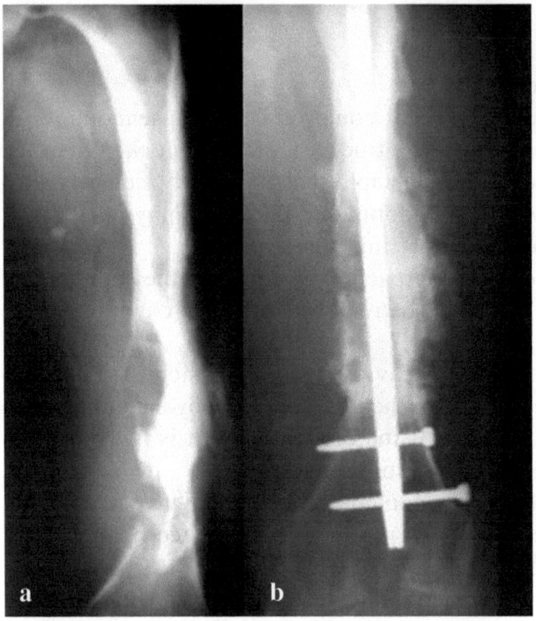

Fig. 34.6 Pseudotumors filled with hydroxyapatite and intramedullary fixation with a locking nail **(a, b)**

- *Internal fixation*: in diaphyseal or diaphymetaphyseal areas with critical damage of the cortex, or in the presence of pathological fracture, additional intramedullary fixation with a locking nail is necessary. The steps are: cavity aspiration, placing of the locking nail, and filling the cavity (Fig. 34.6).
- Patients with a very large epiphyseal or epiphymetaphyseal pseudotumor with cortical erosion will require post-operative orthosis.
- *Wound closure*: the wound is closed by separated nylon stitches. In patients with more than 3 cm cavities, a suction drain should be placed in position for 24 h.
- *External intermittent compression system (vacuum system)*: this device should be used to achieve collapse of the cavities. It is used for 1 week.
- *Rehabilitation*: one day after surgery, the patient can start to actively and passively exercise the areas that are unaffected by the pseudotumor. Rehabilitation of the affected area will depend upon the size and location of the lesion, post-operative immobilization, post-operative bleeding, and the absence or presence of a compromised proximal or distal joint. The physiotherapist plays a key role in evaluating all these variables to design the rehabilitation plan.

Suggested Readings

Rodríguez-Merchán EC (2002) The haemophilic pseudotumor. Haemophilia 8(1):12-16

Caviglia HA, Fernandez-Palazzi F, Gilbert MS (2002) Haemophilic pseudotumours of the limbs and their percutaneous treatment. Haemophilia 8(3): 402-406

Chakal F, Viso R, Fernandez-Palazzi F (2005) Percutaneous treatment of haemophilic digital pseudo tumours. Int Orthop 29(3):197-198

Section VII

Traumatology

Chapter 35

Treatment of Closed Fractures in Hemophiliac Patients

Ömer Taşer

Introduction

A fracture is defined as a disruption in the integrity of a bone. Most bones have the capacity to heal. However, healing of the fracture should not be perceived as only the union of the fractured bone, because when a trauma has the strength to break a bone, it inevitably damages adjacent tissues and joints. In most cases, even though the fracture may heal, the patient cannot go back to pre-fracture functional status if the adjacent tissues do not recover completely.

The aim of modern fracture treatment is both the union of the fractured bone in the correct anatomic position, and the functional healing of the adjacent soft tissues and joints. In other words, its aim is to ensure that the patient goes back to pre-trauma quality of life as fast as possible.

The Incidence of Fractures in Patients with Hemophilia

According to Rodríguez-Merchán [1], fracture is not frequent in patients with hemophilia, as they are less ambulant compared to the general population. This low level of ambulation is correlated to the severity of their illness [1]. On the other hand, osteoporotic bones, joint deformation, and poor musculature increase the fracture risk in hemophiliac individuals, and fractures can sometimes appear after a trivial trauma in these patients [2].

The incidence of fracture in our hemophiliac patient population is also very low. There were only five fractures in our sample of 800 registered patients between 2002 and 2005. In our opinion, this low incidence is related to both the lower rates of daily activities and the slower movements (walking slower, less-nimble turns) that go hand in hand with the condition of the muscles and joints.

H.A. Caviglia, L.P. Solimeno (eds.), *Orthopedic Surgery in Patients with Hemophilia.*

Diagnosis of Fractures

Fractures are diagnosed during physical examination by establishing their classic symptoms and signs (Box 35.1).

Box 35.1 Classic symptoms and sign of a fracture
- Pain, edema
- Increase of pain with active and passive motions
- Acute deformation
- Pathologic motion
- Crepitation
- Dramatically impaired function/function loss

X-rays are crucial in order to confirm the fracture diagnosis, and are also needed to determine the type of fracture and to plan treatment.

X-rays taken on two different planes 90° orthogonal to each other, anteroposterior (AP) and lateral (LAT) planes, are usually sufficient. The joint above and the joint below the fracture should be added to the radiographic area. It is especially important to provide comparative graphs of the contralateral extremity in children with epiphyseal plate injuries.

Treatment is planned after clinical and radiological diagnosis of the fracture. If a conservative (non-operative) treatment is decided on, closed reduction is carried out when necessary, and the extremity is immobilized with a splint or plaster cast. It is important not to forget the control radiograph in the post-plaster period.

Initial Management of Fractures

During the first examination of a fracture, the extremity should be carefully inspected and palpated. The neurological and vascular status of the region distal to the fracture should be monitored and recorded before and after dealing with the fracture. Treatment begins with re-alignment of the fracture and immobilization of the related extremity with a splint (Box 35.2).

Box 35.2 Reasons for and benefits of splinting
- Maintenance and protection of the fracture reduction
- Prevention of pain due to movement of the fracture's edges and periosteal friction
- Prevention of potential neurological and/or vascular damage
- Avoiding more damage to the soft tissues surrounding the fracture that are already damaged
- If there is an indication for surgical treatment, immobilizing the related extremity prior to surgery

However, in hemophiliac patients, temporary splinting and administration of the appropriate dose of factor replacement should be performed, and the necessary analgesia and sedation provided, before fracture reduction. Ibuprofen or paracetamol can be safely used for analgesia in hemophiliac patients.

Unacceptable reduction, or a shift in the alignment of a fracture that was initially in the right position, constitute unsuccessful non-operative treatment. If this is the case, surgery will be necessary.

Hematologic Treatment

The appropriate dose of factor changes according to the patient's weight and factor level. The deficient factor level should be raised to above 50% during closed reduction of the fracture, and should be kept above 50% in the first 48 h, when the risk of bleeding is higher. The factor level should be kept above 40% between days 3 and 8, and above 30% between days 9 and 15. During the later period of immobilization with plaster, it will be sufficient to keep the factor level above 20%.

If surgical treatment is going to be used, then the factor levels should be raised above 50% during the operation, and kept above 50% during the first 4 days after the operation, above 40% in the next 4–8 days, and above 30% in the following 8–15 days. After that, prophylaxis should be applied.

Non-fibrinolytic drugs such as tranexamic acid can be used as an adjunct therapy during the operation as intravenous perfusion, and can be used orally at other times. Tranexamic acid treatment should begin 12 h prior to the operation and be continued for 5–7 days; 10 mg/kg tranexamic acid is given in a single intravenous dose during the operation.

If there is no factor, fresh-frozen plasma can be used in emergency situations.

Acute Compartment Syndrome

Fractures are more common in longer bones in hemophiliac patients. Fracture hematoma tends to be larger in hemophiliac patients than in other patients, and may cause acute compartment syndrome [3].

A fracture hematoma occurs when damaged periosteal and endosteal vessels fill the fracture space. When large vessels around the fracture are torn, the hematoma grows faster. If the fascia around the fracture compartment is still sound, the pressure in the compartment increases. The muscles, nerves, and vessels in the compartment are put under pressure. If this pressure lasts for a long time, irreversible damage such as muscle necrosis, nerve palsies, and peripheral circulation disorders, can occur (Volkmann ischemic contracture).

The crucial point in acute compartment syndrome is diagnosis, and particularly immediate diagnosis. A patient with compartment syndrome will have far more severe pain than the expected fracture pain.

Compartment syndrome can be diagnosed through the measurement of elevated tissue pressure. As peripheral pulses can be palpated in many cases with compartment syndromes, tracing only peripheral pulses can cause a delay in diagnosis.

There is no difference in the treatment of compartment syndrome for hemophiliac and non-hemophiliac patients. The most effective method of decreasing the pressure within the compartment in acute compartment syndrome is surgical fasciotomy [4].

Orthopedic Treatment

The principles of fracture treatment are the same for hemophiliac patients as for the rest of the population, as long as the appropriate factor replacement is performed. The time for the union of a fracture that is treated accurately is the same for hemophiliac and non-hemophiliac patients.

General fracture treatment principles are valid in deciding whether to use conservative or surgical treatment methods in hemophiliac patients. For both methods, it is important to prevent further bleeding during the process of fracture healing in hemophiliac patients. Apart from this, it is important to keep in mind the possibility of serious inactivity osteoporosis in severely deformed patients. An osteoporotic bone can be so fragile that it will not allow stabilization by either internal or external fixation [5].

Infection rates after osteosynthesis or endoprosthesis operations are known to be higher in hemophiliac patients than in the general population [6]. In our opinion this situation is related to the poor vasculature in the muscles, and extensive arthrofibrosis in the joints due to previous local bleeding. In addition to these, the lower stamina levels in hemophiliac patients, espccially in developing countries, play an important role in these higher infection rates.

Operative treatment is a new trauma for the patient. Apart from this, surgical dissection can cause further vascular destruction to the already traumatized tissues. The muscles' flexibility around the fracture is likely to have decreased, and the scar tissue after the surgical dissection can therefore further negatively affect the muscles' flexibility in that area. Taking all of these factors into consideration, one has to be careful when applying surgical treatment in hemophiliac patients. It is important to stay within the internervous planes and avoid transection of the muscles during surgical dissection.

Some additional factors should be taken into consideration when applying surgical treatment in a hemophiliac patient. Percutaneous pins might loosen prematurely because of minor bleeding around the pins [1]. Pin tract infections in external fixators can cause more serious problems for hemophiliac patients. Use of an external fixator was indicated less frequently in the past due to the greater factor requirement. However, today the use of the external fixators is increasing.

We did not use external fixators in our series because there were no indications for them. However, in order to correct a 70° knee ankylosis in one patient and to correct the tibial deformity and shortening that were caused by older fractures in two patients, we used an Ilizarov circular external fixator. In these patients we used the hemostasis protocol for surgical treatment (Table 35.1), and just applied prophylaxis starting from the sixth week. None of the patients had any bleeding complications, loss of the correction, or infection. Because the application time of the external fixator for fracture treatment is generally shorter, its use in the treatment of fractures in hemophiliac patients constitutes a safe alternative [7].

Table 35.1 Hemostasis protocol in surgical treatment for closed fractures

	Severe hemophilia A/B	Mild, moderate hemophilia A/B and von Willebrand's disease	
–12 h + day 5/7	Tranexamic acid 25–40 mg/kg/day, three or four times a day		
–2 h	FVIII: 25 u/kg, FIX: 40u/kg	F VIII and vWF: 20 u/kg, F IX: 40 u/kg	Fresh frozen plasma
Days 1–4	FVIII and vWF: 25u/kg, FIX: 50 u/kg		
Days 4–8	FVIII: 20 u/kg, FIX: 40 u/kg	FVIII: 15 u/kg + DDAVP: 0.3 \mu;g/kg, FIX: 30 u/kg	
Days 8–15	F VIII: 15 u/kg, FIX: 30 u/kg	FVIII: 10 u/kg, FIX: 25 u/kg	

vWF: von Willebrand's factor
FVIII: factor VIII
FIX: factor IX
DDAVP: 1-desamino-8-D-arginine vasopressin (desmopressin)

Interlocking intramedullary devices should be favored in hemophiliac patients with a long bone fracture whenever possible. Plate-screw application should be used only when there is no other alternative [8]. Plate-screw application requires a larger exposure, which means more bleeding and also more scar tissue that will complicate rehabilitation.

Along with the issues discussed above, most hemophiliac patients have some degree of osteoporosis. For patients with severe osteoporosis, a long period of non-weight-bearing may be needed, especially after plate-screw application. This may not be tolerated by all patients. In addition, the extended use of crutches has the potential to cause problems in the elbow and shoulder joints in hemophiliac patients, especially in patients who previously had even a minor arthropathy.

Rehabilitation

Rehabilitation is crucial in all fractures. In hemophiliac patients, rehabilitation is a "sine qua non" due to associated factors like hemophilic arthropathy and muscle contractures.

When treating fractures in hemophiliac patients, rehabilitation should be slow enough not to negatively affect the healing of the fracture and cause further bleeding. It should, however, be fast and aggressive enough to avoid joint adherence and muscle atrophies.

Conclusion

The factors that are peculiar to hemophilia should be taken into consideration when treating fractures in hemophiliac patients. All of the general principles of fracture treatment are relevant for the treatment of fracture in these patients, as long as the conditions stated above are followed, and the appropriate factor replacement carried out.

References

1. Rodríguez-Merchán EC (2002) Bone fractures in the haemophilic patient. Hemophilia 8(2): 104–111
2. Rodríguez-Merchán EC (2003) Orthopaedic surgery for persons with haemophilia: General principles. In: Rodríguez-Merchán EC (ed) The Haemophilic Joints – New Perspectives. Blackwell Publishing, Oxford, pp 3–11
3. Rodríguez-Merchán EC, Caviglia H, Perez-Bianco R, Beeton KS (2001) Principles of surgery in haemophilic patients: Guidelines for developing countries. In: Sohail MT, Heijnen L (eds) Comprehensive Haemophilia Care in Developing Countries. Ferozsons Ltd., Lahor, pp 75–85
4. Amendola A, Twaddle BC (1998) Compartment syndromes. In: Browner BD, Jupiter JB, Levine AM, Trafton PG, eds. Skeletal trauma, WB Saunders Co, pp 365–389
5. Christian CA (1998) General Principles of Fracture Treatment. In: Canale ST (ed) Campbell's Operative Orthopaedics Vol 3, Mosby, pp 1993–2041
6. Rodríguez-Merchán EC, Luck Jr JV, Silva M et al (2003) Total knee replacement in the haemophilic patient. In: Rodríguez-Merchán EC (ed) The Haemophilic Joints – New Perspectives. Blackwell Publishing, Oxford, pp 116–124
7. Kocaoglu M, Zülfikar B, Türker M et al (2004) Osteotomies around the knee and elbow. Haemophilia World Congress, Thailand, Bangkok pp 17–21
8. Duthie RB (1997) Musculoskeletal Problems and Their Management. In: Rizza C, Lowe G, (eds) Haemophilia & Other Inherited Bleeding Disorders. WB Saunders Company Ltd, London-Philadelphia-Toronto-Sydney-Tokyo, pp 227–274

Chapter 36

Treatment of Exposed Fractures in Hemophiliac Patients

S.M. Javad Mortazavi

Introduction

The incidence of fracture in patients with hemophilia is controversial. Some believe that it is infrequent because these individuals are less ambulant due to the gravity of their illness and because their daily activities are reduced due to associated arthropathy and contractures [1–3]. Others hold that fractures may occur frequently and after trivial trauma because of poor musculature, osteoporosis, limited range of motion in the affected joint, and hemophilic changes in the bone [4]. The incidence of open fractures in hemophiliacs is not yet well known, but it seems that it is lower in the hemophiliac population than in the general population. If we accept the idea that fractures are more frequent in patients with hemophilia, they are not open fractures, because according to this opinion, low-energy trauma is the main cause of fracture and the possibility of open fracture is low in the presence of such trauma. On the other hand, thanks to preventive treatment, hemophiliac patients no longer need to restrict their activities, so they are exposed to risks in a similar way to the normal population. This suggests that open fractures *could* occur in hemophiliac patients.

An open fracture is one in which a break in the skin and underlying soft tissues leads directly into, or communicates with, the fracture and its hematoma. Diagnosis of an open fracture can be difficult, so when there is a wound in the same limb segment as the fracture, the fracture should be considered open until proved otherwise [5]. The ultimate goal in the treatment of open fractures is to restore limb and patient function as early and as fully as possible [5, 6]. To achieve this objective, the surgeon managing an open fracture must prevent infection, restore soft tissue, obtain bone union, avoid malunion, and start early joint range of motion and muscle rehabilitation. Of these, the primary concern is prevention of infection, because infection is the most common complication leading to non-union and loss of function.

The two major determinants of the outcome in open fractures are the amount of energy absorbed by the limb at the time of injury, and the level and type of bacterial contamination. The greater the amount of energy absorbed, the greater

H.A. Caviglia, L.P. Solimeno (eds.), *Orthopedic Surgery in Patients with Hemophilia.*

the devitalization of the soft tissue. These two determinants are more important than the fracture configuration itself; however, the latter is a good indicator of whether a fracture is the result of high-energy or low-energy forces [7].

Three major steps in the management of an open fracture are classification, initial emergency management, and formal treatment of the open fracture in the operating room.

Classification

Classification of open fractures is important both for prognosis and to recommend treatment [8, 9]. Classification is the first step in managing an open fracture. The most widely accepted classification of open fractures is Gustilo and Anderson's wound classification system [8], later modified by Gustilo et al [9]. In spite of significant interobserver variation in this classification [10], most authors prefer to use it after clarifying how they apply it [5, 6]. Although the size of the skin wound is one of the critical factors in their classification, it is a mistake to consider it the overriding factor in determining classification, because this alone cannot show the degree of soft tissue damage. The classification of an open fracture before thorough débridement and assessment of the wound and soft tissue injury can be misleading.

A type 1 open fracture is caused by low-energy trauma, and the wound is usually less than 1 cm long. It is generally caused by bone piercing the skin rather than by a penetrating object. A type 1 classification implies minimal crushing or muscle damage and a low level of bacterial contamination.

In a type II open fracture, the wound is more than 1 cm long, is caused by high-energy trauma, and is usually an outside-to-inside injury. The amount of soft tissue damage is moderate, and usually confined to one compartment. All in all, a type II open fracture is considered to be transitional between type I and type II open fractures.

A type III open fracture is usually associated with wounds more than 10 cm long. It results from a high-energy trauma and involves extensive muscle damage. Type III open fractures can be further classified into three subgroups. In type IIIA open fractures, there is limited periosteal and muscle stripping from the bone, and bone coverage is possible without flaps or other major plastic reconstructive procedures. A type IIIB open fracture is one in which there is extensive periosteal and muscle stripping from the bone, so that bone coverage requires a local flap or free tissue transfer. In a type IIIC fracture, there is major vascular injury which requires repair to salvage the limb.

Several factors modify open fracture classification regardless of the size of the wound. Extensive wound contamination due to exposure to soil, water, fecal material, and oral flora, or due to a delay of more than 12 h in treatment, indicates that the fracture should be classified as type III. In addition, any sign of a high-energy mechanism as a cause of fracture, such as displaced segmental fracture, bone loss, severe comminution, compartment syndrome, or crush mechanism, should be considered an indication that the fracture is at least type IIIA. The presence of hemorrhagic diathesis may be considered a modifying factor in type III open fractures, especially when factor substitution is delayed

Initial Emergency Management

Assessing patients for vital functions and stabilizing them is the first step in the emergency room [11]. This should be followed, as soon as possible, by a careful examination to document the neurologic and vascular function of the involved extremity. Compartment syndrome is more likely to occur in hemophiliac patients, so documenting the neurovascular function is vital [12]. Five important principles should be followed in the emergency department after primary evaluation and stabilization of the patient; they are discussed under the following headings.

Normalization of the Coagulation Process

In hemophiliac patients with open fracture, early establishment of good hemostasis is extremely important [1–4, 13], as it prevents excessive blood loss from the wound. It also prevents enlargement of the hematoma at the fracture site, which can cause serious complications such as necrosis of the soft tissue, formation of a hemophilic pseudotumor, and compartment syndrome. Overall, data in the literature suggest that with bolus infusion, adequate surgical hemostasis can be achieved to 80–100% levels during surgery, and >30% levels in the first 2–3 weeks of the post-operative period until wound healing, with perhaps slightly higher levels of 40–50% in the first 3–5 days [14]. Administration of antifibrinolytic drugs such as ε-aminocaproic acid is of utmost importance. They not only help maintain coagulation at the beginning, but also limit fibrinolytic action which results in the activation and liberation of proteolytic enzymes that are harmful for the consolidation process [1, 4]. These drugs should be continued for at least 30 days after reduction and stabilization of the fracture [1, 4]. Several operations are usually indicated in hemophiliac patients with open fractures. It is obvious that the factor levels should be 80–100% during each operation.

Coverage of the Wound with Sterile Dressing

The skin around the wound or wounds should be examined. It is necessary to examine the entire circumference of the extremity, because it is not uncommon for significant wounds in the posterior aspect of the extremity to be overlooked. Foreign bodies and obvious debris such as leaves, stones, or grass found in open wounds should be manually removed with sterile forceps. Then, if the patient will be undergoing immediate surgical débridement in the operating room within

2 h, the wound should be covered with a sterile bandage during transportation to the operating room. If the operating room will not be available for several hours, the wound should be irrigated with 1–2 l of saline fluid before placing the sterile bandage, and the dressing immediately adjacent to the wound soaked with a dilute povidone-iodine solution [6, 15]. Application of povidone-soaked dressings directly over the wound is not recommended because it has been suggested that povidone interferes with osteoblast function [16]. Recent data suggest that pre-débridement cultures have little value, so they are no longer recommended [17]. After the sterile dressing is placed, the wound should not be further inspected until the patient is in the operating room.

Splinting of the Injured Limb

The limb should be appropriately splinted in the emergency room. This not only reduces the patient's pain, but also prevents further movement at the fracture site, which in turn decreases the risk of more hemorrhage and neurovascular damage.

Patients who arrive in the emergency room with an appropriately splinted extremity and a sterile dressing over the wound of an open fracture, and who show no sign of vascular damage, should be taken to the operating room without any manipulation of the wound and its dressing in the emergency room.

Administration of Systemic Antibiotics

Intravenous bactericidal antibiotics with gram-positive coverage — usually a first-generation cephalosporin, e.g., cephazoline sodium — should be started as soon as possible in the emergency room for type I and type II open fractures [18, 19]. For an adult, a loading dose of 2 g, followed by 1 g every 8 h, is effective. In type III open fractures, an intravenous aminoglycoside, e.g., gentamicin — 3–5 mg/kg of lean body weight per day — is given in divided dose every 8 h, and adjusted according to the serum level. In open fractures in which there is a strong risk of significant anaerobic infection, 4–5 million units of penicillin are administered every 6 h as well. Antibiotics should be taken 48–72 h after initial and subsequent débridements, as well as after wound closure. If any signs of infection or drainage occur at any time, the wound should be cultured, and treatment should be based on those cultures [20].

Considering Tetanus Prophylaxis

Recommendations for tetanus prophylaxis are generally based on the condition of the wound and the patient's immunization history. There are clinical features in wounds that predispose them to tetanus. If the wound is old (>6 h), deep, stellate or avulsion type, infected, and contains devitalized tissue, it will be considered tetanus prone. Patients with a history of three doses of adsorbed tetanus toxoid do not need tetanus immune globulin at all. In the presence of a tetanus-prone wound, a toxoid should be administered if more than 5 years have elapsed since the last adsorbed toxoid dose. In a non-tetanus-prone wound, an injection is only needed if it is more than 10 years since the last dose. Toxoid should be administered in all patients with unknown history of vaccination or less than three doses of adsorbed toxoid injection. Tetanus immune globulin should be given concurrently with a separate syringe, and in a separate site, but only if the wound is tetanus prone [21].

Formal Treatment of Open Fractures

All open fractures must be formally treated in the operating room on an urgent basis, with meticulous irrigation and thorough but judicious débridement of devitalized soft tissue and devascularized bone fragments [15]. The patient's medical history should be obtained and any associated co-morbidities elicited. Radiographic evaluation of the injured extremity is essential for diagnosis and planning, and can be helpful in classification. Three important principles should be considered in the treatment of an open fracture: thorough irrigation and débridement, stabilization of the bone, and wound management.

Irrigation and Débridement

Usual surgical preparation and draping is necessary. During preparation, gross debris should be removed from the wound using copious amount of preparation solution [6]. In extremity wounds, a tourniquet is placed, but should not be inflated unless hemorrhage cannot be controlled [5, 6]. For types I to IIIA open fractures, the wound is irrigated with a total of 6 l of normal saline. Bacitracin 50,000 U is added to each of the last 2 l. For highly contaminated type IIIB and IIIC open fractures, four more liters of irrigation is essential. Two liters of irrigation is often used before débridement, in addition to the irrigation used at regular intervals throughout the débridement process [5, 6, 22].

Débridement should be started with enlargement of the wound as needed. Crossing the wound is the incision of choice for wound extension, as this method results in the smallest flap and minimizes the risk of flap necrosis. All ragged, contaminated skin edges should be removed to establish a surgical wound edge that is at right angles to the skin. The surgeon must be conservative in skin débridement, as skin coverage can be a problem in certain areas. As subcutaneous fat and fascia have a poor blood supply, all devascularized or contaminated fat and fascia must be removed. A fasciotomy of the involved myofascial compartment of the open fracture is always indicated as a part of débridement. In hemophiliac patients with type II or worse open tibial fractures, a formal four-compartment fasciotomy is recommended. The best determinants for muscle viability are the muscle's response to a stimulus, and its ability to rebound to normal appearance after being pinched gently with a pair of forceps. The safest approach for muscle débridement is "when in doubt, take it out". As a tendon can retain significant functionality even if only 10% of muscle belly is attatched, it seems logical to leave some marginal muscle at the time of initial débridement in severe open fractures, returning within 24–48 h for re-débridement, when the muscle's viability is clearer. Tendons should be copiously irrigated and preserved. Soft tissue coverage is essential for tendon survival, and preservation of peritenon becomes very important if this is not possible. The most difficult part of débridement is deciding what is to be done with bone fragments. As a general rule, bone débridement can be conservative initially. However, if infection intervenes, early aggressive re-débridement of all non-viable bone is important [23]. Like tendons, bone without periosteum and not covered by soft tissue quickly desiccates and dies, so it is better to thoroughly irrigate periosteum that is attached, rather than débride it, if soft tissue coverage cannot be obtained [15].

Fracture Stabilization

Fracture stability is essential for initial wound care and for fracture union, and after débridement, stabilization has priority. For type I fractures with stable configuration, a cast can be used. Special attention to compartment syndrome is essential in hemophiliac patients. In doubtful cases, the use of a posterior splint in first few days is recommended. Immediate internal fixation of open fractures seems to be called for in many patients. The surgeon's judgment is very important in this regard. Open fractures in the shafts of the femur and tibia can be stabilized with reamed or unreamed intramedullary nails [24–28]. Open fracture of the humeral shaft can be fixed with intramedullary nails or plates [29]. For the radius and ulna, plate fixation remains the first choice. Primary open reduction and internal fixation in open intra-articular fractures has shown good results [30, 31], but in doubtful severe cases, limited internal fixation of the articular surface should be the first part of staged surgery [32]. The primary indication for external fixation is very severe, highly contaminated, type III open fractures, where plating or nailing is either contraindicated or not feasible. An external fixator can be used safely in hemophiliac patients who do not have inhibitors and do not require prolonged factor replacement [13].

Wound Management

Primary closure of a traumatic wound is occasionally indicated. It is safer to leave traumatic wounds open and only close the elective portion of the wound [5, 6]. Special attention should be paid to primary coverage of tendon without peritenon, and bone without periosteum, because desiccation results in the death of these structures [33]. Type I and II wounds are not exposed for inspection until the time of delayed primary closure, 2–5 days after injury. In type III open fractures, early return to the operating room for wound inspection and repeat irrigation and débridement is recommended. The objective is to achieve coverage of bone in 5–10 days. Wounds requiring local flaps or free microvascularized flaps are often ready for flap coverage within 5–10 days.

Amputation versus Limb Salvage

In severe open fractures, salvage may require repeated operation and prolonged disability for 2 years or more, and of course affects the patient's quality of life [6, 34]. In hemophiliac patients with such fractures, amputation will probably be the best option [1].

Rehabilitation

Rehabilitation is the cornerstone of treatment. It should start as soon as possible with the aims of preventing muscle atrophy and preserving mobility of the joints and avoiding their contracture. It should be continued until fracture union and complete restoration of the limb function. It is obvious that coverage with adequate replacement therapy is necessary during the entire rehabilitation period [1, 4].

References

1. Rodríguez-Merchán EC (2002) Bone fractures in the hemophilic patient. Haemophilia 8:104–111
2. Feil E, Bentley G, Rizza CR (1974) Fracture management in patients with haemophilia. J Bone Joint Surg Br 56:643–649
3. Wolff LJ, Lovrien EW (1982) Management of fractures in hemophilia. Pediatrics 70(3):431–436
4. Quintana M, Quintana M, Rodríguez-Merchán EC (2000) Musculoskeletal Aspects of Haemophilia, Chap. 21. Blackwell Science, Oxford, p 148
5. Olson S, Finkemeier CG, Moehring HD (2001) Open fractures. In: Bucholz RW and Heckman JD, Rockwood and Green's Fractures in Adults, Lippincott, Williams & Wilkins, Philadelphia
6. Chapman MW (2001) Open fractures. In: Chapman MW et al Chapman's Orthopedic Surgery, Lippincott, Williams & Wilkins, Philadelphia, pp 381-393
7. Byrd HS, Cierny G III, Tebbetts JB (1981) The management of open tibial fractures with associated soft-tissue loss: external fixation with early flap coverage. Plast Reconstr Surg 68:73–82
8. Gustilo RB, Anderson JT (1976) Prevention of infection in the treatment of one thousand and twenty five open fractures of long bones: retrospective and prospective analyses. J Bone Joint Surg Am 58:453–458
9. Gustilo RB, Mendoza RM, Williams DN (1984) Problems in the management of type III

(severe) open fractures: a new classification of type III open fractures. J Trauma 24:742–746
10. Brumback RJ, Jone AL (1994) Interobserver agreement in the classification of open fractures of the tibia: the results of a survey of 245 orthopaedic surgeons. J Bone Joint Surg Am 76:1162–1166
11. Alexander RH, Proctor HJ (1993) Advanced trauma life support (ATLS) program for physicians, 5th ed. American College of Surgeons, Chicago
12. Olson SA (1997) Open fractures of the tibial shaft. Instr Course Lect 46:293–302
13. Lee V, Srivastava A, PalaniKumar C et al (2004) External fixators in haemophilia. Haemophilia 10(1):52–57
14. Srivastava A (2004) Dose and response in haemophilia-optimization of factor replacement therapy. Br J Haematol 127(1):12–25
15. Olson SA (1996) Open fractures of the tibial shaft. J Bone Joint Surg Am 78:1428–1436
16. Kaysinger KK, Nicholson NC, Ramp WK et al (1995) Toxic effects of wound irrigation solutions on cultured tibiae and osteoblasts. J Orthop Trauma 9:303–311
17. Lee J (1997) Efficacy of cultures in the management of open fractures. Clin Orthop 339:71–75
18. Gustilo RB (1987) Current concepts in the management of open fractures. Inst Course Lect 36:359–366
19. Wilkins J, Patzakis M (1991) Choice and duration of antibiotics in open fractures. Orthop Clin North Am 22:433–437
20. Perry CR, Pearson RL, Miller GA (1991) Accuracy of cultures of material from swabbing of the superficial aspect of the wound and needle biopsy in the preoperative assessment of osteomyelitis. J Bone Joint Surg Am 73:745–749
21. Ross SE (1995) Prophylaxis against tetanus management in wound management. American College of Surgeons, Committee on Trauma. In: www.facs.org/trauma/publications/tetanus.pdf
22. Anglen J, Apostoles S, Christensen G et al (1997) The efficacy of various irrigation solutions in removing slime-producing staphylococcus. J Orthop Trauma 8:390–396
23. Kindsfater K, Jonassen EA (1995) Osteomyelitis in grade II and III open tibial fractures with late debridement. J Orthop Trauma 9:121–127
24. Grose A, Christie J, Taglang G et al (1993) Open adult femoral shaft fractures treated by early intramedullary nailing. J Bone Joint Surg Br 75:562–565
25. Brumback RJ, Ellison PS Jr, Poka A et al (1989) Intramedullary nailing of open fractures of the femoral shaft. J Bone Joint Surg Am 71:1324–1331
26. Olson SA (1996) Open fractures of the tibial shaft. J Bone Joint Surg Am 78:1428–1436
27. Henley MB, Chapman JR, Agel J et al (1998) Treatment of type II, IIIA, and IIIB open fractures of the tibial shaft: a prospective comparison of unreamed interlocking intramedullary nails and half-pin external fixators. J Orthop Trauma 12:1–7
28. Bonatus T, Olson SA, Lee S et al (1997) Nonreamed locking intramedullary nailing for open fractures of the tibia. Clin Orthop 339:58–64
29. Vander Griend R, Tomasin J, Ward EF (1986) Open reduction and internal fixation of humeral shaft fractures: results using AO plating techniques. J Bone Joint Surg Am 68:430–433
30. Franklin JL, Johnson KD, Hanse ST (1994) Immediate internal fixation of open ankle fractures. J Bone Joint Surg Am 66:1349–1356
31. Benirschke SK, Agnew SF, Mayo KA et al (1992) Immediate internal fixation of open, complex tibial plateau fractures. J Orthop Trauma 6:78–86
32. Sirkin M, Sanders R, DiPasquale T et al (1999) A staged protocol for soft tissue management in the treatment of complex pilon fractures. J Orthop Trauma 13:78–84
33. Greene TL, Beatty ME (1988) Soft tissue coverage for lower extremity trauma: current practice and techniques. A review. J Orthop Trauma 2:158–173
34. Georgiadis GM, Berhrens FF, Joyce MJ et al (1993) Open tibial fractures with severe soft tissue loss: limb salvage compared with below-the-knee amputation. J Bone Joint Surg Am 75:1431–1441

Conclusions

Chapter 37

Orthopedic Surgery in Hemophiliac Patients: a Physiotherapist's Point of View

Kathy Mulder

Hemophilia is an ancient disease, but the ability to perform orthopedic surgery safely on people with hemophilia is a recent development. Prior to the discovery of cryoprecipitate in 1965, death was an almost-guaranteed complication of surgery in a hemophiliac patient. In 1890, in keeping with the current state of surgical knowledge, König opened the knee joints of two patients "to relieve painful swollen joints". The positive outcome of this was the world's first published description of hemophilic arthritis. However, both patients died from the ensuing blood loss [1].

A PubMed search of articles published prior to1967 and using key words "Surgery and Hemophilia" produces 104 articles. When the search is refined to "Orthopedic Surgery and Hemophilia", only four articles appear [2–5]. With the development of clotting factor concentrates, the orthopedic surgical procedures that helped people with rheumatoid arthritis and osteoarthritis soon became treatment options for people with hemophilia. Synovectomy, arthrodesis, and joint replacements became commonplace. Forty years later, we can plan elective surgery for people with hemophilia, and even for patients with inhibitors [6, 7].

The working relationship between surgeons and physiotherapists varies widely around the world. This often reflects the education and autonomy provided to therapists in different countries. Some jurisdictions acknowledge physiotherapists as independent practitioners, capable of performing comprehensive assessments and planning treatment programs, while others consider them to be technicians who follow the orders of a practitioner empowered to prescribe therapy (usually a physician or surgeon).

While most surgeons acknowledge that a good outcome relies heavily on proper post-operative rehabilitation, physiotherapists also believe that a successful outcome is even more likely if the physiotherapist — and the patient — is actively involved during the pre-operative planning [8–10]. In many hemophilia treatment centers, it is the physiotherapist who is most familiar with the patient's overall functional status, his bleeding tendencies, and the state of his muscles and joints. In fact, it may be the physiotherapist who recognizes that non-surgical measures are no longer sufficient, and who initiates the referral to the surgeon.

H.A. Caviglia, L.P. Solimeno (eds.), *Orthopedic Surgery in Patients with Hemophilia.*

A physiotherapist can assist the surgeon to determine:

- What are the goals of the surgery? (The patient's goals and the surgeon's goals may not always be the same [11])
- Are the patient's expectations of the surgery realistic?
- How will the proposed surgery affect the other joints?
- Will the patient be able to use walking aids post-operatively if required?
- Should a program of "prehabilitation" be undertaken to prepare adjacent joints and muscles?
- Is there any advantage in performing multiple procedures simultaneously?
- Does the patient understand what the rehabilitation process will entail? And is he able to commit to this process?
- Does the patient have adequate support in place to prepare for and recover from the surgery? For example, if he lives far away from the hemophilia center, is there somewhere for him to stay for the duration of the rehabilitation process?

If for some reason pre-operative communication is not possible, the therapist *must* be familiar with the details of the surgery that has been performed. In fact, it can be extremely useful for the physiotherapist to go to the theater and observe the surgery first hand. This knowledge will allow the therapist to determine realistic and acceptable limits for pain, swelling, range of motion, and muscle function, and to consult with the surgeon and the hematologist if these limits are exceeded during the post-operative period.

Despite the huge strides that have been made in the ability to perform surgery safely in individuals with hemophilia, the ultimate goal of surgeons and physiotherapists alike should be to *prevent* the need for surgery on patients with hemophilia.

In 1963, CB Kerr wrote:

When the final history of Hemophilia is written it will be divided into three parts. The first part will describe the era of clinical observation and ineffectual treatment. The second part will deal with an age of increasingly effective medical management and better understanding of the underlying mechanisms of hemophilia. The third and final chapter has yet to come. Not until the disease can be permanently suppressed . . . will the hemophiliac face life on equal terms with his healthy colleagues [12].

Donna Boone quoted Kerr in her Preface to *Comprehensive Management of Hemophilia* in 1976, and expressed the hope that "during the next decade this [third] chapter will be completed with control or permanent suppression of these disorders and their medical, psychological, and social ramifications" [13].

In 2002, Carlos Rodríguez-Merchán wrote:

Although continuous prophylaxis could avoid the development of the orthopaedic complications of hemophilia that we still see in the 21st century, such a goal has not been achieved so far, not even in developed countries [14].

While temporary hematological control can be achieved relatively easily by the use of clotting factor concentrates and recombinant products, these are not available universally.

Until we get to the "third chapter", close cooperation between orthopedic surgeons, rehabilitation physicians, and physiotherapists will continue to be essential for obtaining satisfactory results after orthopedic procedures that are performed on people with hemophilia.

References

1. König F (1890) Die Gelenkerkrankungen bei Blutern mit besonderer Berücksichtigung der Diagnose, Chirugie I, p 232
2. Brown DL, Hardisty RM, Kosoy MH, Bracken C (1967) Antihaemophilic globulin: preparation by an improved cryoprecipitation method and clinical use. BMJ 2(5544):79–85
3. Jordan HH (1967) Hemophilia-rehabilitation and prophylaxis. Proc Rudolf Virchow Med Soc City NY 26:35–38
4. Jordan HH (1967) Conservative orthopaedic approach to rehabilitation of the severely crippled hemophiliac. Wiederherstellungschir Traumatol 9:95–106
5. Jordan HH (1965) Orthopedic aspects of hemophilia. Acta Orthop Belg 31(4):640–647
6. Solimeno LP, Perfetto OS, Pasta G, Santagostino E (2006) Total joint replacement in patients with inhibitors. Haemophilia 12(Suppl 3):113–116
7. Rodríguez-Merchán EC, Wiedel JD Jr, Wallny T et al (2004), Elective orthopedic surgery for hemophilia patients with inhibitors: New opportunities. Semin Hematol 41(1 Suppl 1):109–116
8. Stephensen D (2005) Rehabilitation of patients with haemophilia after orthopaedic surgery: a case study. Haemophilia 11(Suppl 1):26–29
9. Jones CA, Beaupre LA, Johnston DWC, Suarez-Almazor ME (2005) Total joint arthroplasties: current concepts of patient outcomes after surgery. Clin Geriatr Med p 21
10. Sharma L, Sinacore J, Daugherty C et al (1996) Prognostic factors for functional outcome of total knee replacement: a prospective study. J Gerontol A Biol Sci Med Sci 51(4):M152–157
11. Mancuso CA, Sculco TP, Wickiewicz TL et al (2001) Patients' expectations of knee surgery. J Bone Joint Surg Am 83-A(7):1005-1012
12. Kerr CB (1963) The Fortunes of Haemophiliacs in the Nineteenth Century, Med Hist 7:359–370
13. Boone DC (1976) Comprehensive Management of Hemophilia. F.A. Davis Company, Philadelphia ISBN 0–8036–1000–10009
14. Rodríguez-Merchán EC (2002) Orthopaedic surgery of haemophilia in the 21st century: an overview. Haemophilia 8(3):360–368

In 2002, Carlos Rodriguez-Merchan wrote:

Although continuous prophylaxis could avoid the development of the musculoskeletal complications of hemophilia that we still see in the 21st century, such a goal has not been achieved so far, or even in developed countries [11].

[illegible]

Chapter 38

Ten Pieces of Advice for an Orthopedic Surgeon

Marvin Gilbert, Luigi P. Solimeno and Horacio A. Caviglia

1. Treatment for hemophiliac patients should be multidisciplinary. It requires specialists such as: hematologists, orthopedists, surgeons, physiotherapists, pediatricians, hepatologists, infectologists, psychologists, nurses, laboratory technicians, and social workers. If hemophiliac patients are treated without including these specialists, the results obtained are not the best.
2. Listen to the patient and perform an adequate physical examination.
3. When evaluating diagnostic complementary tests of the patient, remember that patients with hemophilia have a medical radiological dissociation: although the patients frequently show a pronounced radiological lesion, they do not feel much pain. Therefore be careful to treat the patient, and not the images.
4. When explaining treatment to a patient, explain the benefits and risks associated with treatment.
5. Always rehabilitate the patient, and do it before the surgery. After rehabilitation, carry out a re-evaluation to see if surgery is still necessary. After surgery, explain the rehabilitation plan, check to be sure that it is being carried out, and record its final result.
6. Make a good database of your patients. Keep images of diagnostic complementary tests in your database for use in multicenter studies.
7. Even if you have a small number of patients you have to record your data so that they can be statistically analyzed. This will enable you to take part in multicenter studies. Participate in these studies whenever possible.
8. Always show both satisfactory and unsatisfactory results. This is the best way to recognize problems in diagnosis and treatment, and to help patients and alert fellow doctors.
9. If you stop working with hemophilia patients do not let the information get lost. The options are:
   - Look for an orthopedic surgeon to replace you in your task, and pass your records on to him.
   - Pass the information on to someone in the treatment center you were working in.

H.A. Caviglia, L.P. Solimeno (eds.), *Orthopedic Surgery in Patients with Hemophilia.*

- Send the records to the Musculoskeletal Committee of the Hemophilia World Federation.

10. Never forget your Hippocratic Oath, and do not allow patients to be discriminated against because of their illnesses.

Subject Index

T

V

W

MIX
Papier aus verantwortungsvollen Quellen
Paper from responsible sources
FSC® C105338

If you have any concerns about our products,
you can contact us on
ProductSafety@springernature.com

In case Publisher is established outside the EU,
the EU authorized representative is:
Springer Nature Customer Service Center GmbH
Europaplatz 3, 69115 Heidelberg, Germany

Printed by Libri Plureos GmbH
in Hamburg, Germany